INNOVATIVE
NEUROMODULATION

INNOVATIVE NEUROMODULATION

Edited by

JEFFREY ARLE

*Director of Functional Neurosurgery, Associate Chief,
Neurosurgery, Beth Israel Deaconess Medical Center, Boston, MA, United States;
Chief, Neurosurgery, Mt Auburn Hospital, Cambridge, MA, United States; Associate
Professor of Neurosurgery, Harvard Medical School, Boston, MA, United States*

JAY SHILS

*Rush University Medical Center, Director of Intraoperative Neurophysiological
Monitoring, Associate Professor, Rush University Medical Center in the Department of
Anesthesiology, Chicago, IL, United States*

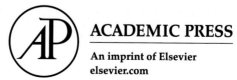

ACADEMIC PRESS

An imprint of Elsevier
elsevier.com

Academic Press is an imprint of Elsevier
125 London Wall, London EC2Y 5AS, United Kingdom
525 B Street, Suite 1800, San Diego, CA 92101-4495, United States
50 Hampshire Street, 5th Floor, Cambridge, MA 02139, United States
The Boulevard, Langford Lane, Kidlington, Oxford OX5 1GB, United Kingdom

Notices
Knowledge and best practice in this field are constantly changing. As new research
and experience broaden our understanding, changes in research methods, professional
practices, or medical treatment may become necessary.

Practitioners and researchers must always rely on their own experience and knowledge
in evaluating and using any information, methods, compounds, or experiments described
herein. In using such information or methods they should be mindful of their own
safety and the safety of others, including parties for whom they have a professional
responsibility.

To the fullest extent of the law, neither the Publisher nor the authors, contributors, or
editors, assume any liability for any injury and/or damage to persons or property as a
matter of products liability, negligence or otherwise, or from any use or operation of any
methods, products, instructions, or ideas contained in the material herein.

British Library Cataloguing-in-Publication Data
A catalogue record for this book is available from the British Library

Library of Congress Cataloging-in-Publication Data
A catalog record for this book is available from the Library of Congress

ISBN: 978-0-12-800454-8

For Information on all Academic Press publications
visit our website at https://www.elsevier.com

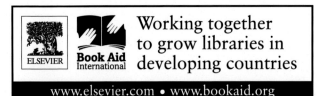

Working together
to grow libraries in
developing countries

www.elsevier.com • www.bookaid.org

Publisher: Mara Conner
Acquisition Editor: Natalie Farra
Editorial Project Manager: Kristi Anderson
Production Project Manager: Chris Wortley
Designer: Mark Rogers

Typeset by MPS Limited, Chennai, India

Contents

I

NEW DIRECTIONS WITH CURRENT THERAPIES

1. Microarrays in the Brain: Can They Be Used for Brain–Machine Interface Control?

W.Q. MALIK AND R. AJEMIAN

2. Feedback-Sensitive and Closed-Loop Solutions

G.P. THOMAS AND B.C. JOBST

3. Directional Deep Brain Stimulation

A. MERCANZINI, A. DRANSART AND C. POLLO

4. Waveform Variation in Neuromodulation

J. ARLE

II

NEW MODES OF THERAPY

5. Ultrasound Neuromodulation

R.F. DALLAPIAZZA, K. TIMBIE AND W.J. ELIAS

III

INNOVATIVE THINKING

10. Neuroprosthetic Advances
W. MAYR, M. KRENN AND M.R. DIMITRIJEVIC

11. Neuromodulation for Memory
D.S. XU AND F.A. PONCE

12. Deep Brain Stimulation for Vegetative State and Minimally Conscious State
D. CHUDY AND V. DELETIS

13. Neuromodulation as a Bypass—Spinal Cord Injury
J. SHILS AND J. ARLE

14. Neuromodulation for Psychiatric Disorders
S. HESCHAM, M. TÖNGE, A. JAHANSHAHI AND Y. TEMEL

Biographies

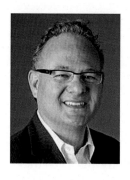

Jeffrey Arle, MD, PhD, FAANS

Dr. Arle is currently the Associate Chief of Neurosurgery at Beth Israel Deaconess Medical Center in Boston, the Chief of Neurosurgery at Mt. Auburn Hospital in Cambridge, and an Associate Professor of Neurosurgery at Harvard Medical School. He received his BA in Biopsychology from Columbia University in 1986 and his MD and PhD from the University of Connecticut in 1992. His dissertation work for his doctorate in Biomedical Sciences was in computational modeling in the cochlear nucleus. He then went on to do a residency in neurosurgery at the University of Pennsylvania, incorporating a double fellowship in movement disorder surgery and epilepsy surgery under Drs. Patrick Kelly, Ron Alterman, and Werner Doyle, finishing in 1999.

He edited the companion text *Essential Neuromodulation* with Dr. Shils, the first edition published by Elsevier in 2011. He has now practiced in the field of functional neurosurgery for 17 years and is experienced in all areas of neuromodulation from deep-brain stimulators to vagus nerve, spinal cord, peripheral nerve, and motor cortex stimulators, contributing frequent peer-reviewed publications and numerous chapters to the literature on many aspects of the neuromodulation field. He currently serves as an associate editor at the journals *Neuromodulation* and *Neurosurgery*, is the co-chair of the Research and Scientific Policy Committee for the International Neuromodulation Society, and is on the Board of Directors for the International Society for Intraoperative Neurophysiology. His longstanding research interests are in the area of computational modeling in the understanding and improved design of devices used in neuromodulation treatments.

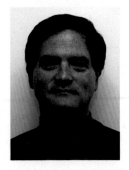

Jay Shils, PhD, DABNM, FASNM, FACNS

Jay Shils was most recently the Director of Intra-operative Neurophysiology in the Department of Neurosurgery at the Lahey Hospital and Health System in Burlington, MA and an Associate Professor in the Department of Neurosurgery at the Tufts University School of Medicine. He received his Bachelor of Science degree in electrical engineering from Syracuse University, and both his masters and PhD in bio-engineering at The University of Pennsylvania using higher-order signal extraction and processing techniques on human EEG data to investigate interactions in the visual system and study EEG in epilepsy.

He began his work in the field of intraoperative neurophysiology in 1994, specializing in single unit recordings during surgery for movement disorders in the Department of Neurology at the University of Pennsylvania School of Medicine. Dr. Shils is presently the Director of Intraoperative Neurophysiology at Rush University Medical Center and an Associate Professor in the Department of Anesthesiology. Dr. Shils' research interests include investigating methods for improving real-time intraoperative neurophysiologic techniques, as well as theoretical research into neuromodulation mechanisms of action. Dr. Shils has published over 30 peer-reviewed papers and multiple chapters on intraoperative neurophysiologic surgical techniques, postoperative management of movement disorder patients, and computational modeling as related to neuromodulation effects on various neural circuits. He has co-edited two books: *Neurophysiology in Neurosurgery: A modern intraoperative approach* with Dr. Vedran Deletis; and *Essential Neuromodulation* with Dr. Jeffrey Arle. Prior to going to graduate school Dr. Shils was an electrical engineer at the Electric Boat division of General Dynamics where he was involved in various modifications to existing electrical systems.

Dr. Shils is the past President of the International Society for Intraoperative Monitoring and was the founding secretary of the society. He is a past board member of and present chairman for the American Society of Neurophysiologic Monitoring ethics committee and is the 2106/2017 President of the ASNM. He is an associate editor for the *Journal of Neurosurgery* and *Journal of Clinical Neurophysiology*.

List of Contributors

R. Ajemian   Massachusetts Institute of Technology, Cambridge, MA, United States

J. Arle   Beth Israel Deaconess Medical Center, Boston, MA, United States; Mt Auburn Hospital, Cambridge, MA, United States; Harvard Medical School, Boston, MA, United States

D. Austin   University College London, London, United Kingdom

N.M. Boulis   Emory University, Atlanta, GA, United States

D. Chudy   University Hospital Dubrava, University of Zagreb, School of Medicine, Zagreb, Croatia

R.F. Dallapiazza   University of Virginia, Charlottesville, VA, United States

V. Deletis   University of Split, Split, Croatia; St Luke's-Roosevelt Hospital, New York, NY, United States

M.R. Dimitrijevic   Foundation for Movement Recovery, Oslo, Norway; Baylor College of Medicine, Houston, TX, United States

A. Dransart   Aleva Neurotherapeutics SA, Lausanne, Switzerland

W.J. Elias   University of Virginia, Charlottesville, VA, United States

F. Fregni   Harvard Medical School, Boston, MA, United States

S. Hescham   Maastricht University Medical Center, Maastricht, The Netherlands

A. Jahanshahi   Maastricht University Medical Center, Maastricht, The Netherlands

B.C. Jobst   Dartmouth-Hitchcock Medical Center, Lebanon, NH, United States; Geisel School of Medicine at Dartmouth, Hanover, NH, United States

P.S.A. Kalanithi[†]   Department of Neurosurgery, Stanford University, Stanford, CA, United States

J.K. Krauss   Medical School Hannover, Hannover, Germany

M. Krenn   Medical University of Vienna, Vienna, Austria

B.J. Mader   Emory University, Atlanta, GA, United States

W.Q. Malik   Harvard Medical School, Boston, MA, United States; Massachusetts Institute of Technology, Cambridge, MA, United States

W. Mayr   Medical University of Vienna, Vienna, Austria

A. Mercanzini   Aleva Neurotherapeutics SA, Lausanne, Switzerland

C. Pollo   Inselspital, Bern University Hospital, Bern, Switzerland

F.A. Ponce   St. Joseph's Hospital and Medical Center, Phoenix, AZ, United States

[†]Deceased

D. Purger   Department of Neurosurgery, Stanford University, Stanford, CA, United States

J. Rothwell   University College London, London, United Kingdom

J. Shils   Rush University Medical Center, Chicago, IL, United States

Y. Temel   Maastricht University Medical Center, Maastricht, The Netherlands

G.P. Thomas   Dartmouth-Hitchcock Medical Center, Lebanon, NH, United States; Geisel School of Medicine at Dartmouth, Hanover, NH, United States

K. Timbie   University of Virginia, Charlottesville, VA, United States

M. Tönge   Maastricht University Medical Center, Maastricht, The Netherlands

T. Wagner   Highland Instruments, Harvard Medical School, and MIT, Cambridge, MA, United States

D.S. Xu   St. Joseph's Hospital and Medical Center, Phoenix, AZ, United States

Preface

The continued success of *Essential Neuromodulation* suggested to us that the field of neuromodulation overall was active, growing, and perhaps seeking an update. The *principles* of electrical stimulation and its interface with the nervous system had not changed appreciably, however. What had changed were the numerous innovations at the cutting edge of the field, and chronicling these immediately seemed to fit the need for an updated view of the field in general and to round out our broader portrayal of neuromodulation we had sought in a follow-up to the first text. Thus was born *Innovative Neuromodulation*.

Whether investigating new waveforms, directional stimulation fields, tweaking the failing function of memory itself, mitigating the scourge of depression, or refining other technologies for modulation using light or high-frequency ultrasound, neuromodulation remains first, still its own field of endeavor, and second, a vibrant fully engaging amalgam of neuroscience, neurosurgery, neurology, pain medicine, physiatry, rehabilitative medicine, psychiatry, biophysics, computer science, bioengineering, electrical engineering, materials science, robotics, and control systems. No other field is at such a nexus.

We quickly noted that virtually all textbooks are just a static window for looking upon what is actually an evolving set of moving targets. We could not possibly hope to capture all of the innovation in neuromodulation, and we knew as well that much of what we might include would be out of date by publication. So the text has tried to accomplish two goals in this context: (1) we include chapters by not only leaders in their respective subfields but also leaders who continue to work within those fields and will likely continue to make advances long after this text needs revision and (2) we cover a variety of topics that gives a broad and in-depth sense of the *range* of innovation currently being pursued in neuromodulation. So, though intriguing, we have not included anything regarding the fascinating area of neuroimmunology and the relationship of stimulation to the inflammatory process, for example. Nor have we included all the potentially innovative uses of deep brain stimulation, such as treatment for addiction and obesity.

Our intent has been to create a comprehensive perspective on the field of neuromodulation that substantively explores both the essential and innovative topics as a double set—whether for the developing bioengineering graduate student hoping to contribute to the field with radical transformations of power supplies, or the experienced neurosurgeon who wants to start understanding the field better and implanting devices. We appreciate your support and hope you find the content helpful and inspiring.

Acknowledgments

We would like to thank all of the contributors to this book—their hard work and time on top of their very busy schedules has now made the field of neuromodulation even better. We specifically wish to give a special acknowledgment to Paul Kalanithi, MD, who even during an illness that recently took his life was still able to contribute a chapter here.

We also now acknowledge our Elsevier cohorts, Kristi Anderson and Natalie Farra, for all of their reminders and work behind the scenes during this process. We have worked with them on two books now and appreciate their endless patience. Finally we want to thank our families, Kelly, Chad, Tyler, Alexis, and Juliane, for all of their support during the editing of this book. We are all busy all of the time it seems, but having them there and in our lives still matters the most.

Introduction—Opportunities and Challenges

J.K. Krauss

Medical School Hannover, Hannover, Germany

Neuromodulation has revolutionized the treatment of various disorders within the past three decades. While the term neuromodulation has been used initially as a synonym for electrical stimulation of different components of the nervous system, as opposed to functional ablation, it has been understood in a much more broad sense in recent years. In that sense, neuromodulation would coincide quite well with the definition of functional neurosurgery as "utilizing dedicated structural and functional neuroimaging to identify and target discrete areas of the nervous system and to perform specific interventions using dedicated instruments and machinery in order to relieve a variety of symptoms of neurological and other disorders and to improve function of both the structurally normal and abnormal nervous system."[1] Nevertheless, electrical stimulation, which might actually result both in stimulation and in inhibition of nervous tissue, is still the major treatment modality with regard to its proven efficiency for many disorders,[2-4] the demonstrated improvement in quality of life, its general availability, its economic aspects, and its continuing spread all over the world. The unparalleled success of electrical stimulation is secondary most likely to its principal reversibility which could be seen as a disadvantage, but which allows to explore new shores, however, with much more ease than with any other currently available technology. We do not know yet and if so how often electrical stimulation of the nervous system may also be a disease-modifying therapy as shown recently in deep brain stimulation (DBS) for dystonia where it might reset altered neuroplasticity which might persist even after discontinuing long-term stimulation.[5-7] With new technology and machinery becoming available neuromodulation, and electrical stimulation in particular, has the potential to foster creativity and innovation like never before.

Neuromodulation, apart from stimulation with fully implanted systems, now also can take advantage of noninvasive techniques such as transcranial magnetic or direct-current stimulation, neuroprotective strategies applying viral vectors or constant infusion of growth factors, and more recently optogenetics. And, undoubtedly, we are facing the early dawn of the renaissance of ablative techniques, which actually have never disappeared completely.[8,9] Fortunately, the times are over when naive minds tried to propagate electrical stimulation as an "augmentative" procedure and to denounce lesioning techniques as "destructive." Certainly, it requires both experience and deliberation to be confident with a technique that might result in irreversible damage when applied indiscriminately. Focused ultrasound might well be a technique to bridge the gap between continuous stimulation and one time ablation once its technical childhood diseases will have been cured, allowing tailored "augmentative lesioning" over several sessions to yield optimal benefit to the affected individual.[10] Neuroprostheses, finally, can act as an interface between the disabled person and the environment, providing an increase in self-sufficiency and autonomy.

Chronic electrical stimulation via implanted electrodes is now being applied not only to the brain (DBS and cortical stimulation) and the spinal cord, but also more frequently to peripheral nerves, such as the occipital nerve for migraine and cluster headache, to the spinal ganglia for relief of neuropathic pain, to cranial nerve ganglia, such as the sphenopalatine ganglion for alleviating cluster headache, and to neuronal structures supplying internal organs. The frequency of DBS, with an exponential increase of numbers worldwide, certainly outnumbers any other neuromodulative approach. It is estimated that about 150,000 patients have undergone DBS up to now, including 120,000 patients with Parkinson disease (PD), 15,000 with tremor, 10,000 with dystonia, 4000 with pain, 2000 with psychiatric disorders, 1000 with epilepsy, and smaller collectives with more rare movement-disorders such as chorea and more experimental indications such as minimally conscious state or addiction. It is not surprising that with regard to the uneven economic global balance DBS has been a privilege to countries with a high economic standard.[9] Only within the past 10 years has DBS also become available for citizens of countries with lower gross national products, although we must keep in mind that in economically less privileged countries neurosurgery, in general, would be considered as luxury, with some African countries still having access to only a single neurosurgeon. It has been shown nicely how the operative treatment of PD depends on the health economics of the region.[9] There are very little solid data about both the exact numbers of DBS surgeries having been performed and on their increase each year in different nations. The analysis of a US database of hospital discharges between 2002 and 2011 indicated that more than 30,000 DBS surgeries had been performed during that time frame in the United States.[11] While the number of PD patients remained rather stable ranging between 2000 and 3000 implantations annually with a slight increase within the past few years, there was a marked increase in DBS surgeries for dystonia (with about 300 surgeries in 2011), and also in "off-label" indications including psychiatric disorders (also with about 300 surgeries in 2011).

In parallel to the increasing number of patients being implanted, there has also been a steep rise in publications on DBS. By using a network approach, more than 7000 papers on DBS published between 1991 and 2014 were identified.[12] There was a steep rise in the number of publications, particularly between 2006 and 2013, with a peak of about 900 publications in 2013. Interestingly, while there was a steady reduction in the fraction of papers on PD related to the overall number of published papers, there was a parallel increase in manuscripts on psychiatric indications, while the publication rate on dystonia remained rather stable. The fact that there is a relative decrease in the number of publications in DBS for PD despite an increase in DBS surgeries, especially on a global level, most likely is multifold. Of course, it is of major importance that DBS has become "routine" in PD. Furthermore, the model of progressive scholarly acceptance has been nicely applied to a similar phenomenon observed in DBS in essential tremor.[13] Progressive scholarly acceptance has been defined as the point when the number of investigations which refine or improve a procedure eclipsed the total number of reports assessing initial efficacy.

The reintroduction of psychiatric surgery taking advantage of the principal reversibility of DBS undoubtedly was a major achievement in the last two decades. There were estimates that psychiatric disorders would be the most frequent indications for DBS. In particular, depression as the most frequent psychiatric disorder was thought to be one of the most frequent indications for DBS. However, data from recent publications have been rather sobering. In the eagerly awaited double-blind randomized controlled multicenter study by Dougherty, DBS of the ventral capsule/ventral striatum was not more efficient than sham stimulation.[14] It remains to be seen whether or not the truly innovative approach of medial forebrain bundle stimulation will revitalize this field in the long term.[15] On the other hand, DBS of the nucleus accumbens or, more recently, of the bed nucleus of the stria terminalis for treatment of obsessive compulsive disorder has shown efficacy in several smaller studies repeatedly, and it is being reimbursed now in several European countries by health insurance carriers.[16] Certainly, it is necessary to proceed with caution in psychiatric neuromodulation, and time will tell what has been hype or hope.[17] As outlined in a recent consensus document, DBS for any psychiatric disorder still remains at an investigational stage, and further research is encouraged to provide more solid evidence for these indications.[18] This document also provided guidelines for the safe and ethical conduct of such studies, in particular also with regard to adequate consent procedures to respect the patient's capacity and autonomy, and to enhance patient safety.

What should be measured when a method is being introduced for a new indication or for a new target? While the classical scientific approach for many years was the demonstration of symptomatic improvement as assessed by objective validated rating scales, in particular for movement disorders such as PD, dystonia, and tremor, many other facets were less explored and achieved more attention only more recently. In particular, studies measuring disability or more subjectively perceived quality of life were pivotal to drive the field forward.[4,19] Such issues are of particular importance in some disorders such as secondary dystonia where sometimes relatively little objective benefit with chronic stimulation is counterbalanced by greater patient satisfaction than, e.g., as seen in PD.[20,21] Future studies will have to consider both, objective demonstration of efficacy but also improvement in the subjective perception of the patient and the personal gain obtained by the intervention. It will be relevant to better define and sort out not only the placebo effects in controlled randomized trials, but the nocebo and lessebo effects as well.[22]

In the past few years there has been a new wave of innovation in DBS technology.[23] While the basic system has remained the same with its components electrode, connecting cable, and pacemaker, several new developments have resulted in more complexity on one hand but also more ease of use on the other.[24] In particular, the exploration of local field potentials recorded from the electrode contacts has furthered our understanding of basal ganglia network activity and the pathophysiology of different movement disorders.[25,26] It has been shown also that enhanced oscillatory activity in certain frequency bands appears to be specific for certain disorders and even states of activity, such as the state of beta oscillatory activity in PD, or that of theta in dystonia. The first proofs-of-principle have demonstrated already that these signals could be used for feedback during stimulation and finally for stimulation on demand or even adaptive stimulation.[23,25,27] While the technology is now at our hands in the form of neurostimulation systems with "sensing and pacing" capabilities, there is still a long way to go to improve recording and decoding and to establish workable algorithms for chronic stimulation. The new developments in pacemaker technology now allow to stimulate more than two electrodes, which opens the way for multifocal DBS, a concept that has been underexplored. Certainly, one of the biggest steps forward was the introduction of new DBS electrodes, leaving the classical quadripolar circular electrode configuration setup behind and allowing more focused or directional stimulation with segmented or multicontact DBS electrodes.[28] These electrodes have already been shown to increase the threshold for side effects with the potential for delivering more targeted energy to the stimulation site. Finally, we have been quite conservative since neurostimulation systems were first introduced. Innovative stimulation paradigms have already been shown to be beneficial in spinal cord stimulation, including chronic stimulation in the 10 kHz range and the use of burst patterns for treatment of chronic pain.[29] Last, though not least, MR-compatible neurostimulation technology has arrived and will be taken for granted in the future.

New targets, apart from thalamus, globus pallidus internus and subthalamic nucleus have been introduced and partially explored. Unfortunately, however, some of these new targets were abandoned before their full range of possibilities was exploited. One such example is the posterior hypothalamic region, which was enthusiastically introduced for treatment of cluster headache but which was only popular for this indication for a few years, before being replaced largely by occipital nerve stimulation which actually now might be replaced by chronic stimulation of the sphenopalatine ganglion in the near future.[30-32] Another example is stimulation of the pedunculopontine region for treatment of freezing and gait ignition failure in PD.[33,34]

The scope of possible new indications for DBS has been outlined in several recent reviews.[35] There are two indications which are of particular interest because of both their high prevalence and their incidence throughout populations worldwide—tinnitus and arterial hypertension. Tinnitus may reduce quality of life significantly. The options of medical treatment are limited, and there has been little new development over the past few years. Neuromodulation, delivered in the form of thalamotomy targeting the centrolateral intralaminar thalamus, was used to treat tinnitus more than two decades ago in the framework of the thalamocortical dysrhythmia concept.[36] Besides the thalamus, also the area light chain within the head of the caudate nucleus, could be a possible site for chronic stimulation.[37] In addition, direct stimulation of primary or secondary cortical hearing areas have been shown to be efficacious in small cohorts of patients, and a novel concept could be intracortical stimulation of the Heschl gyrus.[38,39] Why should we consider arterial hypertension a possible indication for neuromodulation? Arterial hypertension is increasing in prevalence worldwide, and it has been estimated that about 10% of patients who are afflicted by arterial hypertension suffer from resistant hypertension defined as having systolic blood pressure higher than 140mmHg despite medication with at least three antihypertensive medications including a diuretic. Catheter-based radiofrequency denervation of the renal arteries has become the therapy of choice in more than 80 countries worldwide, however, a recent prospective, single-blind, randomized, sham-controlled trial including 535 patients failed to show a significant reduction of blood pressure 6 months after renal denervation.[40] Although the main conclusion from this study was that further evaluation of clinical trials or the validation of alternative methods of renal denervation would be necessary, this unexpected finding clearly also stimulates exploration of other options, including modulation of the central nervous system. It has been demonstrated that stimulation in the periventricular gray for treatment of neuropathic pain may alter blood pressure in the acute stimulation setting.[41] Depending on electrode location it is possible either to decrease or to increase arterial blood pressure. After successful demonstration of the proof-of-principle that periventricular gray DBS can indeed be applied in resistant arterial hypertension,[42] pilot trials are now underway.

The constant increase in knowledge, the improved understanding of pathophysiological processes, and the technological innovation should theoretically enable us to enhance therapy like never before in the history of mankind. Yet, despite all this progress the introduction of new and revolutionary treatments might actually slow down in the near future for a variety of reasons including societal, economic, administrative, and ethical aspects. Experimental research with animal models most likely will become more restricted in many countries, imposing severe limitations on the classical bench-to-bedside approach. At least, the timeline for this approach will become much longer than previously anticipated. The trial-and-error approach which has been a major driving force in particular in functional neurosurgery for decades will also face many more restrictions, and when looking back to the history of the superspeciality of functional neurosurgery we must realize that many trials which have successfully established new therapies could probably not be conducted in current environments. Funding is becoming more limited in many countries and we can only hope that use-led basic research and applied research will be more in the future focus. One problem we have to face in that regard is that many phase II trials which require large investments of funds turn out negative despite the therapy showing promise in the early pilot trials. Sometimes it might well be that we get the wrong answer to the wrong questions, and the concept of primary versus secondary endpoints should be reconsidered. However, other issues which have to be taken into account as well are timing of the studies and long-term perspectives.

Finally, noninvasive neuromodulation is a new field that is expanding rapidly. New technology now allows stimulation of deep brain structures as well[43] and some of these methods could even be combined with invasive techniques. Noninvasive neuromodulation will also challenge concepts on the ethical limits of what could be done. While, e.g., most would consider invasive neuromodulation for cognitive enhancement unethical, this would most likely not be the case with noninvasive methods for cognitive enhancement. Nevertheless, it has to be realized also that the latter, while more acceptable for most, would still constitute an option which would be available for the more privileged and ethical issues would need to be reconsidered under these aspects.

This volume *Innovative Neuromodulation* is a logical step into the future development beyond essential neuromodulation. My congratulations to the editors for the achievement of putting such a comprehensive overview on this field in motion and setting up a new milestone.

References

1. Gildenberg PL, Krauss JK. History of stereotactic surgery. 2nd ed. Lozano A.M. Gildenberg PL, Tasker RR, editors. *Textbook of Stereotactic and Functional Neurosurgery,* vol. 1. Berlin Heidelberg: Springer; 2009.

2. Fasano A, Aquino CC, Krauss JK, Honey CR, Bloem BR. Axial disability and deep brain stimulation in patients with Parkinson's disease. *Nat Rev Neurol.* 2015;11:98–110.

3. Volkmann J, Mueller J, Deuschl G, Falk D, Kuehn A, Kupsch A, et al. Pallidal neurostimulation in patients with medication-refractory cervical dystonia—a sham-controlled randomized trial. *Lancet Neurol.* 2014;13:875–884.

4. Deuschl G, Schade-Brittinger C, Krack P, Volkmann J, Schäfer H, Bötzel K, et al. A randomized trial of deep-brain stimulation for Parkinson's disease. *N Engl J Med.* 2006;355:896–908.

5. Ruge D, Cif L, Limousin P, Gonzalez V, Vasques X, Hariz MI, et al. Shaping reversibility? Long-term deep brain stimulation in dystonia: the relationship between effects on electrophysiology and clinical symptoms. *Brain.* 2011;134:2106–2115.

6. Cheung T, Zhang C, Rudolph J, Alterman RL, Tagliati M. Sustained relief of generalized dystonia despite prolonged interruption of deep brain stimulation. *Mov Disord.* 2013;28:1431–1434.

7. Cif L, Ruge D, Gonzalez V, Limousin P, Vasques X, Hariz MI, et al. The influence of deep brain stimulation intensity and duration on symptoms evolution in an OFF stimulation dystonia study. *Brain Stimul.* 2013;6:500–505.

8. Gross RE. What happened to posteroventral pallidotomy for Parkinson's disease and dystonia? *Neurotherapeutics.* 2008;5:281–293.

9. Jourdain VA, Schechtmann G. Health economics and surgical treatment for Parkinson's disease in a world perspective: results from an international survey. *Stereotact Funct Neurosurg.* 2014;92:71–79.

10. Lipsman N, Mainprize TG, Schwartz ML, Hynynen K, Lozano AM. Intracranial applications of magnetic resonance-guided focused ultrasound. *Neurotherapeutics.* 2014;11:593–605.

11. Youngerman BE, Chan AK, Mikell CB, McKhann GM, Sheth SA. A decade of emerging indications: deep brain stimulation in the United States. *J Neurosurg.* 2016;125(2):461–471.

12. Ineichen C, Christen M. Analyzing 7000 texts on deep brain stimulation: what do they tell us? *Front Integr Neurosci.* 2015;9(52):1–18.

13. Schnurman Z, Kondziolka D. Evaluating innovation. Part 2: development in neurosurgery. *J Neurosurg.* 2016;124:212–223.

14. Dougherty DD, Rezai AR, Carpenter LL, Howland RH, Bhati MT, O'Reardon JP, et al. A randomized sham-controlled trial of deep brain stimulation of the ventral capsule/ventral striatum for chronic treatment-resistant depression. *Biol Psychiatry.* 2015;78:240–248.

15. Schlaepfer TE, Bewernick BH, Kayser S, Hurlemann R, Coenen VA. Deep brain stimulation of the human reward system for major depression—rationale, outcomes and outlook. *Neuropsychopharmacology.* 2014;39:1303–1314.

16. Alonso P, Cuadras D, Gabriëls L, Denys D, Goodman W, Greenberg BD, et al. Deep brain stimulation for obsessive-compulsive disorder: a meta-analysis of treatment outcome and predictors of response. *PLoS ONE.* 2015;10:e0133591.

17. Hariz MI, Hariz GM. Hyping deep brain stimulation in psychiatry could lead to its demise. *BMJ.* 2012;345:e5447.

18. Nuttin B, Wu H, Mayberg H, Hariz M, Gabriels L, Galert T, et al. Consensus on guidelines for stereotactic neurosurgery for psychiatric disorders. *J Neurol Neurosurg Pyschiatry.* 2014;85:1003–1008.

19. Mueller J, Skogseid IM, Benecke R, Kupsch A, Trottenberg T, Poewe W, et al. Pallidal deep brain stimulation improves quality of life in segmental and generalized dystonia: results from a prospective, randomized sham-controlled trial. *Mov Disord*. 2008;23:131–134.

20. Krauss JK, Loher TJ, Weigel R, Capelle HH, Weber S, Burgunder JM. Chronic stimulation of the globus pallidus internus for treatment of non-dYT1 generalized dystonia and choreoathetosis: 2-year follow up. *J Neurosurg*. 2003;98:785–792.

21. Vidailhet M, Yelnik J, Lagrange C, Fraix V, Grabli D, Thobois S, et al. Bilateral pallidal deep brain stimulation for the treatment of patients with dystonia-choreoathetosis cerebral palsy: a prospective pilot study. *Lancet Neurol*. 2009;8:709–717.

22. Schuepbach WM, Rau J, Knudsen K, Volkmann J, Krack P, Timmermann L, et al. Neurostimulation for Parkinson's disease with early motor complications. *N Engl J Med*. 2013;368:610–622.

23. Priori A. Technology for deep brain stimulation at a gallop. *Mov Disord*. 2015;30:1206–1212.

24. Fasano A, Lozano AM. Deep brain stimulation for movement disorders: 2015 and beyond. *Curr Opin Neurol*. 2015;28:423–436.

25. Eusebio A, Thevathasan W, Doyle Gaynor L, Pogosyan A, Bye E, Foltynie T, et al. Deep brain stimulation can suppress pathological synchronisation in parkinsonian patients. *J Neurol Neurosurg Psychiatry*. 2011;82:569–573.

26. Silberstein P, Kuhn AA, Kupsch A, Trottenberg T, Krauss JK, Wohrle JC, et al. Patterning of globus pallidus local field potentials differs between Parkinson's disease and dystonia. *Brain*. 2003;126:2597–2608.

27. Barow E, Neumann WJ, Brücke C, Huebl J, Horn A, Brown P, et al. Deep brain stimulation suppresses pallidal low frequency activity in patients with phasic dystonic movements. *Brain*. 2014;137:3012–3024.

28. Pollo C, Kaelin-Lang A, Oertel MF, Stieglitz L, Taub E, Fuhr P, et al. Directional deep brain stimulation: an intraoperative double-blind pilot study. *Brain*. 2014;137:2015–2026.

29. Grider JS, Manchikanti L, Carayannopoulos A, Sharma ML, Balog CC, Harned ME, et al. Effectiveness of spinal cord stimulation in chronic spinal pain: a systematic review. *Pain Physician*. 2016;19:E33–54.

30. Jürgens TP, May A. Role of sphenopalatine ganglion stimulation in cluster headache. *Curr Pain Headache Rep*. 2014;18:433.

31. Bartsch T, Pinsker MO, Rasche D, Kinfe T, Hertel F, Diener HC, et al. Hypothalamic deep brain stimulation for cluster headache: experience from a new multicase series. *Cephalalgia*. 2008;28:285–295.

32. Schwedt TJ, Vargas B. Neurostimulation for treatment of migraine and cluster headache. *Pain Med*. 2015;16:1827–1834.

33. Hamani C, Aziz T, Bloem RB, Brown P, Chabardes S, Coyne T, et al. Pedunculopontine nucleus region deep brain stimulation in Parkinson disease: surgical anatomy and terminology. *Stereotact Funct Neurosurg*. 2016;94:298–306.

34. Hamani C, Lozano AM, Mazzone PAM, Moro E, Hutchison W, Silburn P, et al. Pedunculopontine nucleus region deep brain stimulation in Parkinson disease: surgical techniques, side effects and postoperative imaging. *Stereotact Funct Neurosurg*. 2016;94:307–319.

35. Hariz M, Blomstedt P, Zrinzo L. Future of brain stimulation: new targets, new indications, new technology. *Mov Disord*. 2013;28:1784–1792.

36. Jeanmonod D, Magnin M, Morel A. Low-threshold calcium spike bursts in the human thalamus. Common physiopathology for sensory, motor and limbic positive symptoms. *Brain*. 1996;119:363–375.

37. Cheung SW, Larson PS. Tinnitus modulation by deep brain stimulation in locus of caudate neurons (area LC). *Neuroscience*. 2010;169:1768–1778.

38. Donovan C, Sweet J, Eccher M, Megerian C, Semaan M, Murray G, et al. Deep brain stimulation of Heschl gyrus: implantation technique, intraoperative localization, and effects of stimulation. *Neurosurgery*. 2015;77:940–947.

39. De Ridder D, Vanneste S. Auditory cortex stimulation might be efficacious in a subgroup of tinnitus patients. *Brain Stimul*. 2014;7:917–918.
40. Bhatt DL, Kandzari DE, O'Neill WW, D'Agostino R, Flack JM, Katzen BT, et al. A controlled trial of renal denervation for resistant hypertension. *N Engl J Med*. 2014;370:1393–1401.
41. Pereira EAC, Wang S, Paterson DJ, Stein JF, Aziz TZ, Green AL. Sustained reduction of hypertension by deep brain stimulation. *J Clin Neurosci*. 2010;17:124–127.
42. Patel NK, Javed S, Khan S, Papouchado M, Malizia AL, Pickering AE, et al. Deep brain stimulation relieves refractory hypertension. *Neurology*. 2011;76:405–407.
43. Kedzior KK, Gierke L, Gellersen HM, Berlim MT. Cognitive functioning and deep transcranial magnetic stimulation (DTMS) in major psychiatric disorders—a systematic review. *J Psych Res*. 2016;75:107e115.

NEW DIRECTIONS WITH CURRENT THERAPIES

1

Microarrays in the Brain: Can They Be Used for Brain–Machine Interface Control?

W.Q. Malik[1,2] and R. Ajemian[2]

[1]Harvard Medical School, Boston, MA, United States; [2]Massachusetts Institute of Technology, Cambridge, MA, United States

OUTLINE

Innovative Neuromodulation.
DOI: http://dx.doi.org/10.1016/B978-0-12-800454-8.00001-X

3

Ever since Hans Berger recorded the first electroencephalogram in 1924,[1] the prospect of using invasive neural implants to record and manipulate brain function was fated to become scientific reality. After all, if electric currents can be detected as far away as the surface of the scalp, then even more detailed neural signals must lurk in the brain itself. It took over a decade for Berger's work to be accepted and roughly three-quarters of a century before the neurotechnology developed to enable clinically acceptable practices for electrode implantation. But once it became established that information processing within the brain leaves coarse electrical signatures that can be detected noninvasively, it was only a matter of time before scientific reductionism led to intracranial neural recording and stimulation.

Turn the clock forward to today, and the field of neural prosthetics (or brain–machine interfacing or brain–computer interfacing) is one of the hottest fields in all of science. We see the confluence of three (hardly independent) factors that generally drive progress in any scientific field: (1) technology development, (2) public interest, and (3) funding availability. In terms of technology development, the last two decades have seen a burst of innovation that has relegated to obscurity techniques for recording from one neuron at a time. Microelectrode arrays with up to 100 channels are commercially available, as are stimulating electrodes with programmable pulses. These tools provide us with an unprecedented ability to record activity from neuronal populations and to stimulate neural circuits in the brain.

In terms of the level of public interest, it is difficult to think of any branch of science which has so effortlessly captured the imagination of the public and with good reason. The history of scientific/technological progress is that of mankind understanding, harnessing, and utilizing one physical resource after the other. Yet, the question of how the mind emerges from the physical processes of the brain remains largely a mystery. In this respect, mentation is something of an untapped frontier, with a longstanding tradition of being explored imaginatively in scientific fiction. Now, perhaps, the day is upon us where the exotic notions of science fiction are realized through the scientific methodology of neural engineering. Hence, it is quite common to see headlines in major news organizations touting the advances of the field through headlines like the following in a 2013 issue of the Daily Mail: "Mind control experiment lets users wag a rat's tail just using brain power." Similarly enticing are the many headlines discussing brain-powered robotic limbs or even brain-powered cars. Brain power does indeed appear to be in vogue.

Finally, regarding financial support levels, the obvious promise of being able to treat neurological injuries and disorders that had previously seemed untreatable (or at least poorly treatable) has ensured a steady flow of health-related research funding from both public and private institutions. Multiple clinical trials are ongoing in the United States that involve invasive neural interfaces, and each of these trials requires millions of dollars of support. Additional uses for neural interfacing may be found in enhancing the natural capabilities of people who are not disabled. For instance, the military, naturally beguiled by the possibility of augmenting human performance with machines, has poured in hundreds of millions of dollars in DARPA programs such as "Revolutionizing Prosthetics," "Reliable Neural-Interface Technology," "Systems-Based Neurotechnology for Emerging Therapies," and "Restoring Active Memory," in addition to support from several other defense research funding mechanisms.

In short, the field of neural prosthetics is characterized by more than ample technology development, public interest, and funding availability; the scientific counterparts to the criminologist's "means, motive, and opportunity" are all present. Yet why are so few people walking around today with chips in their brains? Is it simply a question of technological inadequacy? If so, in 30 years will there be lots of individuals walking around with chips in their brains for a variety of reasons? Or are there more profound scientific barriers to the furtherance of this technology that center around our ability to decipher the complex patterns of neural activity—even when we can observe them—distributed across billions of neurons by means of quadrillions of synapses? The brain is, by many accounts, the most intricately designed pattern of matter extant in the known universe. How much better do we need to understand its function before we can faithfully embark upon feats of neural engineering which will result in all manner of brain-powered contrivances that improve the quality of our lives?

We cannot answer all of these questions, since they are active and ongoing research issues scattered across many scientific disciplines and subdisciplines. But we can provide an overview to the field of neural prosthetics in which brain–machine interfaces are powered by the signals from microarrays in the brain. Specifically, we attempt to offer perspective and context to the discussion by addressing the following three issues:

I. NEW DIRECTIONS WITH CURRENT THERAPIES

- What types of neural signals are currently available using microarrays, how are they processed, and what technological advances may be ahead?
- What is the general design for a brain–machine interface? What are the control requirements for using neural signals to operate or "power" such a device? What control strategies are capable of producing high performance levels?
- What information is contained in neural signals? What information processing paradigms can be used to extract that information? Are there any fundamental limitations on our ability to identify the information contained in neural circuits?

For the most part, this chapter is intended to be about motor neuroprosthetic devices in which a microarray is implanted in the motor cortex of an animal or person, and those signals are used to drive assistive technology, with an emphasis on arm movements as opposed to leg movements. The chapter also does not focus on deep brain stimulation in the case of Parkinson's disease and other pathologies, as other chapters within this compilation do so.

BUILDING A BRAIN–MACHINE INTERFACE

We now present an overview and discussion of some of the major design components of a brain–machine interface system.

Neural Signal Resolution

It has been known since Ramon y Cajal's pioneering work that individual neurons are the fundamental information processing unit in the brain and an action potential, or spike, is the fundamental unit of information. Neurons communicate, in most instances, by sending spikes out through axons and receiving spike-induced signals through dendrites. Importantly, in most areas of the brain, particularly the cortex, the neural circuits are highly distributed in that each neuron is contacted by many other neurons. It is estimated that each cortical neuron is contacted by roughly 10,000 other cortical neurons (although there are certain regional variations). Given all this, from a purely information-processing point of view, the gold standard for neural signal acquisition is to record the time-series of individual spikes from as many individual neurons as possible. This signal-processing ideal, however, must be tempered by the practical costs and complications of recording so densely from inside the brain. Below is a brief discussion of the state-of-the-art technology available for recording spikes from individual neurons, including the advantages and disadvantages of implanting microarrays in the brain.

Over the last decade, there has been an explosion of interest in motor neuroprosthetic devices that rely on microelectrode arrays directly implanted chronically into cortical tissue (e.g., Refs. [2–5]). These arrays consist of multiple elements, each of which provides an independent neural signal channel. The array is therefore capable of recording the activity of an ensemble of neurons, as opposed to just a single-neuron recorded with a single electrode; the former approach is considered necessary for obtaining higher quality of control. Two of the most popular intracortical microelectrode array architectures, with extensive use in the last two decades, are the Utah array[6] and the Michigan array.[7] The Utah array consists of 100 microelectrodes, arranged in a 10 × 10 element grid (see Fig. 1.1). Each electrode, with a micrometer-scale recording surface, is capable of acquiring the activity of a small population of neurons, or single units, in its proximity. The voltage waveform recorded by the electrode therefore represents multiunit activity, typically consisting of a population of 3–4 individually separable single units.[8] Standard signal analysis techniques, such as clustering and principal components analysis, can be used to identify the putative single units from the multiunit recordings through the process of spike sorting.[9]

The central rationale for these intracortical microelectrode devices is the neurophysiology doctrine that neurons are the fundamental unit of information processing,[10] so information at the level of single-unit spikes should, in theory, provide the highest-quality signal.[11] Most neurons generate a spike about a millisecond long in duration, with wide-bandwidth frequency content extending up to several kHz. Neurons spike at various

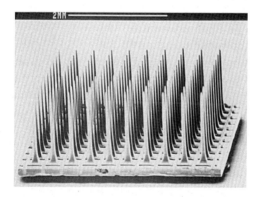

FIGURE 1.1 The commonly used Utah intracortical electrode array with 100 individually addressable microelectrodes. This array is one of the few neural-interface devices that has been approved for use in multiple ongoing clinical trials. *Source: Reprinted from Maynard EM, Nordhausen CT, Normann RA. The Utah intracortical electrode array: a recording structure for potential brain-computer interfaces. Electroencephalogr Clin Neurophysiol. 1997;102(3):228–239.*

rates ranging from under 1 spike/second up to 100–300 spikes/second. It is generally believed that neuronal information is encoded primarily in the spike rate, although the rate coding versus temporal coding debate is still ongoing. In most practical analyses, the spike rate is usually derived as the number of spikes within a time interval, typically around 50 or 100 ms, divided by the width of the interval. The spike rates of neurons in motor-related areas of the brain reflect various aspects of movement planning, initiation and/or execution, as discussed in more detail later in this chapter.

Alternate Signal Types and Risk Factors

Although single-unit spike analysis is well established in classical neurophysiology, various other intracortical signals also provide useful information about the underlying neural activity and offer some practical advantages in a range of neuroengineering applications. A closely related class of signals is the discrete multiunit activity or multiunit spike-train (MSP), which represents a series of events similar to a single-unit spike-train, but reflects the activity of a small set of neurons as opposed to an individual neuron. MSP is usually obtained by detecting threshold-crossing events within the voltage waveform recorded from a microelectrode, after bandpass filtering and other necessary preprocessing steps.[12] The event threshold should be defined carefully to jointly minimize the false alarm rate and the probability of misdetection. A commonly used threshold is −3 to −4.5 times the root mean square voltage.[13,14]

There are three main motivations for the increasing popularity of MSP in neurophysiological analyses, especially those related to brain–machine interfaces. First, processing raw neural data to obtain MSP is a far less complex process than the laborious and computationally intensive steps required to obtain sorted single-unit spike-trains.[15] Second, unlike single-unit recordings that are highly nonstationary, MSPs are relatively stable for much longer periods of time, with important design implications and operational advantages for brain–machine interface design and other applications.[16] Third, even though multiunit spikes lack single-neuron resolution, their performance when used as the input to a neural decoding algorithm is only slightly inferior to that obtained with a single-unit spike-based decoder.[13]

Another manifestation of neural activity that can also be recorded using microelectrode arrays consists of continuous signals referred to as local field potentials (LFPs).[17] LFPs are slower cortical rhythms, centered at a few Hertz frequency, that contain information potentially complementary to that contained in single-unit and multiunit spikes. Besides being derived from much larger neuronal ensembles and spatial span than spikes, LFPs also reflect generative processes that fundamentally differ from those that give rise to spikes.[18] Significantly, because LFPs embody neural activity pooled over a larger spatial scale, these signals are stable over extremely long time periods due to the averaging effect; this property is particularly useful for designing robust brain–machine interfaces based on motor cortical LFP decoding.[19]

Given that action potentials and field potentials may contain nonoverlapping movement information—along with clear differences in signal resolution and robustness—there has also been some interest in using them simultaneously within a brain–machine interface. This idea is practically feasible because these two types of signals are already available from the recording array, and only the decoding algorithms require appropriate modifications. Some recent studies have reported that hybrid decoding of spikes and LFPs offers little improvement over a spike-only decoder, but the improvement is significant once spikes are removed.[20–22] Further investigation of this topic may shed more light on ways to implement the intuitively appealing idea of using all possible information sources available from the recording array.

Before leaving this section, we must discuss the practical concerns of implanting these microelectrodes in the brain,[23,24] which will contribute to decision-making regarding their clinical use. First, there is the mechanical trauma of insertion. Second, the electrode is viewed by the brain as a foreign body, and an immunological response is initiated against it. Third, the risk of infection is serious (and always will be in any scenario that exhibits wires extending from inside the brain to outside). Fourth, because the electrode does not move along with the brain, single units are not stably held across days, and there is no guarantee that the same neuron is being recorded on the same channel from one day to the next. Finally, "these signals fade and disappear after a few months and therefore the current technology is not reliable for extended periods of time."[24] Therefore, before using this technology in humans, one must carefully consider the significant health risks that are incurred for potentially only a few months of device operation. These reasons do not necessarily speak against their clinical use, but they do suggest the need for a critical assessment of the advantages and disadvantages on a condition-by-condition and case-by-case basis. Of course, future technological developments—such as fully wireless transmission and electrode fabrication with new biocompatible materials—have the potential to mitigate several of these risk factors.

THE ARCHITECTURE OF A BRAIN–MACHINE INTERFACE

Once neural signals are being reliably recorded from a typical microarray, such as the Utah microarray, they can be used to help control an external device. A generic description of the main architecture is illustrated in

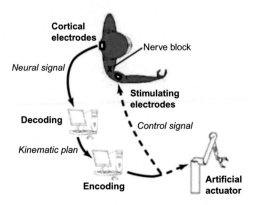

FIGURE 1.2   The basic processing stages for a brain–machine interface (here illustrated with a nonhuman primate). In this case, the goal is either to control an artificial actuator or to activate stimulating electrodes placed in a paralyzed limb.

Fig. 1.2. The architecture contains four distinct stages as discussed below. For reasons to be articulated later in this chapter, we may refer to this specific brain–machine interface design strategy as "indirect decoding."

Signal Acquisition/Processing

As described earlier, a microarray implanted in the brain transmits signals out of the brain through a wired or wireless connection, which are ultimately relayed to an amplifier. After the neural signals are acquired, they are high-pass filtered until spikes are identified. These spikes are usually aggregated over time-bins on the order of about 50 ms, optionally with smoothing, and the resulting firing rate is taken as the instantaneous neural signal. Other brain–machine interface embodiments may use alternative signal representations as discussed in the preceding section.

Decoding

The firing rates are subsequently "decoded" into an underlying kinematic movement intention through use of a specialized computational algorithm. For example, if the neural signals are for controlling the motion of the hand, the neural firing rates over time can be decoded to reveal an underlying kinematic trajectory. This step is where the "magic" happens, in that a transformation is produced which converts brain activity into something tangible in the real world, like a hand trajectory. In philosophical terms, decoding is where Descartes' supposedly inviolable separation of mind and body is irrevocably bridged.

Command Recoding

Once a movement intention has been ascertained through the decoding stage, it remains to be instantiated via the end-effector, which may assume many possible forms, such as an onscreen computer cursor, a robotic limb, or a functional electrical stimulation controller. To instantiate the desired movement command (such as to move in a straight line to the left with a bell-shaped velocity profile), control commands must be computed and sent to the actuation system for the end-effector in whatever form is appropriate. For example, if the end-effector is a robotic limb powered by electrically driven torque motors, the command signals would be the appropriate voltages for the motors.

End-Effector Actuation

The transduced command for evoking the movement intention actuates the end-effector, resulting in brain-controlled movement. This movement is subsequently perceived by the agent and can influence future behavior in the standard perception–action closed loop.

As indicated above, decoding is the key stage in this architecture, for that is the stage at which neural activity is converted into a "usable" form, presumably through our scientific knowledge of how the brain operates, i.e., our understanding of what certain patterns of neural activity imply for behavior. Therefore, a brain–machine interface relying upon this decoding architecture will perform only as well as its decoder, which in turn can perform only as well as our understanding of how the brain works. Ultimately, in order to build a brain–machine interface, there is no escaping the question of somehow interpreting activity in the brain.

WHAT DOES THE MOTOR CORTEX DO?

In this section, we trace the long scientific history of the quest to understand the meaning of neural activity in the motor cortex, given its fundamental importance for brain–machine interface design for neuromotor rehabilitation.

Movements Versus Muscles Debate in the Distant Past

This seemingly innocuous question belies a long and turbulent history of scientific inquiry. To this day, the question remains unsettled, although not from any shortage of claims or counterclaims. In 1870, the German physiologists Fritsch and Hitzig made the seminal discovery that, when a particular region of a dog's cortical surface was stimulated, small twitches of functionally related muscles were subsequently observed.[25] This discovery, occurring well before Penfield's seminal studies on humans which led to the notion of a motor topography,[26] suggested to Fritsch and Hitzig that the motor cortex operates as a kind of structured repository for upper-motor neurons: when a region is stimulated, neighboring cortical neurons excite functionally linked muscles by activating the corresponding spinal interneuronal circuits and/or alpha motor neurons. Just 3 years later, the British physiologist Ferrier performed a similar set of experiments and determined that stimulation of the motor cortex does not merely trigger a correlated cascade of muscle fiber twitches; rather, stimulation of the motor cortex engages circuits responsible for portions of natural motor behaviors that are more complex and abstract in their structure.[27] Thus was born the famous "movements versus muscles debate," which has played out over the last 145 years without resolution.[28–30]

In simplest terms, the basic point of the debate is the following: does the motor cortex represent movement behavior at the low level of muscular details or at some higher and more abstract level of movement plans/goals? Ultimately, all movement commands must be expressed at the level of muscular details in order to be instantiated by the motor system. The question is where the motor cortex fits in this overall hierarchy of the sensorimotor transformation.[31] If the motor cortex represents low-level muscular details of movement, then much of the "heavy-lifting" of the computations needed to effect the sensorimotor transformation (converting a kinematic movement intention into an underlying set of muscle commands) has already been performed upstream of the motor cortex. These computations may be executed in areas such as parietal and premotor cortex (putting aside for the moment subcortical regions like the cerebellum and the basal ganglia). Under this interpretation, motor cortical neurons act like upper-motor neurons, which relay their signals to corresponding alpha motor neurons in the spinal cord, without undergoing significant additional transformations at this stage.

If, on the other hand, the motor cortex represents movements from a more ecological perspective, such as high-level kinematic movement intentions or segments of learned behaviors (independent of muscular details), then one's interpretation of motor cortical function is different. The processing stage from the motor cortex to the spinal cord would indeed effectuate a significant portion of the remaining computations inherent in the sensorimotor transformation. One can imagine that these two different interpretations bear strongly on our ability to faithfully interpret motor cortical activity.

Part of the reason why Fritsch and Hitzig obtained results that differed from Ferrier is that electrical current was used to stimulate small portions of the motor cortex. Given that current spreads and that electrical stimulation will stimulate not just neurons but their fibers as well, it is hard to quantify—particularly using the technology of that era—the extent to which a stimulation protocol engages the motor cortex. Are merely a few individual neurons recruited or are elements of functional neural circuits engaged? One can imagine a scenario whereby a lower level of current might recruit a relatively small number of neighboring neurons, leading to homonymous muscle twitches, while higher levels of current engage both neurons and synaptic circuitry that may correspond to some aspect of a learned behavior. In this latter case, the delivery of electrical current taps into these preconfigured circuits, sculpted through motor learning, to give the false impression that the motor cortex represents high-level details of movement commands simply because the input pulse is more diffuse than focal. This and other scenarios illustrate the difficulty of drawing definitive conclusions from stimulation studies, without being able to precisely control the level of current and its field of spread, something which is hard to achieve even today, and clearly unimaginable before the turn of the 20th century.

Movements Versus Muscles Debate in the Recent Past

The movements versus muscles debate remained dormant for several decades until the advent of acute single-neuron recording technology, first in visual cortex by Hubel and Wiesel[32] and then in the motor cortex of awake behaving nonhuman primates through the pioneering work of Edwin Evarts.[33] The basic concept behind these studies is very simple and has not substantively changed over the last half century.[34] A nonhuman primate performs a well-rehearsed motor task for which the movement parameters are tightly controlled. The firing rates of individual motor cortical neurons (often, but not always, pyramidal tract output neurons in layer 5) are recorded during task performance, from which one can construct response histograms based on multiple repetitions of the same motor behavior. Having simultaneously recorded both the movement parameters of the behavior and the response properties of the neurons, one can subsequently correlate the two quantities—i.e., see which movement parameter best correlates with the observed neural response. In the case of Evarts' initial study,[33] the behavioral paradigm was carefully designed to tease apart the movement covariates of force and position (i.e., under the usual circumstances, force and position are positively correlated to a significant degree). What Evarts found by means of this dissociation is that most neurons correlated better with force (or its rate of change) than position, an observation that comports better with a muscle interpretation for motor cortical activity than a movement interpretation. This work was performed using wrist flexion/extension movements.

Fifteen years later, a pioneering study was performed by Georgopoulous and colleagues that changed the field.[35] In this experimental paradigm, illustrated by Fig. 1.3, a monkey makes whole-arm center-out reaching

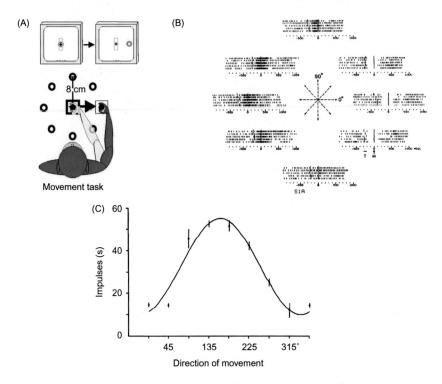

FIGURE 1.3   The experimental paradigm of Georgopoulos et al.[35] (A) A nonhuman primate makes planar reaching movements of 8 cm in response to onscreen visual cues. (B) The activity elicited during movement can be tabulated and visualized by means of a raster plot over trial repetitions. (C) For an example neuron, the cosine function fits the average movement-related activity across the eight different movement directions.

movements in one of eight different directions uniformly interspersed around the circle by means of a planar manipulandum which is grasped at the handle (see Fig. 1.3A). Neural activity is recorded from single neurons before, during, and after both target presentation and movement onset. Each movement direction is repeated multiple times for the construction of a raster plot for the task (see Fig. 1.3B). Since direction is the controlled movement parameter which differs across conditions and since the speed profiles are fairly consistent in the different directions, it makes sense to regress movement-related neural activity against the direction of movement. When this analysis was performed, they[35] found that individual neural activity was quite well fit (see Fig. 1.3C) by the following mathematical model:

$$r_i(\theta) = b_0 + b_1 \cos(\theta - \theta_0)$$

where r_i is the average firing rate of the ith neuron during the movement-related epoch, b_0 is the baseline level of movement-related firing activity across all directions, b_1 is a scaling factor, and θ_0 is the preferred direction for that particular neuron. The preferred direction is the critical concept, which means that the neuron fires maximally in one movement direction (analogous to orientation tuning in neurons in primary visual cortex). The firing rate decreases in a gradual fashion as one moves in directions that increasingly misalign with the preferred direction, an observation usually described as "broad tuning."

The conclusion from this study that was further developed in the papers that followed (e.g., Georgopoulos et al.[36]) was that individual neurons in the motor cortex conveniently encode movement direction of the hand in Cartesian space, i.e., the direction in space with reference to an invariant body-centered coordinate system. Furthermore, one can decode the direction of arm movement from the firing rates of a population of neurons. These ideas, if true, comport with the idea of the motor cortex as representing high-level attributes of movement, such as the direction in space of an end-effector.

The Representational Approach and Encoding Versus Decoding

Before continuing, it behooves us to formally introduce two concepts: *encoding* and *decoding*. These critical concepts underlie the *representational approach* to understanding neural activity, an approach which remains the dominant one in the field to this day due to its simplicity.

Encoding: The idea behind encoding is that a cell's activity in time can be expressed as a function of the value of a specific movement variable(s) in time. More precisely, a cell's firing rate can be well-approximated by a mathematical function that takes as input the value of a movement variable(s). The general formulation is as follows:

$$r_i(t - \tau, \vec{M}(t)) = f(t, \vec{M}(t), \vec{A}) \tag{1.1}$$

where $r_i(t - \tau)$ is the firing rate of the ith neuron at time $t - \tau$, $\vec{M}(t)$ is a vector of movement variables evaluated at time t, f is a mathematical function that (for whatever scientific reason) describes the neuron's response, and $\vec{A}$ is a vector of parameters that parameterizes the function f. The term τ is a temporal offset parameter which signifies that the neural activity causes the movement of the end-effector and not the other way around. In the case of the cosine-tuning model described above, the function f is the cosine function.

To summarize, encoding expresses the activity of an individual neuron (or a neuronal population) as a function of movement variables. Thus, what the neuron encodes intuitively embodies something about the aspect of movement to which that neuron somehow directly contributes. Encoding models are almost always chosen empirically through correlative analysis of the data taken from motor neurophysiological experiments, where neural activity and movement variables are monitored simultaneously.

Decoding: The complementary or inverse operation to encoding is decoding. Whereas encoding represents the activity of single neurons as a function of movement variables, decoding represents the value of a movement variable as a function of the firing rates of a population of recorded neurons.

$$M_j(t, \vec{r}(t - \tau - \Delta t : t - \tau)) = g(t, \vec{r}(t - \tau - \Delta t : t - \tau), \vec{B}) \qquad (1.2)$$

where M_j is the jth movement variable that is being decoded (it could, e.g., be the horizontal position of the hand or the vertical component of hand velocity), $\vec{r}$ is the vector of firing rates taken for the population of motor cortical neurons being simultaneously recorded, $(t - \tau - \Delta t : t - \tau)$ is the time interval of magnitude Δt over which the firings rates contribute, g is a mathematical functional that describes the mathematical procedure used to fit firing rates to the movement variables, and $\vec{B}$ is the vector of parameters used to obtain the best-fitting functional.

There are a couple of points to make about the definition of decoding. The movement variable M_j is a function not just of the firing rates at an instant in time, but the firing histories of the neurons over a temporal interval Δt. Often this time window is on the order of 100–500 ms, and the neural activity throughout this interval is considered to influence the behavioral output. This means that g is a functional which maps functions (or their vector approximations) to values, as opposed to a function which maps values to values. The approach provides significantly more information for the decoder to use and, concomitantly, increases the number of parameters in $\vec{B}$; it also implicitly assumes that some period of neuronal dynamics is involved with determining instantaneous behavioral output. In the case of encoding, f is usually a function of a movement variable (or variables) at a fixed point in time, as opposed to a time history (though it could be otherwise). Decoding models, like encoding models, are constructed empirically through data fitting from trials in which the movement behavior and neural firing rates are both monitored (in some contexts, imagined movements, rather than actual movements, are all that is available). To summarize, the goal behind decoding is to express the value of a movement variable as a function of the firing histories of a population of recorded neurons.

It is critical to note that decoding and encoding are complementary or inverse operations—they both relate neural activity and movement variables to each other, only from slightly different perspectives. Specifically, they make different assumptions about which variable is considered the independent one and which is the dependent one (i.e., which set of variables is causal to the other set of variables). From the point of view of movement execution, the neural activities are dependent and the movement variables are independent, since the goal is to generate the intended movement with whatever neural activities are required. From the point of view of movement planning, the movement variables are independent and the neural activities are dependent, since the goal is to generate the neural activities needed to implement whatever movement is intended. Fig. 1.4 illustrates this duality.

When the motor system functions properly, f and g are inverses of each other since the executed movement equals the planned movement. The important point is that one cannot exist without the other: given an encoding model for individual neurons, the optimal decoder can be straightforwardly constructed; given a decoding model, the representations used in the encoding model are determined a priori. Importantly, in either case, one has to make an assumption about what movement variables are represented in the activity of motor cortical neurons, and to the extent that assumption is incorrect, model performance is compromised.

Finally, we note that meaningful decoding was not possible in realtime until the advent of microelectrode array technology such as the Utah array. Without such technology, one could only record a single (or a few) neurons at a time. This level of information does not suffice for making good estimates of movement variables, especially since neurons are noisy and often broadly tuned (see later discussion on sampling). For this reason, the first brain–machine interface for movement control in a nonhuman primate was developed by Nicolelis and colleagues[2] when chronic microelectrode array implants came of age.

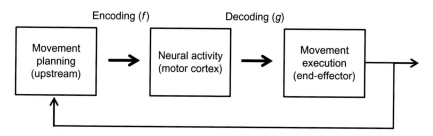

FIGURE 1.4   The sensorimotor transformation converting a movement plan into appropriate commands for muscles which subsequently implement the desired movement plan. Encoding is used to capture the former, and decoding the latter. When all goes well, the movement plan and the executed movement are identical, and encoding/decoding are exactly inverse operations, when taken over the entire motor system. Usually the movement plan and the executed movement differ due to noise, as discussed below, implying that feedback is critical to the system.

Movements Versus Muscles Versus Other Stuff: The Debate Continues Endlessly

The critical yet elusive question of what movement variables are represented in the motor cortex—a question defined both qualitatively and quantitatively above—remains yet to be answered. After Georgopoulos et al.[35] dozens of single-neuron studies have been published that investigate what types of movement variables are encoded in the activity of single neurons. Similarly, after Wessberg et al.[2] dozens of microelectrode array studies have been published that investigate which movement variables can best be decoded by the activity of a recorded population of motor cortical neurons. The results have, at best, been mixed.

Beginning in the late 1980s, perhaps as a counterweight to the success of Georgopoulos's cosine-tuning encoding model, a series of studies showed that the responses of motor cortical neurons do appear to be heavily influenced by several variables that embody low-level implementational details of movement. For example, multiple investigations have shown that joint torques,[37–40] dynamic muscle force,[41,42] and postural configuration [43–47] are significant determinants of neural activity. Other studies still maintained that what matters are high-level Cartesian representations of hand position,[48,49] hand direction/velocity,[50–52] hand acceleration,[53] movement amplitude,[54,55] end-effector force direction,[56–58] and/or target location or direction.[59–61] Still other studies have provided, alternatively, evidence for the encoding of muscle activity,[62,63] muscle synergies,[64] joint angular velocities,[65] joint trajectories in reach-and-grasp movements,[66,67] preferred trajectories,[68] movement curvature,[69] temporally extended and curvilinear movement fragments,[70] end-posture of the arm,[71] and many other variables related to muscles or movements. A set of stimulation studies, drawing upon the earlier findings of Ferrier,[27] has suggested that motor cortical neurons are organized to encode a small set of ecologically salient behaviors.[72] In short, single-neuron activity in motor cortex appears to relate to a plethora of potential variables that fully span the sensorimotor spectrum.

Nor have these citations exhausted all the encoding possibilities for which evidence has been adduced. Even though the motor cortex is viewed as a motor structure (for good reason given its direct projections to the spinal cord), investigators have implicated a variety of sensory/cognitive variables as major determinants of neural response. These include elements of movement preparation,[73,74] movement sequence information,[75,76] task mode,[77] cue-dependent sensorimotor processing[59,78]; action observation,[79] and even representation of color.[80] Another study found that putting behavioral variables aside, the spiking history of a neuron and its neighbors contributed significantly to the ability to predict whether or not a neuron would itself spike.[81] Finally, in a sharp departure from a pure representational point of view, a new line of research suggests an even more exotic interpretation of the activity of a population of motor cortical neurons. Specifically, the work of Churchland, Cunningham, Shenoy, and colleagues argues that the activity of motor cortical neurons is not intended to reflect the dynamics of any motor variable (intrinsic or extrinsic), but rather reflects the internal dynamics of connected neural circuits that have been shaped to achieve a functional outcome regardless of the initial state of the network.[82,83]

Turning our attention to motor cortical decoding, where a comprehensive survey of all of the relevant literature exceeds the scope of this chapter, we simply note that the results are equally ambiguous. Many studies have reconstructed muscle-related variables from the activity of a population of neurons.[84–89] Yet even more studies have reconstructed higher-level kinematic movement variables related to spatial trajectory, particularly in the context of brain–machine interfaces operating in real-time.[2–4,90–94] Additional studies have decoded hybrid kinetic-kinematic state,[95] hand configuration,[96] future movements,[97,98] state of rest versus motion,[99] and many other variables of all imaginable types.

It seems highly unlikely that the motor cortex could be simultaneously representing all of the implicated variables in an explicit fashion. Thus, the conclusion from any serious review of the literature is inescapable: after nearly 150 years of neurophysiological research on the motor cortex, nothing approaching a consensus exists as to what the motor cortex does. There are almost as many interpretations of motor cortical function as there are motor neurophysiologists. The question is: why?

Confounded Variables Embedded Within Distributed Neural Circuits

There are two separate, though related, questions that need to be addressed. The first is: why is it so difficult to tease apart the type of variables that are represented in the activity patterns of motor cortical neurons? The second is: how good are the existing encoding and decoding models overall—i.e., to what extent can neural activity be explained or movement behavior predicted? These questions are putatively related in that if we discern the "true" representation, presumably the fits to the data will be as good as they can be (i.e., however good). This section addresses the first question, while the next section addresses the second one.

Two factors conspire to obscure the type of movement information represented in the activity patterns of motor cortical neurons.

1. *Variable confounds*: The first factor is that the different variables of movement are highly interrelated through the physical equations of motion, the physiological mechanisms of force production, and

the geometry of coordinate transformations. For example, joint torques are converted into forces at the hand through the dynamical equations of motion formulated through either Lagrangian or Hamiltonian mechanics (e.g., Asada and Slotine[100]). Muscle activities can be converted into muscle forces through a state-dependent Hill-type muscle model.[101] System state variables can be rendered in end-effector coordinates, joint angle coordinates, or muscle-space coordinates.[102] And so it goes for any movement-related variable. This is especially true when the experiments are performed under movement contexts that do not vary significantly (e.g., the workspace is narrow relative to limits of behavior), as is usually the case for pragmatic reasons. This means that correlations of some kind invariably exist between all pairs of movement variables; therefore, if neural activity correlates with one movement variable, it will invariably correlate with other movement variables, a fact which has been known for some time.[29,103–106] To determine which variable is the "true" variable being encoded in the activity of motor cortical neurons becomes an exceedingly difficult task.

2. *Deficiency of the representational approach in distributed neural circuits*: The idea that the brain represents movement information in terms equivalent to those used by a roboticist in conveniently formulating an engineering problem embodies an anthropomorphic bias that fails to respect the distinctions between a neurobiological control system and an engineering one. To be sure, both systems are obligated to solve similar computational problems, but the means by which they do so differs dramatically. In particular, neural circuits in the brain are highly distributed and parallel in their processing of information, while conventional control algorithms are serial and modular. (Relatedly, the architecture for neurobiological control developed incrementally through evolutionary means, while conventional control algorithms are optimized on the basis of global computational considerations.) It is well-known from the study of connectionism (e.g., Ref. [107]) that neural networks provide an extreme redundancy of solutions to any problem; more specifically, the same functionality can be achieved by a multitude of network configurations that depend on somewhat arbitrary factors, such as the initial network configuration, presentation order during the learning phase, and assorted network parameters. Given the a priori indeterminate nature of parallel computing, the simple correlative approach used in motor neurophysiology to infer underlying representations may lead to conflicting or misleading conclusions.

These points were eloquently articulated over two decades ago in a famous article by Eberhard Fetz provocatively entitled: "Are movement parameters recognizably coded in the activity of single neurons?"[104] In it, he prophetically concluded that "the search for explicit coding may be diverting us from understanding distributed neural mechanisms that operate without literal representation." The intervening time may have only borne out his original supposition. That said, drawing attention to the problems posed by the representational approach does not necessarily point us in the direction of the answers we seek. Even within the confines of parallel computing, there still exist a multitude of potential architectures utilizing a variety of different operating principles, each of which is capable of implementing sensorimotor transformations. To figure out which mechanisms are actually employed by the brain on the basis of signatures present in the neural and behavioral data remains a wide-open problem, one whose solution will not come easily. In a conceptually immature field like neuroscience,[108] it is always easier to criticize an existing idea than to propose a new one.

To conclude this section, the failure to ascertain an answer to the question of what the motor cortex does may reflect a deep-seated teleological inadequacy endemic to correlative neurophysiological inquiry. At the level of observation/measurement, the broad spectrum of relevant movement variables might be unavoidably confounded to such an extent as to deny the possibility of reductionist disentanglement. At the level of the underlying neurobiological mechanisms, there may be little reason to expect the canonical correlations presupposed by the representational approach, let alone find them.

LOW PERFORMANCE LEVEL AND LIMITED ABILITY TO GENERALIZE

The fact that we do not know what the motor cortex does, though suggestive, does not explicitly address our ability to build models that either explain motor cortical activity or predict movement variables. Perhaps despite the overriding uncertainty, we can still construct algorithms that decipher a user's movement intention to a high enough precision to replace or substitute for natural movement behavior by means of an artificial device. Is this currently possible? Unfortunately, the short answer to this question is "no": by any common engineering metric, we are not able to decode movement intentions well enough to imitate the known characteristics of biological movement control. Similarly, our ability to explain neural activity as a function of behavior is limited. Our capacity for encoding and decoding remains mired at the proof-of-concept stage, whereby we can clearly discern some relationship between neural activity and movement behavior, but we cannot pinpoint that relationship with the precision required for effective reverse systems engineering.

So how can we quantify performance in state-of-the-art encoders/decoders? We begin with encoding where the idea is to explain a neuron's response as a function of movement variables (such as in the cosine-tuning model). A standard metric in these cases is the coefficient of determination or R^2 value, which lies between 0 and 1, with 1 being a perfect fit. (For non-linear and other more complex models, it is more appropriately labeled pseudo-R^2 with various mathematical extensions.) Generally speaking, the inclusion of three to eight free model parameters leads to fits of R^2 ~0.7 as reported in a large number of recent studies. This appears to be the case regardless of what specific movement variables one incorporates into the encoding model. More specifically, one can use either extrinsic or intrinsic variables or a combination without significantly impacting the fit. In fact, the best determinant of goodness-of-fit is the number of variables that are included in the model, as opposed to the identity of those variables. Even when one overfits with a higher number of movement variables, the R^2 value saturates well below one. Sometimes these fits are inappropriately produced by training and testing the model on the same data. More usually, the models are trained and tested on different trials of the same movement type through cross-validation, which is an improvement. However, the true manner by which to test these or any other models is to evaluate the model's ability to generalize to novel movement contexts (such as a movement in a different part of the workspace or under the influence of exogenous forces). On rare occasions when true generalization is tested, the R^2 value drops precipitously, suggesting that model construction is more likely an exercise in curve-fitting than it is a step toward systems identification.

The story is quite similar for evaluating the quality of the fits obtained by state-of-the-art decoders, where the goal is to explain or predict the activity of movement variables, such as the position and/or velocity of the end-effector, on the basis of the firing rates of a population of recorded motor cortical neurons. Motor decoding can be studied in conventional motor neurophysiology experiments, where an animal makes movements while both the neural signals and behavioral variables are monitored. Brain–machine interface with humans or nonhuman primates also involve motor decoding algorithms to directly convert the recorded neural signals into the movement of some external device (see Fig. 1.2). (The brain–machine interface experiments can also be run in two different modalities, either open-loop which correspond to purely feed-forward movements without error correction, or closed-loop where the user can adjust the output on the basis of feedback.) Here our brief discussion of motor decoding lumps together these different studies, since the results are fairly similar in terms of the performance ranges achieved.

A variety of metrics are used to evaluate reconstructed behavioral performance in the case of motor decoding. Without getting into the details of different metrics, suffice it to say that the decoding of intended motor output generally falls far short of being able to generate naturalistic movement behavior. For example, the defining characteristics of primate point-to-point reaching movements are: (1) essentially straight-line paths and (2) a relatively smooth unimodal bell-shaped speed profile. While it is easy to imagine many control strategies generating straight-line arm reaches, the second characteristic is more demanding, since it requires the control system to plan and/or compensate for a variety of posture-dependent factors, including interaction torques.[109] Yet neurotypical reaching behavior effortlessly generates such smooth trajectories on every trial and, moreover, when reaching movements are perturbed with exogenous forces, individuals very quickly reestablish these highly stereotypical kinematics.[110] In sharp contrast, the online movements performed by state-of-the-art brain–machine interfaces in conditions of full visual feedback generally manifest 3–5 different velocity peaks in order to acquire a target. This observation suggests that state-of-the-art performance in brain–machine interfaces usually entails making multiple movements to the same target, guided by online visual feedback, rather than a single movement. Interestingly, the movements made by stroke patients are similarly fractionated and, during neurorehabilitative recovery, gradually become blended.[111] Movement duration is also significantly longer, often by a factor of 2–3 or more, in large part because of the accumulation of submovements.

In summary, current brain–machine interface technology lags significantly in being able to generate realistic movement trajectories, even when the decoding model is trained and tested on similar movement types. The ultimate goal of movement generalization—producing realistic trajectories in novel movement contexts outside of the training set—appears to fall outside the realm of current possibility.

Noise, Feedback, and Sparse Sampling

Are there additional factors that lead to such poor performance in motor encoding and decoding, beyond those that have been stated? We would argue that there are at least three related factors.

Noise: Neurons are noisy information-processing elements.[112,113] Their axon hillocks are noisy signal processors, their synapses are noisy signal transducers, and the level of noise relative to signal may be high.[114,115] By extension, neural circuits are impacted by this noise. The presence of noise implies that the circuit behavior will differ even in circumstances where the input to the circuit is nearly identical. Consistent with this idea, it is well-known that the neural responses of visual cortical neurons differ significantly upon presentation of the same stimulus (e.g., Ref. [116]). Using acute recording techniques for single neurons in the motor cortex, many have similarly shown that the activity of motor cortical neurons differs on trials even when the motor output is observed to be the same (e.g., Refs. [117,118]). The noise invariably corrupts the patterns of recorded neural activity, thereby lowering the performance of any encoding or decoding scheme. How much performance is lowered as a result of noise remains an entirely open question, since little is known about the amount and type of noise inherent in neural systems.

Feedback: In biological motor control, it has long been known that feed-forward control does not operate perfectly. Even when relatively simple or well-rehearsed movements are performed by experts, movement precision requires multimodal feedback[119,120] for a variety of reasons, including the presence of noise in the system. Although few attempts have been made to quantify the degree of feedback present in typical movements, one study estimated that feedback control accounted for roughly 10% of the torque production in the context of perturbation correction.[121] To whatever extent motor cortical activity arises as feedback compensation for online disturbances, the goodness-of-fit of any encoding or decoding model will necessarily be compromised (since the activity corresponds to an arbitrary and unknown course correction).

Sparse sampling: Current neurotechnology allows for the implantation of one (or at most a few) microarrays, meaning that ~100 neurons are typically being recorded simultaneously. This number is a tiny fraction of the millions of neurons that constitute the entire motor cortex in the human brain (as a general rule of thumb, there are approximately 100,000 neurons in every mm^3 of cortex). With respect to motor decoding, how do we know whether or not this small sample adequately reflects the information contained in the circuit? Should we be concerned about a potential sampling bias in the recorded neurons on the basis of topographic considerations or the fact that there exist multiple distinct classes of neurons? Why are millions of neurons needed in the first place, i.e., is it a scaling requirement, a noise-averaging requirement, or some other requirement emblematic of underlying neural processing mechanisms? These questions remain unanswered to date, and without definitive answers, there are more reasons than not to suspect that sparse sampling significantly compromises the performance of decoding models.

Can Anything Be Done to Improve Performance?

In order to improve the performance of online brain–machine interface devices, an enormous amount of work over the last 15 years has gone into crafting better decoding algorithms. Perhaps better decoding algorithms, so the thinking went, will yield performance improvements sufficient to make these devices clinically relevant. Early explorations of neural decoding for primary motor cortical neuronal ensembles involved a population vector algorithm, which assumes that neurons are cosine-tuned to movement direction, and the preferred directions of neurons in an ensemble are uniformly distributed.[4,52] A linear filter relating neural activity to movement kinematics was reported to provide somewhat better performance and was used in several monkey and human brain–machine interface studies.[3,68,93,122]

A widely used refinement, based on incorporating the dynamics of movement variables into the mathematical description, was obtained through the use of state-space models and Kalman filtering algorithms.[15,21,22,123–130] Direct comparisons of closed-loop neural decoding performance with linear and Kalman filtering have suggested that the latter approach provides superior performance.[124,131] The alternative framework of neural networks has also been used for continuous decoding,[2] although this approach has been significantly more popular in discrete classification as opposed to continuous decoding or proportional control. Recurrent neural networks have also been explored for neural decoding, with some attractive properties such as internal network dynamics, the capability of capturing nonlinear input–output relationships, and the incorporation of feedback.[132,133] Training a recurrent neural network is a highly complex task, although some computational modifications have been attempted for overcoming this challenge.[134,135] This brief survey is intended to provide only a flavor of the vast arsenal of computational techniques that have been brought to bear on the problem of motor decoding.

What has been the net effect of recruiting multiple branches of advanced mathematics into this area of neural engineering? The short answer is: not much. Performance has improved slightly, though often at the cost of overfitting leading to a lack of generalization. Even these slight improvements appear to be trailing off, as overall performance throughout the field has appeared to plateau at a level well below what is needed for widespread clinical use (and even further below the level of naturalistic movements). Even with regard to performance improvements throughout the field, the following general observation can be made: the number of parameters used in a decoder is a far better indicator of decoder performance than the representation chosen or the algorithm used. This observation, together with the apparent plateauing of performance, once again suggests that what is being achieved is mere statistical curve fitting, rather than genuine systems identification.

The inability to improve motor decoding by ratcheting up the sophistication of complex mathematical algorithms is explained quite straightforwardly through inspection of Eq. (1.2). The function, g, represents (along with the time interval over which it is collected) a formula for relating neural activity to an unidentified movement variable(s). That is one component of the decoding equation. There are other components: one is obtaining a representative sample of neural activities sufficient to construct such a function; another is actually choosing the specific movement variable that the equation is intended to represent. Even if one has identified the perfect functional expression, it does one very little good without identifying the correct variables, because failure to identify the correct variables automatically leads to poor generalization. From this point of view, the field might be better served by resisting the temptation to improve performance slightly by using different algorithms that require more parameters, and instead investigate which set of variables leads to the lowest drop-off in performance in novel movement contexts independent of the baseline level of performance.

SO THE ANSWER TO WHAT THE MOTOR CORTEX DOES IS...

We simply do not know. In the sections above, we outlined two fundamental limitations of the conventional methodology that call into question the whole concept of motor encoding/decoding: (1) movement variables are inextricably confounded to a high degree (particularly when movement contexts do not span the space of possible movements) and (2) the neural mechanisms mediating the sensorimotor transformations may not be consistent with the existence of widespread canonical correlations, as predicted by the representational approach. Even to the extent that the representational approach does hold, we outlined three constraints which severely limit its efficacy: noise, feedback, and sparse sampling. It has been known for some time that there exists no consensus on what the motor cortex does. But without directly addressing the fundamental limitations and constraints described above, it may be impossible to build a brain–machine interface based on motor decoding which performs well enough to be used clinically.

While this view may seem pessimistic, we note that brain–machine interfaces guided by motor decoding do not have to be used only for continuous control of an end-effector. Instead, motor decoding can be used to choose between one of a small set of possible behavioral options. For example, suppose a person with tetraplegia is presented with the possibility or changing the television channel, turning on a light, or taking a sip of water. It is quite conceivable that the activity patterns of ~100 recorded neurons will suffice in distinguishing which of those three motor intentions is being envisioned by the user. Here the motor decoder is only being asked to perform discrete classification among a finite alphabet of desired goals or action plans. The actual implementation of these high-level goals can be relegated to some assistive technology, suitably designed to respond to high-level commands. This approach has been adopted by Andersen and colleagues[136] by using neural signals emanating from the parietal cortex, an area upstream of the motor cortex, where higher-level and more abstract movement goals and/or motor imagery might be generated. Therefore, while continuous control may be the holy grail of the field due to the extraordinary behavioral flexibility it provides, a more limited discrete control paradigm offers a better chance for success, at least in the near future.

Finally, on an even more optimistic note, if one does want to achieve continuous control, there exists another potential and relatively unexplored approach described below.

FUTURE POSSIBILITIES

Let us reconsider the "indirect" decoding architecture of Fig. 1.2. The recorded neural signals are processed by a decoding algorithm to reveal, as accurately as possible, the underlying movement intention. (This decoding algorithm must be calibrated with training data in a way that depends on the specific paradigm.) During use, once the neural signals are decoded into a movement plan, the command recoder converts this plan into the form appropriate for the output device using conventional control methods. For example, if the output device is a torque motor, the movement command is converted into the electrical activity necessary to actuate the motor so that the proper movement occurs. Note that movement intention and neural control are decoupled in this approach, since the brain does not directly exert a control function. Also note that the sole limiting factor in this approach is the performance of the decoder, since once the movement command is decoded, it is separately implemented by a robotic control system/actuator that performs the desired movement to roughly 100% accuracy (depending on the performance range of the system in question). Within the confines of this architecture, the "learning" takes place in the decoding algorithm, which effectuates a learned mapping between recorded signals and movement plans. As our discussion in the previous sections indicated, this approach is only as good as the decoder, and the serious limitations inherent in decoding limit the ultimate efficacy of this approach. Is there a way to have brains operate machines without any decoding whatsoever?

Direct Control

Indeed, an entirely different architecture is possible, as depicted in Fig. 1.5. Here signals from the cortex are converted directly into inputs that control some end-effector (e.g., a body part or an artificial device), without any effort to extract a movement intention from those signals. Hence, the

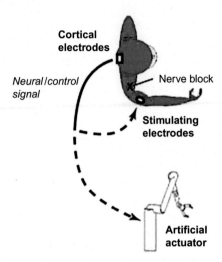

FIGURE 1.5   The "direct control" approach illustrated with a nonhuman primate. In this design, the link from the brain to the actuator is fixed and unchanging. Furthermore, the neural signals are used purely for control purposes as opposed to inferring movement intention.

approach may be referred to as direct control (both the decoding and command recoding stages are eliminated). The mapping from the neural signals to the actuator is fixed (in analogy to the idea that the wiring from the brain to the spinal cord is considered fixed). Obviously, the neural signals must be converted, by means of some transducer, into a form that makes them compatible as input signals for the output device. Other than signal transduction, however, no processing of the neural signals takes place: all of the mapping and learning must occur within the cortex of the user, upstream of the output neurons. In other words, the brain must adapt its activity to learn to control the output pathway through trial and error.

What are the central differences between these approaches? Phrased in colloquial terms, the decoding stage of the indirect decoding approach performs the function of a "mind reader," discerning an underlying movement intention, which is then converted into a control signal by conventional means. The direct control approach, however, better resembles a process of "telekinesis," whereby neural signals themselves are the substrate for control. But, one might ask, is not a scheme for transducing really just a decoder by a different name? It could be, except that the following two conditions are imposed on transduction which distinguish it from decoding: (1) the mapping is not formed with regard to minimizing behavioral error during training and (2) the variable into which the neural activity is transduced must be an input to a system with some intrinsic dynamics, as opposed to the desired output of the system.

With regard to this last point, most brain–machine interfaces rely on decoding schemes whereby neural activity is converted directly into the desired form, i.e., the position and velocity of the end-effector. However, in reality, neural commands do not directly result in an end-effector trajectory, but act through a variety of transformations (through the spinal cord to muscles to joints to movements). Therefore, relating neural activity to an input of a dynamical system better reflects reality. Furthermore, this approach offers a computational advantage: in a feedback control system where end-effectors have significant inertia and viscosity (as biological musculoskeletal systems do), the stable control approach is to convert the command signal into a dynamical input.[137] If the command signal is somehow instantaneously converted into an end-effector state, the result will be a high loop gain that, especially with temporal delays in a noisy system, leads to control instability.

The primary challenge for the indirect decoding scheme is the fidelity with which neural signals can be converted into movement plans. In contrast, the primary challenge for the direct control scheme is whether the brain can learn to adapt its activity to effectively control a newly established artificial pathway. Is there any evidence that such a capacity exists? The phenomenon known as cortical operant conditioning, studied for almost a half-century,[138] offers such evidence. In the original studies of operant conditioning, the experimenter would link the firing rate of a single motor cortical neuron in a nonhuman primate to a desirable external contingency, such as making a light brighter or a sound louder to obtain a reward. Remarkably, even though the animal has no explicit knowledge of this linkage, the firing rate of the individual motor cortical neurons increases from 50% to 500% within minutes of the contingency being established. The natural question is: how can the brain possibly know which specific neuron is being linked to the outside world? The answer is that the brain does not know which neuron is being so wired and, in fact, the firing rates of many neighboring neurons will also increase. But this body of work demonstrates that the brain is quite capable of detecting correlations between activity patterns within its own neural circuits and external events. In a certain sense, this conclusion is not surprising, since all sophisticated behaviors are learned through the developmental processes of motor babbling and circular reactions.[139]

All this being said, establishing a link between ~100 neurons on a cortical array and an external device is quite different from the operating mechanisms of the brain's natural sensorimotor circuitry. Even these operant conditioning studies only show that the individual motor cortical neurons can generally modulate their response properties, either up or down, to obtain more reward. They do not establish—nor have any other studies established—that the neurons can precisely modulate their activity to control some sort of external variable continuously with precision. It thus remains a completely open question as to whether or not this approach can work in constructing a brain–machine interface with today's technology. The section below discusses some advantages and disadvantages of the two different design approaches.

DIRECT CONTROL VERSUS INDIRECT DECODING

The vast majority of neuroprosthetic devices based on the firing rates of an ensemble of single neurons operate on the principle of indirect decoding, with the exceptions of the devices in Refs. [140,141]. Why is this approach so widely adopted? The main advantage of indirect decoding is one of expediency in that it "learns" over extremely short timescales. The methodology of decoding converts the learning problem into a problem of function approximation under the constraint of error minimization—i.e., a function is fit from the recorded neural signals to high-level movement kinematics with minimum error. Function approximation problems can be solved rapidly with computer algorithms, meaning that the interface can be up and running quickly. Furthermore, with the indirect decoding approach, if the performance drops because, e.g., certain recorded units have been lost, the decoder can simply be recalibrated quickly in the new condition.

In contrast, if the mapping is left fixed and only intrinsic learning mechanisms are used for learning, as in direct control, the learning will take considerably longer, on the order of weeks to months to years (as an illustration, one may think of how long it takes to learn movement control over the course of motor development or posttraumatic rehabilitation). New motor behaviors are not naturally learned rapidly, since the learning requires modification of a large and highly distributed neural sensorimotor control circuit. As a result of this extended learning time, the direct control approach suffers from additional disadvantages: (1) the technology does not exist to record stably from many individual neurons over the requisite length of time and (2) neither animals nor humans can likely to maintain the necessary motivation to learn with such a system over that timescale.

Despite the enormous practical advantages of indirect decoding, there are several reasons why the indirect decoding approach may be fundamentally limited in the performance it can achieve. Most of these reasons can be traced back to the problems of decoding described earlier.

Representational mismatch. In order to implement a decoder, a representation must be imposed upon the brain, i.e., one must assume that neurons are encoding something specific, like the position and/or velocity of the hand. To the extent that the assumptions of the decoder are wrong—and given the lack of certainty on this question, they almost certainly will be—the performance of the system will be limited to a suboptimal level, particularly in its ability to generalize to novel movement contexts.

Coadaptation problem. In many instances with an adaptive motor decoding scheme, both the decoder and the brain are adapting at the same time at different rates (the decoder faster than the brain), while neither system has access to the internal states of the other. This problem, known as "coadaptation" in the literature,[142] limits performance by "confusing" the hybrid system, as the brain and decoding algorithm are not coordinated in trying to find a unified control solution and may even be competing with each other. Without knowing what representations exist at what levels in the motor system, this problem is insoluble due to its ill-posed nature.

Prevention of neural exploration for finding robust solutions. Decoder recalibration is always intended to minimize behavioral error, which presumably is desirable. In the short term, this is true. However, frequent optimization interferes with the brain's natural capacity for long-term motor learning, a capacity that requires extensive trial-and-error exploration of a vast control space (vast because of the huge number of synapses and neurons contained in neural circuits) to gradually converge upon robust solutions through discovering the structure of that control space. Indeed, it is well documented in the kinesiology and sports science literature[143]—with analogies in learning theory (e.g., reinforcement learning[144])—that motor learning for robustly acquiring skills is a process that takes time (due to the fact that synapses change slowly), requires extensive practice (due to the large number of units in the control space), and inevitably leads to short-term performance dips to realize more robust long-term solutions (due to the complicated and nonlinear error surface in the control space, the structure of which must be discovered). This basic paradigm of biological motor learning has a principal requirement—the control space (i.e., the brain) must be allowed to interact with the environment through a relatively fixed interface to project changes in the control space into predictable environmental consequences. In a healthy person, this stable interface could be considered the peripheral nervous system from the spinal motor neurons to the muscles (this system too changes, though on slower timescales). The act of regular decoder calibration thus precludes any brain–interface system from exploiting the innate mechanisms of motor learning for robust skill acquisition, just as the coadaptation problem undermines accurate sensorimotor map formation.

Cortical nonstationarity. Up until now, it has been assumed that whatever information is encoded by a cortical neuron, the encoding scheme does not change over time. There is a growing body of work, however, that suggests that this representation might change over time depending on task requirements and other factors.[22,117,145,146] Such representational nonstationarity would only further complicate the indirect decoding approach.

These pitfalls are avoided by using the direct control approach. Since a single autonomous system (i.e., the brain) self-organizes on the basis of a fixed interface, no coadaptation problem results. Since the system is fully autonomous (no decoder to contend with), the brain learns the effects it generates—it does not have to "chase" a decoder representation that is constantly updated—so no representational mismatch can occur, and the capacity for task generalization emerges naturally. Finally, a fixed interface to the outside world will afford ample opportunity for the brain to explore configurations of its internal control space for the purpose of converging upon effective and robust solutions.

In summary of the comparison of the two approaches, the indirect decoding approach is "quick-and-dirty," meaning that a brain–machine interface can be made to function, albeit at a low level, on a fairly rapid timescale. The direct control approach has several theoretical advantages, but it is not practical using current technology given the need for significantly longer learning periods. It remains to be seen if there are certain specialized circumstances in which the problems of extended learning can be overcome and direct control can be used to obtain superior performance in brain–machine interface applications.

CONCLUDING REMARKS

Although microarray-based brain–machine interfaces are currently limited in their performance capabilities, many of the limiting factors may be resolved given the pace of technological change. For example, two-photon microscopy and other techniques may soon provide us with the ability to record the activity of thousands of neurons simultaneously. In fact, a recent DARPA program announcement seeks applications that propose to "design, build, demonstrate, and validate a neural interface platform capable of recording from more than 1,000,000 neurons and stimulating more than 100,000 neurons in proposer-defined regions of the human auditory, visual and somatosensory cortex." It seems only a matter of time before our ability to observe and manipulate neural circuits becomes greatly enhanced.

Nonetheless being able to observe and to manipulate does not imply being able to understand. Without a better understanding of how the brain works, we will be unable to harness our technological prowess for the construction of clinically useful devices. As always, scientific certainty must precede engineering possibility, and so the neuroscientists yet have some work to do before the neuroengineers can usher forth transformative brain–machine interface neurotechnology.

Acknowledgments

The authors would like to thank Emilio Bizzi for many helpful comments and conversations about the manuscript. This work was funded in part by the Craig H. Neilsen Foundation and the Wings for Life Spinal Cord Research Foundation.

References

1. Berger H. Über das Elektrenkephalogramm des Menchen. *Archives für Psychiatrie.* 1929;87:527–570.
2. Wessberg J, Stambaugh CR, Kralik JD, et al. Real-time prediction of hand trajectory by ensembles of cortical neurons in primates. *Nature.* 2000;408(6810):361–365.
3. Serruya MD, Hatsopoulos NG, Paninski L, Fellows MR, Donoghue JP. Instant neural control of a movement signal. *Nature.* 2002;416(6877):141–142.
4. Taylor DM, Tillery SI, Schwartz AB. Direct cortical control of 3D neuroprosthetic devices. *Science.* 2002;296(5574):1829–1832.
5. Pohlmeyer EA, Oby ER, Perreault EJ, et al. Toward the restoration of hand use to a paralyzed monkey: brain-controlled functional electrical stimulation of forearm muscles. *PLoS ONE.* 2009;4(6):e5924.
6. Maynard EM, Nordhausen CT, Normann RA. The Utah intracortical electrode array: a recording structure for potential brain-computer interfaces. *Electroencephalogr Clin Neurophysiol.* 1997;102(3):228–239.
7. Kipke DR, Vetter RJ, Williams JC, Hetke JF. Silicon-substrate intracortical microelectrode arrays for long-term recording of neuronal spike activity in cerebral cortex. *IEEE Trans Neural Syst Rehabil Eng.* 2003;11(2):151–155.
8. Nordhausen CT, Maynard EM, Normann RA. Single unit recording capabilities of a 100 microelectrode array. *Brain Res.* 1996;726(1–2):129–140.
9. Rey HG, Pedreira C, Quian Quiroga R. Past, present and future of spike sorting techniques. *Brain Res Bull.* 2015;119(Pt B):106–117.
10. Stevens CF, Zador A. Neural coding: the enigma of the brain. *Curr Biol.* 1995;12:1370–1371.
11. Schwartz AB. Cortical neural prosthetics. *Annu Rev Neurosci.* 2004;27:487–507.
12. Fraser GW, Chase SM, Whitford A, Schwartz AB. Control of a brain-computer interface without spike sorting. *J Neural Eng.* 2009;6(5):055004.
13. Christie BP, Tat DM, Irwin ZT, et al. Comparison of spike sorting and thresholding of voltage waveforms for intracortical brain-machine interface performance. *J Neural Eng.* 2015;12(1):016009.
14. Humphrey D, Schmidt EM, Thompson WD. Predicting measures of motor performance from multiple cortical spike trains. *Science.* 1970;170(959):758–762.
15. Todorova S, Sadtler P, Batista A, Chase S, Ventura V. To sort or not to sort: the impact of spike-sorting on neural decoding performance. *J Neural Eng.* 2014;11(5):056005.
16. Chestek CA, Gilja V, Nuyujukian P, et al. Long-term stability of neural prosthetic control signals from silicon cortical arrays in rhesus macaque motor cortex. *J Neural Eng.* 2011;8(4):045005.
17. Andersen RA, Musallam S, Pesaran B. Selecting the signals for a brain-machine interface. *Curr Opin Neurobiol.* 2004;14(6):720–726.
18. Donoghue JP, Nurmikko A, Black M, Hochberg LR. Assistive technology and robotic control using motor cortex ensemble-based neural interface systems in humans with tetraplegia. *J Physiol.* 2007;579(Pt 3):603–611.
19. Flint RD, Wright ZA, Scheid MR, Slutzky MW. Long term, stable brain machine interface performance using local field potentials and multiunit spikes. *J Neural Eng.* 2013;10(5):056005.

20. Stavisky SD, Kao JC, Nuyujukian P, Ryu SI, Shenoy KV. A high performing brain-machine interface driven by low-frequency local field potentials alone and together with spikes. *J Neural Eng.* 2015;12(3):036009.

21. Bansal AK, Truccolo W, Vargas-Irwin CE, Donoghue JP. Decoding 3D reach and grasp from hybrid signals in motor and premotor cortices: spikes, multiunit activity, and local field potentials. *J Neurophysiol.* 2012;107(5):1337–1355.

22. Perge JA, Zhang S, Malik WQ, et al. Reliability of directional information in unsorted spikes and local field potentials recorded in human motor cortex. *J Neural Eng.* 2014;11(4):046007.

23. Polikov VS, Tresco PA, Reichert WM. Response of brain tissue to chronically implanted neural electrodes. *J Neurosci Methods.* 2005;148(1):1–18.

24. Durand DM, Ghovanloo M, Krames E. Time to address the problems at the neural interface. *J Neural Eng.* 2014;11(2):020201. http://dx.doi.org/10.1088/1741-2560/11/2/020201.

25. Fritsch GT, Hitzig E. Über die elektrische Erregbarkeit des Grosshirns. *Arch Anat Physiol Med Wiss.* 1870:300–332. Translation in Von Bonin G. 1960. Some papers on the cerebral cortex. Springfield (IL): Charles C Thomas.

26. Penfield W, Jasper H. *Epilepsy and the Functional Anatomy of the Human Brain.* Boston: Little, Brown; 1954.

27. Ferrier D. Pathological illustrations of brain function. *West Riding Lunatic Asylum Medical Reports.* 1874;4:30–62.

28. Taylor CS, Gross CG. Twitches versus movements: a story of motor cortex. *Neuroscientist.* 2003;9(5):332–342.

29. Kalaska JF. From intention to action: motor cortex and the control of reaching movements. *Adv Exp Med Biol.* 2009;629:139–178.

30. Phillips CG. Laying the ghost of 'muscles versus movements'. *Can J Neurol Sci.* 1975;2:209–218.

31. Kalaska JF, Crammond DJ. Cerebral cortical mechanisms of reaching movements. *Science.* 1992;255(5051):1517–1523.

32. Hubel DH, Wiesel TN. Receptive fields of single neurones in the cat's striate cortex. *J Physiol.* 1959;148:574–591.

33. Evarts EV. Relation of pyramidal tract activity to force exerted during voluntary movement. *J Neurophysiol.* 1968;31:14–27.

34. Schmidt EM. Single neuron recording from motor cortex as a possible source of signals for control of external devices. *Ann Biomed Eng.* 1980;8(4–6):339–349.

35. Georgopoulos AP, Kalaska JF, Caminiti R, Massey JT. On the relations between the direction of two-dimensional arm movements and cell discharge in primate motor cortex. *J Neurosci.* 1982;2(11):1527–1537.

36. Georgopoulos AP, Schwartz AB, Kettner RE. Neuronal population coding of movement direction. *Science.* 1986;233:1416–1419.

37. Cheney PD, Fetz EE. Functional classes of primate corticomotoneuronal cells and their relation to active force. *J Neurophysiol.* 1980;44:773–791.

38. Ajemian R, Green A, Bullock D, Sergio L, Kalaska J, Grossberg S. Assessing the function of motor cortex: single-neuron models of how neural response is modulated by limb biomechanics. *Neuron.* 2008;58(3):414–428.

39. Herter TM, Kurtzer I, Cabel DW, Haunts KA, Scott SH. Characterization of torque-related activity in primary motor cortex during a multijoint postural task. *J Neurophysiol.* 2007;97:2887–2899.

40. Kalaska JF, Cohen DAD, Hyde ML, Prud'homme M. A comparison of movement direction-related versus load direction-related activity in primate motor cortex, using a two-dimensional reaching task. *J Neurosci.* 1989;9:2080–2102.

41. Sergio LE, Hamel-Paquet C, Kalaska JF. Motor cortex neural correlates of output kinematics and kinetics during isometric-force and arm-reaching tasks. *J Neurophysiol.* 2005;94:2353–2378.

42. Todorov E. Direct cortical control of muscle activation in voluntary arm movements: a model. *Nat Neurosci.* 2000;3:391–398.

43. Scott SH, Kalaska JF. Reaching movements with similar hand paths but different arm orientations. I. Activity of individual cells in motor cortex. *J Neurophysiol.* 1997;77:826–852.

44. Sergio LE, Kalaska JF. Systematic changes in motor cortex cell activity with arm posture during directional isometric force generation. *J Neurophysiol.* 2003;89:212–228.

45. Caminiti R, Johnson PB, Urbano A. Making arm movements within different parts of space: dynamic aspects in the primate motor cortex. *J Neurosci.* 1990;10:2039–2058.

46. Ajemian R, Bullock D, Grossberg S. Kinematic coordinates in which motor cortical cells encode movement direction. *J Neurophysiol.* 2000;84:2191–2203.

47. Ajemian R, Bullock D, Grossberg S. A model of movement coordinates in the motor cortex: posture-dependent changes in the gain and direction of single cell tuning curves. *Cereb Cortex.* 2001;11:1124–1135.

48. Georgopoulos AP, Caminiti R, Kalaska JF. Static spatial effects in motor cortex and area 5: quantitative relations in a two-dimensional space. *Exp Brain Res.* 1984;54:446–454.

49. Kettner RE, Schwartz AB, Georgopoulos AP. Primate motor cortex and free arm movements to visual targets in three-dimensional space. III. Positional gradients and population coding of movement direction from various movement origins. *J Neurosci.* 1988;8:2938–2947.

50. Schwartz AB. Direct cortical representation of drawing. *Science.* 1994;265(5171):540–542.

51. Schwartz AB, Kettner RE, Georgopoulos AP. Primate motor cortex and free arm movements to visual targets in 3-d space. I. Relations between single cell discharge and direction of movement. *J Neurosci.* 1988;8:2913–2927.

52. Moran DW, Schwartz AB. Motor cortical representation of speed and direction during reaching. *J Neurophysiol.* 1999;82(5):2676–2692.

53. Ashe J, Georgopoulos AP. Movement parameters and neural activity in motor cortex and area 5. *Cereb Cortex.* 2004;6:590–600.

54. Fu Q-G, Suarez JI, Ebner TJ. Neuronal specification of direction and distance during reaching movements in the superior precentral premotor area and primary motor cortex of monkeys. *J Neurophysiol.* 1993;70:2097–2116.

55. Fu Q-G, Flament D, Coltz JD, Ebner TJ. Temporal encoding of movement kinematics in the discharge of primate primary motor and premotor neurons. *J Neurophysiol.* 1995;73:836–854.

56. Taira M, Boline J, Smyrnis N, Georgopoulos AP, Ashe J. On the relations between single cell activity in the motor cortex and the direction and magnitude of three-dimensional static isometric force. *Exp Brain Res.* 1996;109:367–376.

57. Boline J, Ashe J. On the relations between single cell activity in the motor cortex and the direction and magnitude of three-dimensional dynamic isometric force. *Exp Brain Res.* 2005;167:148–159.

58. Georgopoulos AP, Ashe J, Smyrnis N, Taira M. The motor cortex and the coding of force. *Science.* 1992;256:1692–1695.

59. Shen L, Alexander GE. Neural correlates of a spatial sensory-to-motor transformation in primary motor cortex. *J Neurophysiol.* 1997;77:826–852.

60. Kakei S, Hoffman DS, Strick PL. Muscle and movement representation in the primary motor cortex. *Science.* 1999;285:2136–2139.

61. Alexander GE, Crutcher MD. Neural representations of the target (goal) of visually guided arm movements in three motor areas of monkey. *J Neurophysiol.* 1990;64:164–178.

62. Townsend BR, Paninski L, Lemon RN. Linear encoding of muscle activity in primary motor cortex and cerebellum. *J Neurophysiol.* 2006;96:2578–2592.

63. Jackson A, Mavoori J, Fetz EE. Correlations between the same motor cortex cells and arm muscles during a trained task, free behavior, and natural sleep in the macaque monkey. *J Neurophysiol.* 2007;97:360–374.

64. Holdefer RN, Miller LE. Primary motor cortical neurons encode functional muscle synergies. *Exp Brain Res.* 2002;146:233–243.

65. Reina GA, Moran DW, Schwartz AB. On the relationship between joint angular velocity and motor cortical discharge during reaching. *J Neurophysiol.* 2001;85:2576–2589.

66. Saleh M, Takahashi K, Amit Y, Hatsopoulos NG. Encoding of coordinated grasp trajectories in primary motor cortex. *J Neurosci.* 2010;30:17079–17090.

67. Vargas-Irwin CE, Shakhnarovich G, Yadollahpour P, Mislow JM, Black MJ, Donoghue JP. Decoding complete reach and grasp actions from local primary motor cortex populations. *J Neurosci.* 2010;30:9659–9669.

68. Paninski L, Fellows MR, Hatsopoulos NG, Donoghue JP. Spatiotemporal tuning of motor cortical neurons for hand position and velocity. *J Neurophysiol.* 2004;91(1):515–532.

69. Hocherman S, Wise SP. Effects of hand movement path on motor cortical activity in awake, behaving rhesus monkeys. *Exp Brain Res.* 1991;83:285–302.

70. Hatsopoulos NG, Xu Q, Amit Y. Encoding of movement fragments in the motor cortex. *J Neurosci.* 2007;27:5105–5114.

71. Aflalo T, Graziano MSA. Partial tuning of motor cortex neurons to final posture in a free-moving paradigm. *Proc Natl Acad Sci USA.* 2006;103:2909–2914.

72. Graziano MS, Taylor CS, Moore T, Cooke DF. The cortical control of movement revisited. *Neuron.* 2002;36(3):349–362.

73. Kettner RE, Marcario JK. Control of remembered reaching sequences in monkey. II. Storage and preparation before movement in motor and premotor cortex. *Exp Brain Res.* 1996;42:223–227.

74. Alexander GE, Crutcher MD. Preparation for movement: neural representations of intended direction in three motor areas of the monkey. *J Neurophysiol.* 1990;64:133–150.

75. Ben-Shaul Y, Drori R, Asher I, Stark E, Nadasdy Z, Abeles M. Neuronal activity in motor cortical areas reflects the sequential context of movement. *J Neurophysiol.* 2004;91:1748–1762.

76. Carpenter AF, Georgopoulos AP, Pellizzer G. Motor cortical encoding of serial order in a context-recall task. *Science.* 1999;283(5408):1752–1757.

77. Matsuzaka Y, Picard N, Strick PL. Skill representation in the primary motor cortex after long-term practice. *J Neurophysiol.* 2007;97(2):1819–1832.

78. Salinas E, Romo R. Conversion of sensory signals into motor commands in primary motor cortex. *J Neurosci.* 1998;18:499–511.

79. Dushanova J, Donoghue J. Neurons in primary motor cortex engaged during action observation. *Eur J Neurosci.* 2010;31(2):386–398.

80. Zach N, Inbar D, Grinvald Y, Bergman H, Vaadia E. Emergence of novel representations in primary motor cortex and premotor neurons during associative learning. *J Neurosci.* 2008;28(38):9545–9556.

81. Truccolo W, Hochberg LR, Donoghue JP. Collective dynamics in human and monkey sensorimotor cortex: predicting single neuron spikes. *Nat Neurosci.* 2010;13(1):105–111.

82. Shenoy KV, Sahani M, Churchland MM. Cortical control of arm movements: a dynamical systems perspective. *Annu Rev Neurosci.* 2013;36:337–359.

83. Churchland MM, Cunningham JP, Kaufman MT, et al. Neural population dynamics during reaching. *Nature.* 2012;487(7405):51–56.

84. Schieber MH, Rivlis G. Partial reconstruction of muscle activity from a pruned network of diverse motor cortex neurons. *J Neurophysiol.* 2007;97:70–82.

85. Ethier C, Oby ER, Bauman MJ, Miller LE. Restoration of grasp following paralysis through brain-controlled stimulation of muscles. *Nature.* 2012;485(7398):368–371.

86. Fagg AH, Ojakangas GW, Miller LE, Hatsopoulos NG. Kinetic trajectory decoding using motor cortical ensembles. *IEEE Trans Neural Syst Rehabil Eng.* 2009;17:487–496.

87. Griffin DM, Hudson HM, Belhaj-Saïf A, McKiernan BJ, Cheney PD. Do corticomotoneuronal cells predict target muscle EMG activity? *J Neurophysiol.* 2008;99(3):1169–1986.

88. Morrow MM, Miller LE. Prediction of muscle activity by populations of sequentially recorded primary cortex neurons. *J Neurophysiol*. 2003;89(4):2279–2288.

89. Oby E, Ethier C, Miller LE. Movement representation in the primary motor cortex and its contribution to generalizable EMG predictions. *J Neurophysiol*. 2013;109(3): 666–678.

90. Velliste M, Perel S, Spalding MC, Whitford AS, Schwartz AB. Cortical control of a prosthetic arm for self-feeding. *Nature*. 2008;453(7198):1098–1101.

91. Carmena JM, Lebedev MA, Crist RE, et al. Learning to control a brain–machine interface for reaching and grasping by primates. *PLoS Biol*. 2003;1:E42.

92. Collinger JL, Wodlinger B, Downey JE, et al. High-performance neuroprosthetic control by an individual with tetraplegia. *Lancet*. 2013;381(9866):557–564.

93. Hochberg LR, Serruya MD, Friehs GM, et al. Neuronal ensemble control of prosthetic devices by a human with tetraplegia. *Nature*. 2006;442(7099):164–171.

94. Hochberg LR, Bacher D, Jarosiewicz B, et al. Reach and grasp by people with tetraplegia using a neurally controlled robotic arm. *Nature*. 2012;485(7398):372–375.

95. Suminski A, Fagg A, Willett F, Bodenhamer M, Hatsopoulos N. Online adaptive decoding of intended movements with a hybrid kinetic and kinematic brain machine interface. *Conf Proc IEEE Eng Med Biol Soc*. 2013:1583–1586.

96. Schaffelhofer S, Agudelo-Toro A, Scherberger H. Decoding a wide range of hand configurations from macaque motor, premotor, and parietal cortex. *J Neurosci*. 2015;35:1068–1081.

97. Shanechi MM, Hu RC, Powers M, Wornell GW, Brown EN, Williams ZM. Neural population partitioning and a concurrent brain-machine interface for sequential motor function. *Nat Neurosci*. 2012;15(12):1715–1722.

98. Willett FR, Suminski AJ, Fagg AH, Hatsopoulos NG. Improving brain-machine interface performance by decoding intended future movements. *J Neural Eng*. 2013;10:026011. http://dx.doi.org/10.1088/1741-2560/10/2/026011.

99. Velliste M, Kennedy SD, Schwartz AB, Whitford AS, Sohn J-W, McMorland AJC. Motor cortical correlates of arm resting in the context of a reaching task and implications for prosthetic control. *J Neurosci*. 2014;34(17):6011–6022.

100. Asada H, Slotine J-JE. *Robot Analysis and Control*. New York: John Wiley and Sons; 1986.

101. Zajac FF. Muscle and tendon: properties, models, scaling, and application to biomechanics and motor control. *Crit Rev Biomed Eng*. 1989;17(4):359–411.

102. Mussa-Ivaldi FA, Morasso P, Zaccaria R. Kinematic networks. A distributed model for representing and regularizing motor redundancy. *Biol Cybern*. 1988;60:1–16.

103. Scott SH. Role of motor cortex in coordinating multi-joint movements: is it time for a new paradigm? *Can J Physiol Pharmacol*. 2000;78(11):923–933.

104. Fetz EE. Are movement parameters recognizably coded in activity of single neurons? *Brain Behav Sci*. 1992;15:679–690.

105. Loeb GE, Brown IE, Scott SH. Directional motor control. *Trends Neurosci*. 1996;19:137–138.

106. Bizzi E, Ajemian R. A hard scientific quest: understanding voluntary movements. *Daedalus*. 2015;144(1):83–95.

107. Haykin S. *Neural Networks: A Comprehensive Foundation*. Upper Saddle River, NJ: Prentice Hall; 1999.

108. Ajemian R, Hogan N. Experimenting with theoretical neuroscience. *J Mot Behav*. 2010;42(6):333–342.

109. Hollerbach JM, Flash T. Dynamic interactions between limb segments during planar arm movement. *Biol Cybern*. 1982;44(1):67–77.

110. Shadmehr R, Mussa-Ivaldi FA. Adaptive representation of dynamics during learning of a motor task. *J Neurosci*. 1994;14(5 Pt 2):3208–3224.

111. Rohrer B, Fasoli S, Krebs HI, et al. Movement smoothness changes during stroke recovery. *J Neurosci*. 2002;22(18):8297–8304.

112. Steinmetz PN, Manwani A, Koch C, London M, Segev I. Subthreshold voltage noise due to channel fluctuations in active neuronal membranes. *J Comput Neurosci.* 2000;9(2):133–148.

113. Bialek W, Rieke F, de Ruyter van Steveninck RR, Warland D. Reading a neural code. *Science.* 1991;252(5014):1854–1857.

114. Simmons PJ, de Ruyter van Steveninck R. Reliability of signal transfer at a tonically transmitting, graded potential synapse of the locust ocellar pathway. *J Neurosci.* 2005;25(33):7529–7537.

115. Czanner G, Sarma SV, Ba D, et al. Measuring the signal-to-noise ratio of a neuron. *Proc Natl Acad Sci USA.* 2015;112(23):7141–7146.

116. Schiller PH, Finlay BL, Volman SF. Short-term response variability of monkey striate neurons. *Brain Res.* 1976;105:347–349.

117. Li C-SR, Padoa-Schioppa C, Bizzi E. Neuronal correlates of motor performance and motor learning in the primary motor cortex of monkeys adapting to an external force field. *Neuron.* 2001;30:593–607.

118. Richardson AG, Borghi T, Bizzi E. Activity of the same motor cortex neurons during repeated experience with perturbed movement dynamics. *J Neurophysiol.* 2012;107(11):3144–3154.

119. Saunders JA, Knill DC. Humans use continuous visual feedback from the hand to control fast reaching movements. *Exp Brain Res.* 2003;152(3):341–352.

120. Gibbs CB. The continuous regulation of skilled response by kinaesthetic feedback. *Br J Med Psychol.* 1954;45(1):24–39.

121. Bizzi E, Dev P, Morasso P, Polit A. Effect of load disturbances during centrally initiated movements. *J Neurophysiol.* 1978;41(3):542–556.

122. Lebedev MA, Carmena JM, O'Doherty JE, et al. Cortical ensemble adaptation to represent velocity of an artificial actuator controlled by a brain-machine interface. *J Neurosci.* 2005;25(19):4681–4693.

123. Gage GJ, Ludwig KA, Otto KJ, Ionides EL, Kipke DR. Naive coadaptive cortical control. *J Neural Eng.* 2005;2(2):52–63.

124. Kim SP, Simeral JD, Hochberg LR, Donoghue JP, Black MJ. Neural control of computer cursor velocity by decoding motor cortical spiking activity in humans with tetraplegia. *J Neural Eng.* 2008;5(4):455–476.

125. Mulliken GH, Musallam S, Andersen RA. Decoding trajectories from posterior parietal cortex ensembles. *J Neurosci.* 2008;28(48):12913–12926.

126. Li Z, O'Doherty JE, Hanson TL, Lebedev MA, Henriquez CS, Nicolelis MA. Unscented Kalman filter for brain-machine interfaces. *PLoS ONE.* 2009;4(7):e6243.

127. Zhuang J, Truccolo W, Vargas-Irwin C, Donoghue JP. Decoding 3-D reach and grasp kinematics from high-frequency local field potentials in primate primary motor cortex. *IEEE Trans Biomed Eng.* 2010;57(7):1774–1784.

128. Malik WQ, Truccolo W, Brown EN, Hochberg LR. Efficient decoding with steady-state Kalman filter in neural interface systems. *IEEE Trans Neural Syst Rehabil Eng.* 2011;19:25–34.

129. Wu W, Gao Y, Bienenstock E, Donoghue JP, Black MJ. Bayesian population decoding of motor cortical activity using a Kalman filter. *Neural Comput.* 2006;18(1):80–118.

130. Malik WQ, Hochberg LR, Donoghue JP, Brown EN. Modulation depth estimation and variable selection in state-space models for neural interfaces. *IEEE Trans Biomed Eng.* 2015;62(2):570–581.

131. Koyama S, Chase SM, Whitford AS, Velliste M, Schwartz AB, Kass RE. Comparison of brain-computer interface decoding algorithms in open-loop and closed-loop control. *J Comput Neurosci.* 2010;29(1–2):73–87.

132. Fetz EE. Volitional control of neural activity: implications for brain–computer interfaces. *J Physiol.* 2007;579(Pt 3):571–579.

133. Maier MA, Shupe LE, Fetz EE. Dynamic neural network models of the premotoneuronal circuitry controlling wrist movements in primates. *J Comput Neurosci.* 2005;19:125–146.
134. Sanchez JC, Erdogmus D, Nicolelis MAL, Wessberg J, Principe JC. Interpreting spatial and temporal neural activity through a recurrent neural network brain–machine interface. *IEEE Trans Neural Syst Rehabil Eng.* 2005;13:213–219.
135. Sussillo D, Nuyujukian P, Fan JM, et al. A recurrent neural network for closed-loop intracortical brain–machine interface decoders. *J Neural Eng.* 2012;9(2):026027.
136. Aflalo T, Kellis S, Klaes C, et al. Neurophysiology. Decoding motor imagery from the posterior parietal cortex of a tetraplegic human. *Science.* 2015;348(6237):906–910.
137. Ben-Pazi H, Ishihara A, Kukke S, Sanger T. Increasing viscosity and inertia using a robotically controlled pen improves handwriting in children. *J Child Neurol.* 2010;25(6):674–680.
138. Fetz EE. Operant conditioning of cortical unit activity. *Science.* 1969;163(870):955–958.
139. Piaget J. *The Origins of Intelligence in Children.* New York: International Universities Press; 1952.
140. Moritz CT, Perlmutter SI, Fetz EE. Direct control of paralyzed muscles by cortical neurons. *Nature.* 2008;456:639–642.
141. Ganguly K, Carmena JM. Emergence of a stable cortical map for neuroprosthetic control. *PLoS Biol.* 2009;7(7):e1000153.
142. Merel J, Fox R, Jebara T, Paninski L. A multi-agent control framework for co-adaptation in brain-computer interfaces. *Neural Inf Process Syst.* 2013.
143. Schmidt RA, Lee TD. *Motor Control and Learning.* Champaign, IL: Human Kinetics; 1999.
144. Sutton RS, Barto AG. *Reinforcement Learning: An Introduction.* Cambridge, MA: MIT Press; 1998.
145. Wise SP, Moody SL, Blomstrom KJ, Mitz AR. Changes in motor cortical activity during visuomotor adaptation. *Exp Brain Res.* 1998;121:285–289.
146. Ajemian R, D'Ausilio A, Moorman H, Bizzi E. A theory for how sensorimotor skills are learned and retained in noisy and nonstationary neural circuits. *Proc Natl Acad Sci USA.* 2013;110:E5078–E5087.

Feedback-Sensitive and Closed-Loop Solutions

G.P. Thomas[1,2] and B.C. Jobst[1,2]

[1]Dartmouth-Hitchcock Medical Center, Lebanon, NH, United States;
[2]Geisel School of Medicine at Dartmouth, Hanover, NH, United States

Innovative Neuromodulation.
DOI: http://dx.doi.org/10.1016/B978-0-12-800454-8.00002-1

INTRODUCTION

Epilepsy affects about 1% of the population, with between 30% and 40% suffering from medically refractory disease and recurrent seizures.[1] Poorly controlled epilepsy directly interferes with many aspects of daily life including driving, working, and recreation, and has pervasive effects on mood and cognition. Epilepsy surgery is an effective treatment of choice in this patient population but is not always feasible due to the risk of a functional deficit.[2] The need for innovative therapies is greatest in this subgroup of epilepsy patients for whom traditional surgery is not an option. Electrical deep brain stimulation, e.g., has proven neuromodulatory effects for advanced Parkinsonism, dystonia, and other movement disorders, and experimental evidence suggests a role in other neurologic conditions including epilepsy. In contrast to epilepsy surgery, electrical brain stimulation offers several advantages; it is reversible, adjustable, and can be used in situations when resection might lead to significant functional or cognitive impairment. Brain stimulation methods can be segregated further into two broad categories: open-loop and closed-loop stimulation. Open-loop systems are programmed to deliver stimulation at specific, predetermined times irrespective of brain state. Closed-loop or responsive neurostimulation in contrast delivers stimulation according to real-time electrophysiologic events recoded from the patient's brain. The aim of this chapter is to discuss closed-loop brain stimulation applications in medically refractory epilepsy.

CRANIAL NERVE ELECTRICAL STIMULATION FOR SEIZURE CONTROL

Open-loop stimulation for seizure control has been in clinical use in the United States since 1997. The vagus nerve stimulator (VNS) consists of a small generator implanted in the anterior chest wall with electrical leads attached to the left vagus nerve. The device provides stimulation according to programmed intervals and intensity, but stimulation can also be triggered by the patient if they note symptoms of an impending seizure. Reports of efficacy reflect responder rates (that is, those with 50% or greater reduction in seizure frequency) in the range of 30–40%.[3] The mechanism by which VNS reduces seizure frequency is not known, but animal evidence suggests that it might modulate neuroinflammation via blocking IL-6 effects on synaptic activity.[4] Changes in functional networks in VNS-treated patients have also been reported, suggesting plasticity effects as well.[5] While VNS appears to offer benefit in terms of reduced seizure frequency, there appears to be an association with the development of sleep apnea.[6,7] The development of hoarseness, coughing, and throat pain are common adverse effects that limit the tolerability of VNS.[8]

Trigeminal nerve stimulation for medically refractory seizures was studied in a double-blind randomized trial.[9] Subjects underwent transcutaneous open-loop stimulation of the bilateral ophthalmic and trochlear branches of the trigeminal nerve for at least 12 hours daily for a period of 18 weeks. This study showed a responder rate (greater than 50% seizure reduction) of 40.5% at the end of the study period. Trigeminal nerve stimulation for epilepsy is not currently FDA-approved for the treatment of epilepsy.

BRAIN STIMULATION FOR EPILEPSY: HISTORICAL PERSPECTIVE

The first description of the effects of electrical stimulation on epileptic brain was in 1954 by Penfield and Jasper who reported decreased amplitude of electrocortigraphic recordings in both normal and epileptic cortex reflecting local inhibition.[10] Subsequent experiments with brain stimulation focused on regions for stimulation that might have widespread effects on electrical activity. As early as 1954 researchers studied cerebellar stimulation for seizure control, reasoning that facilitation of inhibitory cerebellar output, mediated by γ-aminobutyric acid (GABA)-ergic Purkinje cells, might provide diffuse inhibition and reduce seizure frequency. Animal models showed mixed results but laid the groundwork for human studies.[11-13] Human studies of chronic cerebellar stimulation initially showed variable influence of stimulation on seizures. Cooper et al. performed cerebellar stimulation for up to 3 years in 15 subjects with intractable seizures, reporting reduced seizure frequency in 10 of these subjects with no reports of adverse events.[14] A subsequent study by this same group showed reduced seizures in 18 of 29 subjects again without adverse events.[15] These early studies however were uncontrolled and further blinded trials were less conclusive and actually showed no efficacy. No seizure reduction was noted after 10 months of cerebellar stimulation in a more scientifically rigorous study of five subjects with epilepsy.[16] Velasco et al. studied cerebellar stimulation for seizure control in a double-blind randomized study of five subjects. They reported a 33% reduction in seizures in the initial 3-month double-blind period with continued improvement specifically in tonic-clonic seizures over the 2 years the subjects were followed, while other seizure types were less responsive.[16] Further work was ultimately abandoned due to lack of evidence.

BRAIN STIMULATION IN VITRO AND IN VIVO

The hippocampus and related pathways have also drawn attention as a potential target for electrical stimulation. Using in vitro hippocampal slices from Sprague–Dawley rats to study the effects of electrical stimulation on penicillin and picrotoxin-induced epileptiform activity, Durand[17] demonstrated not only the effects of stimulation but also the complex effects of stimulation on neuronal activity. Extracellular recordings were made from the CA1 layer, with stimulating electrodes in the striatum radiatum for orthodromic stimulation and in the alveus for antidromic stimulation. It was found that orthodromic stimulation led to a decrease in epileptiform spikes. The degree of amplitude attenuation however was related to several factors including waveform, charge, and timing of the stimulation. The polarity of stimulation also influenced the response, with cathodic stimulation leading to approximately twice as much inhibition as anodic stimulation. In another study using rat hippocampal slice preparations, it was shown that repetitive stimulation at a low frequency (1 Hz) was most effective at reducing epileptiform activity in the entorhinal cortex. In this preparation Schaffer collaterals, which inhibit epileptiform activity in the entorhinal cortex, were transected. Bursts of epileptiform activity were induced by single electrical shocks in 4-aminopyridine treated hippocampal slices. Repetitive stimulation ranging from 0.2 to 10 Hz at strengths from 10 to 20 µA was applied, with stimulation at 1 Hz the most effective at inhibiting the induced epileptiform activity.[18] Stimulation of hippocampal afferent pathways,[19] hippocampus proper,[20–22] and hippocampal efferent pathways[23] have all been described with encouraging results, but the power requirements of the open-loop designs of these methods precluded translation beyond the experimental stage.

THALAMIC BRAIN STIMULATION

Given its location in the Papez circuit and potential role in seizure propagation and spread, the thalamus has been identified as a potential target for stimulation for seizure control. The centro-median nucleus of the thalamus in particular exhibits wide excitatory cortical projections that might mediate generalized seizure spread. In a study of centro-median nucleus stimulation in seven patients with epilepsy, Fisher et al.[24] found that continual rather than scheduled electrical stimulation was effective in reducing seizures. Stimulation voltage was set according to each patient's sensory threshold, and delivered in 90-µs pulses at a frequency of 65 pulses per second for 1 minute every 5 minutes. The initial total duration of stimulation was limited to 2 hours/day, which was well tolerated but did not reduce seizure frequency. When the stimulation was changed to run continually however there was a 50% reduction in seizure frequency. Thus while perhaps clinically effective, the power requirements of this method presented a barrier to clinical translation.

Due in part to variable results with stimulation of the centro-median nucleus of the thalamus several studies focused on the anterior nucleus of the thalamus (ANT). The anterior thalamic nucleus has extensive connections to medial temporal lobe structures, occupying a key place in the limbic system and therefore might be involved in the propagation and spread of seizures. Using deep brain stimulation, Osorio et al.[25] showed consistent mesial temporal lobe evoked potentials in response to ANT high-frequency stimulation, and a 75% mean reduction in seizure frequency in four human subjects. Stimulation of the ANT for epilepsy was rigorously studied in a multicenter double-blind randomized study, the SANTE trial. Deep brain stimulation electrodes were implanted in 110 study participants. Stimulation consisted of 5V delivered in 90-μs pulses at 145 pulses per second, delivered for 1 minute every 5 minutes. During the blinded phase the stimulation group exhibited a significant reduction in clinical seizures of 35%, while the nonstimulation group showed 14.1% fewer clinical seizures. It should be noted that since both groups underwent lead placement, the differences in response reflect the effects of stimulation alone and not microthalotomy. In the extended open phase the overall group showed 41% fewer seizures versus baseline at 13 months and 56% fewer at 25 months.[26] There are however reports of psychiatric side effects of thalamic brain stimulation for epilepsy, and depression was a concern in SANTE.[27] This adds to the already existing burden of depression in patients with epilepsy, which is a comorbid condition.[28]

LOCATION OF BRAIN STIMULATION

Numerous studies mentioned earlier in this chapter describe stimulation at specific anatomic structures with the intent of exploiting their widespread projections to mediate the effects of electrical stimulation. This method is attractive in cases without a focal zone of seizure onset (i.e., primarily generalized seizures) at least in theory. Stimulation of the zone of seizure onset when known has also been explored. The basis for this comes in part from animal studies that show the ability of electrical stimulation to inhibit the kindling process[29,30] and increase the threshold for afterdischarges in kindled rats.[29,30] In humans with temporal lobe epilepsy, direct stimulation of the hippocampus with high-frequency (130–190 Hz) current was shown to reduce interictal epileptiform activity as well as seizure frequency.[31,32] Velasco et al.[22] reported their impressive results of high-frequency hippocampal stimulation in seven patients with temporal lobe epilepsy undergoing evaluation for epilepsy surgery. Electrical stimulation (130 Hz, 450 μs duration, 200–400 mA) delivered 23 of 24 hours/day stopped clinical seizures in the seven patients that completed the entire observation period of 2–3 weeks. They also noted reduction of interictal abnormalities and normalization of background electroencephalogram (EEG) activity. Subsequent histopathologic examination of resected tissue showed no difference between the stimulated and nonstimulated tissue.[22]

Afterdischarges occurring after cortical stimulation during mapping procedures are common and it has been shown that these can be terminated by shorter-duration repeat stimulation.[33] Further study of the effects of cortical stimulation for seizure abatement have shown that timing of stimulation to coincide with a negative peak early in the course of an afterdischarge seems to be most effective.[34] Using subdural electrodes for seizure monitoring, high-frequency stimulation reduced epileptiform discharges by about 25%, while low-frequency stimulation led to about 19% fewer discharges.[35,36]

ELECTRICAL PARAMETERS FOR BRAIN STIMULATION

Our understanding of electrical current flow through the brain includes that electrical current does not flow uniformly, rather the current density is distributed over numerous pathways influenced by local variability in impedance as well as regional variation in cytoarchitecture. Furthermore, the diffusion of electrical current is dependent on the electrical state of the network related to recent activity.[37] Given that electrical activity in the brain is not static but rather a dynamical system, the timing and location of an ideal stimulation is likely not fixed. The results of stimulation therefore might differ based on the excitability at the location of stimulation.[38] Stimulation intensities between 0.4 and 12.0 mA have been reported to be effective in modulating local electrical activity[39] and charge densities of less than 30–60 $\mu C/cm^2$ per phase are generally considered safe, with increased risk of tissue damage at higher energies. While most research has been conducted using high-frequency stimulation, currently there is no definite evidence which stimulation is most ideal to exhibit an antiepileptic effect. A summary of commonly accepted parameters for brain stimulation in epileptic patients is presented in Table 2.1.

POSSIBLE MECHANISMS OF ACTION

Early observations of the effects of electrical stimulation describe attenuation of electrical activity in response to electrical stimulation,[10] and early formal studies in humans focused on stimulation of regions with widespread inhibitory projections.[16,43–45] Using rat hippocampal slice preparations suspended in a hypocalcemic, hyperkalemic solution treated with

TABLE 2.1 Stimulation Parameters Used in Different Types of Brain Stimulation in Humans for Epilepsy. Values in Brackets Are the Ranges to Which the Respective Devices Can Be Adjusted. The Listed Values Are the Most Commonly Applied Values

	Pulse duration	Frequency	Amplitude	Pulse width
Standard functional mapping for epilepsy[10]	5 s	50 Hz	1–10 mA (1–25 mA)	500 μs
Direct cortical stimulation motor evoked potential monitoring[40]	5 single pulses	250 Hz	1–20 mA	500 μs
Deep brain stimulation: Device Kinetra medtronics, Inc.[26]	1 min ON 5 min OFF	130 Hz (2–250 Hz)	5 V (0–10.5 V)	90 μs (60–450 μs)
Responsive neurostimulation: RNS, NeuroPace Inc.[41]	200 ms hippocampal 100 ms neocortical (10–100 ms)	100–200 Hz (1–333 Hz)	0.5–12 mA	160 μs (40–1000 μs)
Cortico-cortical evoked potentials[42]	20–100 single pulses	1 Hz	10–20 mA	300 μs

picrotoxin, they show that high-frequency (50 Hz) stimulation blocked bursting as recorded in the extracellular CA1 region for up to 4 minutes. They conclude that this inhibition via application of a broad electrical field reflects a nonsynaptic mechanism. They further noted that this stimulation abolished activity in the alveus, suggesting that electrical stimulation also inhibits axonal conduction.[46] High-frequency stimulation (greater than 100 Hz) has been shown to promote local inhibition by upregulation of glutamic acid decarboxylase while downregulating calmodulin-dependent protein kinase II.[47] In a study to explore the mechanisms underlying CA3 inhibition by mossy fibers, Thompson and Gahwiler showed that repetitive electrical stimulation led to increased intracellular chloride which was thought to reflect GABA effects.[48–50] Thus, electrical stimulation might lead to hyperpolarization via GABA-mediated increases in intracellular chloride. Local stimulation of epileptogenic regions appears to disrupt synchronous activity preceding seizures,[17,51,52] preventing evolution into clinical seizures. Electrical stimulation also appears to modulate activity in larger networks, including the mouse limbic system,[18] reduce afterdischarge duration,[53] and alter seizure threshold.[54] Induction of short- and long-term depression, changes in receptor expression and injection of electrical noise that disrupts seizure propagation with electrical stimulation[38] have also been postulated to mediate the effects of electrical stimulation on seizures. At the moment it is not clear which if any one or a combination of these observations is the most relevant in seizure control with electrical stimulation.

CLOSED-LOOP BRAIN STIMULATION

As open-loop stimulation is a general and nonspecific approach to modification of seizure activity, a more tailored approach that specifically targets the seizure onset zone might be more desirable. The studies discussed thus far describe stimulation of brain remote from the epileptogenic site, but stimulation of the zone of seizure onset has also been explored. The earliest experiences with local brain stimulation arose in the setting of brain mapping for epilepsy surgery; the generation of afterdischarges (electrical phenomena that share some similarity with spontaneous rhythmic epileptiform discharges) with cortical stimulation are well known, as is the observation that repeat stimulation can cause their termination. This phenomenon was formally studied in 1999 by Lesser et al.[33] who described the occurrence of afterdischarges with brief bursts of 50-Hz cortical stimulation, which were terminated with further electrical stimulation. Thus, in a very basic manner, the potential of local responsive neurostimulation in seizure control was demonstrated experimentally. Such local stimulation specifically at the site of electrical epileptiform activity avoids widespread neuromodulation and therefore might be preferable in terms of avoiding complications such as depression with brain stimulation.[39]

Closed-loop or responsive brain stimulation differs from open-loop systems in that closed-loop systems deliver stimulation based on real-time evaluation of brain electrical activity. The ideal brain stimulator would deliver the right stimulation at the right time and therefore would be the most efficacious and energy-efficient. This might also reduce the incidence of neuropsychiatric side effects seen with open-loop stimulation.

As mentioned earlier, the termination of spontaneous or induced epileptiform activity during brain mapping procedures with additional electrical stimulation reflects the key principles of "responsive" brain stimulation.[33] In this model however, there is no automation and the stimulation is dependent entirely on constant human intervention. These observations led to further innovative development of responsive neurostimulation. Early experiments with responsive neurostimulators at the bedside showed promise and laid the groundwork for development of a feasible clinical solution. Using responsive cortical stimulation triggered by simple detection methods, Peters et al.[55] showed effectiveness in reducing seizure frequency in four subjects undergoing epilepsy surgery evaluation. This early demonstration of responsive stimulation required the integration of a commercial EEG device, two personal computers, two neurostimulators, and custom-built interfaces to integrate these discrete components,[55] underscoring the complexity of designing such a system and the challenges in translating this technique to an implantable device.

In contrast to earlier studies that relied on stimulation of regions with widespread inhibitory connections, most work with responsive neurostimulation has focused on stimulation of cortex directly, specifically the epileptogenic zone related to seizure onset. Kossoff et al.[56] studied the safety and efficacy of a bedside responsive system in four patients undergoing evaluation for epilepsy surgery. Seizure detection was based on EEG pattern recognition (half-wave tool), and complexity (line length and area tools). Stimulation consisted of biphasic, charge-balanced pulses of 1–200 Hz and 0.5–12 mA in intensity delivered via subdural electrodes. They noted that this was well tolerated with only mild sensory symptoms in two patients that resolved with decreased stimulation intensity. Clinical seizure occurrence was reduced during the simulation period. Osorio et al.[38] reported in 2005 their results with an external responsive brain stimulation in eight subjects. They used high-frequency (100–500 Hz) electrical stimulation applied directly to the epileptogenic zone in four subjects, comparing the effects of anterior thalamus stimulation in an additional four subjects. The local stimulation group exhibited a 55.5% reduction in seizure rate, while the remote stimulation group showed a 40.8% reduction in seizures. Thus while both remote and local stimulation appear to have benefit in seizure control, direct stimulation of the epileptogenic site when known appears to be at least as effective.

Smith et al.[57] reported on their experience with a single patient with medically refractory epilepsy who had previously undergone resection but continued to have frequent seizures. Further resection was not feasible because the presumed seizure focus lay near eloquent cortex. The patient underwent implantation of a responsive neurostimulator targeted to the left insula. Detection methods were limited to EEG complexity and energy (line length and half-wave tools), with stimulation of 20 Hz and current of 8 mA. This resulted in a 60% reduction of seizure frequency. This case underscores the potential benefits for epilepsy patients who are not candidates for resection.

Although beyond the focus of this chapter, it should be mentioned that responsive brain stimulation is not limited to electrical energy; devices for local cooling as well as drug delivery have shown a neuromodulatory effect.[58–61] While still experimental, this suggests alternatives to electrical stimulation for seizure management, and the modalities that might be considered in closed-loop systems.

CLINICAL APPLICATIONS

An effective implantable closed-loop neurostimulator must be able to detect seizures, and deliver an appropriate stimulation at the right time and at the right place. These functions are discussed next, followed by a description of the first FDA-approved brain stimulation devise for epilepsy, the Responsive Neurostimulator System, NeuroPace Inc.

Seizure Detection

Current closed-loop stimulators analyze several features of cortical electrical recordings to determine when to deliver stimulation. The most basic trigger is spike detection signaling an epileptic seizure or ongoing epileptiform activity, but such simple methods are prone to false detections related to artifacts. Detection of rhythmic activity offers better discrimination of real events than simple spike detection. By decomposing EEG data into bands based on frequencies between 3 and 20 Hz, Gotman et al.[62] were able to detect seizures in extended surface EEG and electrocortography recordings, but still noted frequent false positive detections. Tzallas et al.[63] showed more robust results using time-frequency analysis that took into account the power density within each discrete band. These computationally efficient methods perform best in defining ictal and nonictal states and therefore are limited in prediction abilities. While stimulation based on these triggers of impending seizure have been shown to lead to shortened seizure duration or symptoms,[38] they do not predict and therefore cannot prevent seizures.

The Responsive Neurostimulator System

The NeuroPace responsive neurostimulator (RNS, NeuroPace Inc., Mountain View, CA, United States) is the first implanted neurostimulator for epilepsy approved for clinical use in the United States. The device consists of a battery-powered seizure detector and stimulation generator implanted in a burr hole in the patient's skull (Fig. 2.1). Up to two leads with four iridium contacts each can be placed in or near the zone of seizure onset, either on the cortical surface or within the brain parenchyma via depth leads. Any combination of the eight contacts can be arranged in up to four channels. The contacts can further be programmed as bipolar leads, or as reference leads with the device case acting as an electrode. Contacts serve to both sense electrical activity and deliver stimulation (see Figs. 2.1 and 2.2). The device continuously screens the electrocorticogram for epileptiform features and significant events are saved for retrieval and analysis by a physician.

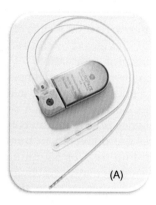 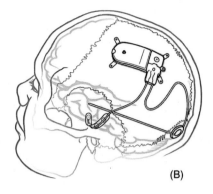

FIGURE 2.1 The NeuroPace RNS device consists of a small battery-powered programmable implanted control unit that serves to sense and record electrical activity and deliver stimulation via both depth and surface electrodes to stop seizures. The device with electrodes (A) and a diagrammatic representation of how the system is implanted (B) are shown. *Source: Images courtesy of NeuroPace Inc., Mountain View, CA, United States.*

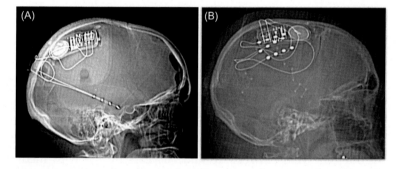

FIGURE 2.2 Implanted NeuroPace RNS. The images show the NeuroPace RNS with bilateral hippocampal depth electrodes (A) and cortical strip electrodes (B).

The RNS system uses three computationally efficient, distinct, real-time algorithms to detect seizures. The first of these, a band-pass tool, characterizes electrocorticography complexity and features by analyzing amplitude and frequency of electrocorticogram readings in specific frequency bands known to be associated with epileptogenesis. The second algorithm, the line-length tool, assesses dynamic changes in EEG amplitude and frequency. Data within a short-term time window (128 ms to 4 seconds) are compared to those of the immediately preceding longer-term window (4 seconds to 16 minutes). The third algorithm measures electrocorticogram energy as a function of area-under-the-curve without regard to frequency, triggering stimulation when a preset threshold is exceeded.

Triggering thresholds are customized, based on each individual's electro-corticogram recordings and their seizure patterns. Several weeks of post-implantation electrocorticogram recordings are reviewed by the patient's epileptologist to determine the optimal settings for stimulation.

The stimulation parameters can be chosen based on effectiveness and tolerability. Stimulation currents between 0.5 and 12 mA can be selected, pulse width can be set between 40 and 1000 μs, burst duration can be programmed between 10 and 5000 ms, and frequency of stimulation between 1 and 333 Hz are available. Triggered pulses are delivered in bursts of up to five pulses that on average summate to a total of 5.9 minutes of stimulation/day. The overall current is low as the energy is delivered in pulses rather than continually. Stimulation is triggered when the line-length value in the short-term window exceeds that in the longer-term window by a preset threshold. The stimulation delivered by the device is programmable with amplitudes from 0.5 to 12 mA, pulse widths from 40 to 1000 microseconds, and frequency from 1 to 333 Hz.[64]

Bidirectional communication between the implanted device and the programming software is accomplished wirelessly. Programmed parameters, saved seizure events, and real-time electrocortography can be downloaded or reviewed from the device. Programming parameters can be uploaded and their effects can be immediately reviewed before ending the session.

THE RNS SYSTEM: PIVOTAL AND LONG-TERM RESULTS

The safety and effectiveness of the RNS were studied over a 2-year period. Subjects were between 18 and 70 years of age with medically resistant partial-onset seizures with one or two identified seizure foci. A total of 191 subjects were implanted with the RNS device, with electrodes placed near or in the epileptogenic zone. Electrocorticograms were recorded for 4 weeks after implantation and stimulation was optimized for another 4 weeks before participants were randomized to either a treatment or sham group for the 12-week blinded portion of the study. All participants received stimulation during the following open-label portion of the study that concluded 24 months after implantation.

Changes in seizure frequency between preimplantation and during the blinded period were compared across the treatment and sham groups. During the open label period seizure change was characterized by the mean percent change in seizure frequency every 3 months compared to the preimplantation seizure frequency. Responder rate (that is, the proportion of subjects demonstrating more than 50% reduction in seizures) during the open label period was also calculated. Adverse events were classified as either mild or serious, and device-related or -unrelated. Quality of life as well as a variety of neuropsychologic metrics including assessment of mood, measures of performance in visual and verbal memory, language, and cognitive flexibility were assessed at baseline as well as at 1 and 2 years.

After implantation, the detection parameters were adjusted based on electrocorticographic patterns in individual patients. The default stimulation settings (200 Hz, pulse width 160 μs, burst duration 100 ms) were used in most patients. Stimulation current was titrated to tolerance. The mean total daily duration of stimulation was 5.9 minutes.

Of the 191 patients initially randomized, 175 completed the full 2 years of study. By the end of the blinded period the treatment group showed 41.5% fewer seizures compared to preimplantation, while 9.4% fewer seizures were seen in the sham group. During the open label period, the subjects in the sham group showed reduced seizure frequency during months 2 through 5 of stimulation. Both groups continued to show reduced seizures during the open label period, with 44% fewer seizures at 1 year and 55% at 2 years. Fifty-four percent of subjects showed greater than 50% reduction in seizures with stimulation. Measurements of quality of life showed improvement at both 1 and 2 years.

The most common adverse events were implant site infection (2.6%) and intracranial hemorrhage (2.1%). No negative effects on neuropsychological function were noted during the 2 years, and mood was not negatively affected.[39] This groundbreaking study showed the long-term safety and efficacy of RNS as an adjunctive therapy for medically refractory epilepsy.

SEIZURE PREDICTION

While clinical seizures seem to be random and unpredictable, analysis of long-term intracranial EEG data suggests that seizures are the culmination of a cascade of electrophysiologic aberrations. Both epileptiform discharge frequency and total EEG energy increase hours before clinical seizures.[65] The complexity of seizure prediction has been likened to other dynamical systems such as weather and earthquakes. Successful prediction therefore must take into account nonstochastic and nonstationary features of seizure physiology.[66]

Linear methods of EEG data analysis, such as Fourier and wavelet transformation, can be used to characterize the signal in terms of frequency and frequency plus time, respectively, and both methods have been used to predict a neurophysiologic environment favoring seizures.[63,67–69] Nonlinear methods based on the theory of dynamical systems have also been used to analyze EEG data for characteristics predictive of seizures.

By estimating the spatial and temporal chaocity of EEG dynamics reflected by the maximum Lyapunov exponent, e.g., Chaovalitwongse et al.[70] demonstrated a viable seizure warning system. In this context, the maximum Lyapunov exponent estimates the stability of a dynamical system. Reports using this method show that changes in electrophysiologic dynamics can be seen several minutes before a clinical seizure[71] and that the spatial coherence of the changes in stability has value in localizing the zone of seizure onset.[72]

Methods collectively leveraging the strengths of these individual methodologies appear to be particularly powerful in accurately predicting seizures. Costa[73] describes a technique integrating signal energy (accumulated energy and energy variation), wavelet transformation, and nonlinear dynamics to classify EEG data from a single patient (from the Freiburg EEG database) into four states (interictal, preictal, ictal, and postictal) with 99% accuracy. Using the same metrics described above with the addition of measurements of moments, spectral band and spectral frequency Moghim and Corne[74] showed accuracy of greater than 97% using data from 14 subjects in the Freiburg EEG database. While these methods have been shown to be effective, the computational requirements of their complex detection algorithms pose a barrier to translation into a small implantable and energy-efficient device.

An implanted seizure advisory system (NeuroVista Inc., Seattle, WA, United States) aims to predict seizure likelihood by analyzing interictal EEG.[75] This system consists of an implanted telemetry unit, intracranial recording electrodes, and a wireless advisory unit. The aim of the device is to provide epilepsy patients with real-time information regarding the likelihood of seizures. After implantation, electrocorticography is recorded for a period of several months. These data are reviewed and compared to clinical events to allow for individualization of the seizure detection algorithm. The algorithm itself categorizes the electrocorticography in real-time with regard to seizure likelihood (i.e., high, moderate, or low) based on signal power.[75–78] Early experimental results show strong negative predictive value in the subset of subjects in whom the "low likelihood" advisory system was activated, but results regarding the clinical usefulness of seizure prediction were less clear. Subjects with high variability in their reported seizure likelihood in particular had trouble responding to the advisories.[75]

ADVERSE EFFECTS AND TECHNICAL CHALLENGES

Years of experience with deep brain stimulation for movement disorders has shown relatively low rates of complications, with mechanical failure (3.1%), hemorrhage/infarction (1.2%), and infection 0.4%) the most common.[79] Similar types of complications have been reported with brain stimulation for seizures.[75,80] There is justifiable concern for electrode heating during MRI scans. At 1.5T these fears appear to be unsubstantiated[81] but are a consideration at higher field strengths.[82] Immune responses to central nervous system implants also pose a challenge to effective neurostimulation therapy. The acute immunologic reaction is characterized by astrocytic response to trauma followed later by the formation of a glial scar that can act as an electrical barrier between the electrode and viable tissue. Long-term viability of implanted leads is influenced in part by the chemical makeup of the implant.[83]

SUMMARY

Electrical brain stimulation in various configurations has been shown experimentally to reduce seizure frequency in medication-resistant epilepsy and might offer options for those patients who are not candidates for traditional epilepsy surgery. Open-loop or scheduled brain stimulation delivers a greater amount of current density to the brain and is relatively nonspecific. Closed-loop or responsive stimulation on the other hand aims to deliver electrical stimulation specifically when epileptiform activity is detected. The primary advantage of this over open-loop stimulation is reduced energy expenditure and therefore longer battery life in implanted devices as well as improved tolerability. While responsive neurostimulation can reduce seizure frequency, further seizure prediction methods are emerging that might enable intervention before clinical signs of a seizure occur.

References

1. Sander JW. The epidemiology of epilepsy revisited. *Curr Opin Neurol*. 2003;16(2):165–170.
2. de Tisi J, Bell GS, Peacock JL, et al. The long-term outcome of adult epilepsy surgery, patterns of seizure remission, and relapse: a cohort study. *Lancet*. 2011;378(9800):1388–1395.
3. Ben-Menachem E, Manon-Espaillat R, Ristanovic R, et al. Vagus nerve stimulation for treatment of partial seizures: 1. A controlled study of effect on seizures. First international vagus nerve stimulation study group. *Epilepsia*. 1994;35(3):616–626.
4. Garcia-Oscos F, Pena D, Housini M, et al. Vagal nerve stimulation blocks interleukin 6-dependent synaptic hyperexcitability induced by lipopolysaccharide-induced acute stress in the rodent prefrontal cortex. *Brain Behav Immun*. 2014;43:149–158.
5. Fraschini M, Demuru M, Puligheddu M, et al. The re-organization of functional brain networks in pharmaco-resistant epileptic patients who respond to VNS. *Neurosci Lett*. 2014;580:153–157.
6. Malow BA, Edwards J, Marzec M, Sagher O, Fromes G. Effects of vagus nerve stimulation on respiration during sleep: a pilot study. *Neurology*. 2000;55(10):1450–1454.
7. Marzec M, Edwards J, Sagher O, Fromes G, Malow BA. Effects of vagus nerve stimulation on sleep-related breathing in epilepsy patients. *Epilepsia*. 2003;44(7):930–935.

8. Hsieh T, Chen M, McAfee A, Kifle Y. Sleep-related breathing disorder in children with vagal nerve stimulators. *Pediatr Neurol.* 2008;38(2):99–103.
9. DeGiorgio CM, Soss J, Cook IA, et al. Randomized controlled trial of trigeminal nerve stimulation for drug-resistant epilepsy. *Neurology.* 2013;80(9):786–791.
10. Penfield W, Jasper H. *Epilepsy and the Functional Anatomy of the Human Brain.* Boston: Little, Brown; 1954.
11. Snider RS, Cooke PM. Cerebral seizures as influenced by cerebellar stimulation. *Trans Am Neurol Assoc.* 1954;13(79th Meeting):87–89.
12. Grimm RJ, Frazee JG, Bell CC, Kawasaki T, Dow RS. Quantitative studies in cobalt model epilepsy: the effect of cerebellar stimulation. *Int J Neurol.* 1970;7(2):126–140.
13. Reimer GR, Grimm RJ, Dow RS. Effects of cerebellar stimulation on cobalt-induced epilepsy in the cat. *Electroencephalogr Clin Neurophysiol.* 1967;23(5):456–462.
14. Cooper IS, Amin I, Riklan M, Waltz JM, Poon TP. Chronic cerebellar stimulation in epilepsy. Clinical and anatomical studies. *Arch Neurol.* 1976;33(8):559–570.
15. Cooper IS, Upton AR. Effects of cerebellar stimulation on epilepsy, the EEG and cerebral palsy in man. *Electroencephalogr Clin Neurophysiol Suppl.* 1978;34:349–354.
16. Velasco F, Carrillo-Ruiz JD, Francisco Brito F, Velasco M, Velasco AL, et al. Double-blind, randomized controlled pilot study of bilateral cerebellar stimulation for treatment of intractable motor seizures. *Epilepsia.* 2005;46(7):1071–1081.
17. Durand D. Electrical stimulation can inhibit synchronized neuronal activity. *Brain Res.* 1986;382(1):139–144.
18. D'Arcangelo G, Panuccio G, Tancredi V, Avoli M. Repetitive low-frequency stimulation reduces epileptiform synchronization in limbic neuronal networks. *Neurobiol Dis.* 2005;19(1–2):119–128.
19. Bragin A, Wilson CL, Engel JJ. Increased afterdischarge threshold during kindling in epileptic rats. *Exp Brain Res.* 2002;144(1):30–37.
20. Sramka M, Fritz G, Galanda M, Nadvornik P. Some observations in treatment stimulation of epilepsy. *Acta Neurochir (Wien).* 1976(suppl 23):257–262.
21. Velasco AL, Velasco F, Velasco M, et al. Electrical stimulation of the hippocampal epileptic foci for seizure control: a double-blind, long-term follow-up study. *Epilepsia.* 2007;48(10):1895–1903.
22. Velasco M, Velasco F, Velasco AL, et al. Subacute electrical stimulation of the hippocampus blocks intractable temporal lobe seizures and paroxysmal EEG activities. *Epilepsia.* 2000;41(2):158–169.
23. Koubeissi MZ, Kahriman E, Syed TU, Miller J, Durand DM. Low-frequency electrical stimulation of a fiber tract in temporal lobe epilepsy. *Ann Neurol.* 2013;74(2):223–231.
24. Fisher RS, Uematsu S, Krauss GL, et al. Placebo-controlled pilot study of centromedian thalamic stimulation in treatment of intractable seizures. *Epilepsia.* 1992;33(5):841–851.
25. Osorio I, Overman J, Giftakis J, Wilkinson SB. High frequency thalamic stimulation for inoperable mesial temporal epilepsy. *Epilepsia.* 2007;48(8):1561–1571.
26. Fisher R, Salanova V, Witt T, et al. Electrical stimulation of the anterior nucleus of thalamus for treatment of refractory epilepsy. *Epilepsia.* 2010;51(5):899–908.
27. Nowell M, Miserocchi A, McEvoy AW, Duncan JS. Advances in epilepsy surgery. *J Neurol Neurosurg Psychiatry.* 2014;85(11):1273–1279.
28. Kanner AM. Depression in epilepsy: a frequently neglected multifaceted disorder. *Epilepsy Behav.* 2003;4(suppl 4):11–19.
29. Weiss SR, Eidsath A, Li XL, Heynen T, Post RM. Quenching revisited: low level direct current inhibits amygdala-kindled seizures. *Exp Neurol.* 1998;154(1):185–192.
30. Weiss SR, Li XL, Rosen JB, et al. Quenching: inhibition of development and expression of amygdala kindled seizures with low frequency stimulation. *Neuroreport.* 1995;6(16):2171–2176.

31. Velasco F, Velasco M, Velasco AL, Menez D, Rocha L. Electrical stimulation for epilepsy: stimulation of hippocampal foci. *Stereotact Funct Neurosurg*. 2001;77(1–4):223–227.
32. Tellez-Zenteno JF, McLachlan RS, Parrent A, Kubu CS, Wiebe S. Hippocampal electrical stimulation in mesial temporal lobe epilepsy. *Neurology*. 2006;66(10):1490–1494.
33. Lesser RP, Kim SH, Beyderman L, et al. Brief bursts of pulse stimulation terminate afterdischarges caused by cortical stimulation. *Neurology*. 1999;53(9):2073–2081.
34. Motamedi GK, Lesser RP, Miglioretti DL, et al. Optimizing parameters for terminating cortical afterdischarges with pulse stimulation. *Epilepsia*. 2002;43(8):836–846.
35. Kinoshita M, Ikeda A, Matsuhashi M, et al. Electric cortical stimulation suppresses epileptic and background activities in neocortical epilepsy and mesial temporal lobe epilepsy. *Clin Neurophysiol*. 2005;116(6):1291–1299.
36. Kinoshita M, Ikeda A, Matsumoto R, et al. Electric stimulation on human cortex suppresses fast cortical activity and epileptic spikes. *Epilepsia*. 2004;45(7):787–791.
37. Sunderam S, Talathi SS, Lyubushin A, Sornette D, Osorio I. Challenges for emerging neurostimulation-based therapies for real-time seizure control. *Epilepsy Behav*. 2011;22(1):118–125.
38. Osorio I, Frei MG, Sunderam S, et al. Automated seizure abatement in humans using electrical stimulation. *Ann Neurol*. 2005;57(2):258–268.
39. Heck CN, King-Stephens D, Massey AD, et al. Two-year seizure reduction in adults with medically intractable partial onset epilepsy treated with responsive neurostimulation: final results of the RNS System Pivotal trial. *Epilepsia*. 2014;55(3):432–441.
40. Szelenyi A, Joksimovic B, Seifert V. Intraoperative risk of seizures associated with transient direct cortical stimulation in patients with symptomatic epilepsy. *J Clin Neurophysiol*. 2007;24(1):39–43.
41. Heck CN, King-Stephens D, et al. Two-year seizure reduction in adults with medically intractable partial onset epilepsy treated with responsive neurostimulation: final results of the RNS System Pivotal trial. *Epilepsia*. 2014;55(3):432–441.
42. Matsumoto R, Nair DR, LaPresto E, et al. Functional connectivity in the human language system: a cortico-cortical evoked potential study. *Brain*. 2004;127(Pt 10):2316–2330.
43. Cooper IS, Amin I, Upton A, et al. Safety and efficacy of chronic cerebellar stimulation. *Appl Neurophysiol*. 1977;40(2–4):124–134.
44. Rosenow J, Das K, Rovit RL, Couldwell WT, Irving S. Cooper and his role in intracranial stimulation for movement disorders and epilepsy. *Stereotact Funct Neurosurg*. 2002;78(2):95–112.
45. Wright GD, McLellan DL, Brice JG. A double-blind trial of chronic cerebellar stimulation in twelve patients with severe epilepsy. *J Neurol Neurosurg Psychiatry*. 1984;47:769–774.
46. Durand DM, Jensen A, Bikson M. Suppression of neural activity with high frequency stimulation. *Conf Proc IEEE Eng Med Biol Soc*. 2006;1:1624–1625.
47. Liang F, Isackson PJ, Jones EG. Stimulus-dependent, reciprocal up- and downregulation of glutamic acid decarboxylase and Ca^{2+}/calmodulin-dependent protein kinase II gene expression in rat cerebral cortex. *Exp Brain Res*. 1996;110(2):163–174.
48. Thompson SM, Gahwiler BH. Activity-dependent disinhibition. II. Effects of extracellular potassium, furosemide, and membrane potential on ECl- in hippocampal CA3 neurons. *J Neurophysiol*. 1989;61(3):512–523.
49. Thompson SM, Gahwiler BH. Activity-dependent disinhibition. I. Repetitive stimulation reduces IPSP driving force and conductance in the hippocampus in vitro. *J Neurophysiol*. 1989;61(3):501–511.
50. Thompson SM, Gahwiler BH. Activity-dependent disinhibition. III. Desensitization and GABAB receptor-mediated presynaptic inhibition in the hippocampus in vitro. *J Neurophysiol*. 1989;61(3):524–533.
51. Sohal VS, Sun FT. Responsive neurostimulation suppresses synchronized cortical rhythms in patients with epilepsy. *Neurosurg Clin N Am*. 2011;22:481–488.

52. Khosravani H, Carlen PL, Velazquez JL. The control of seizure-like activity in the rat hippocampal slice. *Biophys J.* 2003;84(1):687–695.
53. Goodman JH, Berger RE, Tcheng TK. Preemptive low-frequency stimulation decreases the incidence of amygdala-kindled seizures. *Epilepsia.* 2005;46(1):1–7.
54. Carrington CA, Gilby KL, McIntyre DC. Effect of focal low-frequency stimulation on amygdala-kindled afterdischarge thresholds and seizure profiles in fast- and slow-kindling rat strains. *Epilepsia.* 2007;48(8):1604–1613.
55. Peters TE, Bhavaraju NC, Frei MG, Osorio I. Network system for automated seizure detection and contingent delivery of therapy. *J Clin Neurophysiol.* 2001;18(6):545–549.
56. Kossoff EH, Ritzl EK, Politsky JM, et al. Effect of an external responsive neurostimulator on seizures and electrographic discharges during subdural electrode monitoring. *Epilepsia.* 2004;45(12):1560–1567.
57. Smith JR, Fountas KN, Murro AM, et al. Closed-loop stimulation in the control of focal epilepsy of insular origin. *Stereotact Funct Neurosurg.* 2010;88(5):281–287.
58. Rothman S, Yang XF. Local cooling: a therapy for intractable neocortical epilepsy. *Epilepsy Curr.* 2003;3(5):153–156.
59. Skarpaas TL, Morrell MJ. Intracranial stimulation therapy for epilepsy. *Neurotherapeutics.* 2009;6(2):238–243.
60. Smith DC, Krahl SE, Browning RA, Barea EJ. Rapid cessation of focally induced generalized seizures in rats through microinfusion of lidocaine hydrochloride into the focus. *Epilepsia.* 1993;34(1):43–53.
61. Eder HG, Stein A, Fisher RS. Interictal and ictal activity in the rat cobalt/pilocarpine model of epilepsy decreased by local perfusion of diazepam. *Epilepsy Res.* 1997;29(1):17–24.
62. Gotman J. Automatic recognition of epileptic seizures in the EEG. *Electroencephalogr Clin Neurophysiol.* 1982;54(5):530–540.
63. Tzallas AT, Tsipouras MG, Fotiadis DI. Epileptic seizure detection in EEGs using time-frequency analysis. *IEEE Trans Inf Technol Biomed.* 2009;13(5):703–710.
64. Sun FT, Morrell MJ. Closed-loop neurostimulation: the clinical experience. *Neurotherapeutics.* 2014;11(3):553–563.
65. Litt B, Esteller R, Echauz J, et al. Epileptic seizures may begin hours in advance of clinical onset: a report of five patients. *Neuron.* 2001;30(1):51–64.
66. Osorio I. Reframing seizure prediction. *Clin Neurophysiol.* 2014;126:425–426.
67. Samiee K, Kovacs P, Gabbouj M. Epileptic seizure classification of EEG time-series using rational discrete short time Fourier transform. *IEEE Trans Biomed Eng.* 2014;62(2).
68. Nesaei S, Sharafat AR. Real-time detection of precursors to epileptic seizures: non-linear analysis of system dynamics. *J Med Signals Sens.* 2014;4(2):103–112.
69. Liu Y, Zhou W, Yuan Q, Chen S. Automatic seizure detection using wavelet transform and SVM in long-term intracranial EEG. *IEEE Trans Neural Syst Rehabil Eng.* 2012;20(6):749–755.
70. Chaovalitwongse W, Iasemidis LD, Pardalos PM, et al. Performance of a seizure warning algorithm based on the dynamics of intracranial EEG. *Epilepsy Res.* 2005;64(3):93–113.
71. Le Van Quyen M, Martinerie J, Baulac M, et al. Anticipating epileptic seizures in real time by a non-linear analysis of similarity between EEG recordings. *Neuroreport Brain Topogr.* 1999;10(10):2149–2155.
72. Iasemidis LD, Sackellares JC, Zaveri HP, Williams WJ. Phase space topography and the Lyapunov exponent of electrocorticograms in partial seizures. *Brain Topogr.* 1990;2(3):187–201.
73. Costa RP, Oliveira P, Rodrigues G, Leita B, Dourado A. Epileptic seizure classification using neural networks with 14 features. 2008; 281–288.
74. Moghim N, Corne DW. Predicting epileptic seizures in advance. *PLoS ONE.* 2014;9(6):e99334.

75. Cook MJ, O'Brien TJ, Berkovic SF, et al. Prediction of seizure likelihood with a long-term, implanted seizure advisory system in patients with drug-resistant epilepsy: a first-in-man study. *Lancet Neurol.* 2013;12(6):563–571.

76. Davis KA, Sturges BK, Vite CH, et al. A novel implanted device to wirelessly record and analyze continuous intracranial canine EEG. *Epilepsy Res.* 2011;96(1–2):116–122.

77. Gardner AB, Krieger AM, Vachtsevanos G, Litt B. One-class novelty detection for seizure analysis from intracranial EEG. *J Mach Learn Res.* 2006;7:1025–1044.

78. Snyder DE, Echauz J, Grimes DB, Litt B. The statistics of a practical seizure warning system. *J Neural Eng.* 2008;5(4):392–401.

79. McGovern RA, Sheehy JP, Zacharia BE, et al. Unchanged safety outcomes in deep brain stimulation surgery for Parkinson disease despite a decentralization of care. *J Neurosurg.* 2013;119(6):1546–1555.

80. Morrell MJ. Responsive cortical stimulation for the treatment of medically intractable partial epilepsy. *Neurology.* 2011;77(13):1295–1304.

81. Nazzaro JM, Lyons KE, Wetzel LH, Pahwa R. Use of brain MRI after deep brain stimulation hardware implantation. *Int J Neurosci.* 2010;120(3):176–183.

82. Nazzaro JM, Klemp JA, Brooks WM, et al. Deep brain stimulation lead-contact heating during 3T MRI: single- versus dual-channel pulse generator configurations. *Int J Neurosci.* 2014;124(3):166–174.

83. Polikov VS, Tresco PA, Reichert WM. Response of brain tissue to chronically implanted neural electrodes. *J Neurosci Methods.* 2005;148:1–18.

3

Directional Deep Brain Stimulation

A. Mercanzini[1], A. Dransart[1] and C. Pollo[2]

[1]Aleva Neurotherapeutics SA, Lausanne, Switzerland; [2]Inselspital, Bern University Hospital, Bern, Switzerland

DEEP BRAIN STIMULATION INHIBITS NEURONAL FIRING

Early surgical management of movement disorders involved lesioning one or more subcortical structures, such as thalamotomy and pallidotomy for Parkinson's disease (PD). More recently, however, deep brain stimulation (DBS) has largely supplanted ablative procedures. DBS has been applied successfully in the past 20 years for the treatment of neurologic movement

Innovative Neuromodulation.
DOI: http://dx.doi.org/10.1016/B978-0-12-800454-8.00003-3

disorder symptoms, refractory to medication.[1] This treatment is approved for use in Europe, the United States, and other locations for PD, essential tremor, and dystonia. DBS is approved for the treatment of refractory epilepsy in Europe, Canada, and Australia. There have been over 120,000 patients treated to date and about 10,000 patients per year worldwide.

High-frequency (>100 Hz) stimulation appears to mimic a subcortical lesion in the targeted region. DBS in the ventral intermediate (VIM) nucleus of the thalamus or VIM thalamotomy both abolish essential tremor, for example. This suggests that high-frequency stimulation may suppress neuronal firing rather than drive it. Yet, while there is indeed evidence that high-frequency stimulation inhibits neuron firing,[2] not all actions of DBS precisely mimic lesioning. An illustrative example is the lesson learned from the surgical treatment of essential tremor. Unilateral thalamotomy is an effective treatment for refractory tremor with relatively few unintended consequences.[3] Bilateral thalamotomy, on the other hand, often causes several unwanted neurologic sequelae including intellectual impairment and dysarthria.[4] In contrast, the standard approach for DBS in the treatment of essential or Parkinsonian tremor is bilateral lead placement into the same subcortical region. Therefore, it is likely high-frequency stimulation does not simply provide a lesioning effect. Indeed, the effect includes features of excitation and inhibition and several effects of DBS are still under investigation and not well understood.[5]

DBS possesses several advantages over ablative procedures. Perhaps the most important are that DBS is modifiable and reversible. The prescribing physician can adjust the amplitude and other variables of stimulation to achieve the desired neurologic effect. Likewise, once neurostimulation is turned off, the effect ceases. VIM DBS seems to be superior to VIM thalamotomy in reducing amplitude, frequency, and regularity of tremor.[6] Unilateral pallidotomy is inferior to bilateral DBS of the subthalamic nucleus (STN) in reducing Parkinsonian symptoms.[7] For these reasons and others, DBS has largely eclipsed ablative surgery for movement disorder treatment.

DBS HARDWARE

DBS hardware consists of three implanted components, the DBS lead, the extension cable, and a battery-powered neurostimulator. The DBS lead is implanted in a subcortical structure of interest using routine stereotactic or frameless neurosurgical techniques.[8] The lead exits the cranium and is connected to an extension cable. The extension cable is placed under the skin of the head and neck via a tunneling procedure, and is ultimately connected to the neurostimulator. The neurostimulator, also called an implantable pulse generator (IPG), is implanted under the subclavicular or abdominal skin. A fourth component, which is not attached to the DBS hardware and is not implanted, is a device used by the neurologist to program the neurostimulator.

Current DBS systems typically include a lead with four (Medtronic Activa, St Jude Brio) to eight (Boston Scientific Vercise) annular electrode contacts that are 1.27–1.4 mm diameter and 1.5 mm in height. This configuration yields 6 mm^2 of surface area per electrode. Electrical stimulation with currently approved DBS systems on the market is carried in all directions (omnidirectional) around the stimulation lead. DBS leads under development may even contain thousands of contacts addressable with sophisticated multiplexing electronics.

DBS target areas are rather small and surrounded by several fiber tracts and other important brain nuclei. Thus, as increasing stimulation is delivered to the target area, omnidirectional stimulation may also affect untargeted, surrounding regions, including axons en passage. The restricted size of the targeted functional areas, the proximity of surrounding structures, and a DBS lead stimulation area greater than required for treatment results in a "spill-over" effect. This unintended stimulation may induce acutely disabling side effects such as tonic muscular contraction, dysarthria, conjugate eye deviation, paresthesia, or gait imbalance.[9,10] Moreover, stimulation of nonmotor portions of the STN may impair behavior and induce limbic effects such as depression, hypomania, and impulsivity.[11,12]

ACCURATE DBS LEAD TARGETING AND PLACEMENT IS CRITICAL FOR SUCCESS OF THE THERAPY

DBS lead placement is the most technically challenging aspect of the surgical procedure. DBS surgeries require high targeting accuracy and electrode placement. Deviations of DBS lead placement as small as 1–2 mm within the STN can alter the spread of current to surrounding structures, causing tetanic muscle contraction, speech disturbance, and ocular deviation.[13] Despite advances in imaging techniques and the accuracy of stereotactic devices, deviations in lead placement can still occur. MR image distortion, imperfect identification of targeted structures, mechanical stereotactic errors, and intraoperative shift of subcortical structures due to cerebrospinal fluid leakage can result in deviations up to 4 mm.[14,15] Furthermore, it is not always possible to predict functional performance on neuroanatomy alone.

To remedy this, many centers apply intraoperative electrophysiological mapping techniques combined with intraoperative clinical testing to refine target localization and optimize placement of the permanent DBS lead.[15–17]

While neuroimaging greatly aids targeting, it is usually not sufficient for final lead placement. The structures targeted in DBS surgery are relatively small and may not provide clear delineation between structures even by magnetic resonance imaging (MRI) or high-resolution computed tomography (CT). Furthermore, it is not always possible to predict functional performance based on neuroanatomy alone. Therefore, intraoperative, in situ testing is performed both to optimize placement of the DBS lead and stimulation parameters.

During intraoperative testing, high-frequency (~130 Hz) impulses are delivered through micro- or semimicroelectrodes or the DBS lead itself to brain tissue. The patient is conscious and can follow commands during testing. A neurologist or neurosurgeon performs repeated neurological testing to assess clinical efficacy of stimulation and monitor for adverse effects. Based on the behavioral outcomes of stimulation, the neurologist and/or the neurosurgeon determine the best position for the permanent DBS lead.

After electrophysiological target refinement the permanent DBS lead is put in place and anchored to the skull; however, small deviations in lead position may occur during anchoring. Commonly, intraoperative imaging (X-ray, fluoroscopy, or CT) is applied to monitor lead position and corrective action can be taken when deviations are observed.[16,18] Nonetheless, despite careful planning, elaborate intraoperative electrophysiological target refinement and accurate stereotactic device technique, placement errors of 1–2 mm are commonly reported with current stereotactic procedures.[19]

The testing physician, and later, the prescribing physician, have control over certain stimulation parameters such as positive or negative stimulation, pulse width, amplitude, and frequency, but have no control on the direction of stimulation. More recently, stimulation features such as interleaved stimulation, or differential stimulation have been introduced to increase the threshold for the appearance of side effects and improve the therapeutic window (TW) (range of stimulation intensities between clinical effect and adverse effect). However, the cylinder-symmetric design of common DBS electrodes implies that the stimulation field is distributed symmetrically around the lead. These DBS systems provide only limited spatial control over stimulus delivery, i.e., coarse field shifts in steps of 2–3 mm along the lead's axis. Millimeter to submillimeter targeting accuracy may be needed for optimal DBS therapy delivery.[13,18] If the lead is placed slightly off the center of the target, omnidirectional current may spread to nontargeted structures with very little room for postsurgical compensation. Once the lead is placed, the spread of current into adjacent structures can only be prevented by reducing the total stimulus intensity. This range of stimulation intensities between clinical effect and adverse effect is known as the TW of DBS. Consequently, the therapeutic effect of DBS may be sacrificed to reduce adverse motor, behavioral, and cognitive effects.[1]

DIRECTIONAL DBS LEADS CONFER SEVERAL BENEFITS

One promising solution to the problem of suboptimal lead placement is the directional delivery of current such that the stimulation can be aimed in one direction from the lead's central axis. Thus, the DBS current is directed toward the target preferentially in a more controlled distribution with less risk of stimulating adjacent, nontargeted areas.

DBS stimulation with a directional lead could confer several benefits. First, current could be delivered more precisely. Higher currents could be administered to the target area to increase and sustain clinical benefit. Simultaneously, nontargeted areas would be comparatively spared from receiving current. In other words, more current is applied to the intended target and less to surrounding structures. Second, directional stimulation would reduce the overall electrical current requirement. For instance, if a directional lead directs current in only one-third of the lead's cylindrical axis, total current could be reduced substantially, resulting in an extended battery life of the neurostimulator. Since the neurostimulator is implanted under the skin, battery replacement requires an additional surgical procedure. Reduced current requirements could extend battery life and reduce the need for surgery to replace the neurostimulator.

Another benefit of directional stimulation is that it makes DBS lead placement significantly more forgiving. The ability to manipulate the direction of the applied current greatly increases the operator's ability to optimize stimulation parameters. In effect, this overcomes technical and functional issues of suboptimal lead placement.

DIRECTIONAL DBS IN PARKINSON'S DISEASE AND ESSENTIAL TREMOR

Most of the DBS surgeries are currently performed in patients with advanced PD and essential tremor. DBS stimulation of the STN and VIM in PD and essential tremor, respectively, reduces symptoms tremor, rigidity, and bradykinesia.[1] In fact, DBS is superior to best medical therapy when compared in head-to-head trials.[20,21] DBS significantly increases "on-time" without causing troubling dyskinesia, provides a higher rate and degree of clinically meaningful motor improvement, and provides higher quality of life than those treated with best medical therapy.

While DBS is effective, current procedures and devices do not fully remove PD motor symptoms. To illustrate this point, consider the principal scale used to evaluate the intensity of these symptoms, the unified PD rating scale (UPDRS). In a review of 18 trials, Benabid and coauthors found that patients only experienced a reduction on the UPDRS

(Sections I, II, or III) of between 28% and 71% compared to baseline, with most exhibiting a reduction between 50% and 60%.[1] Moreover, the rate of serious adverse events is higher in DBS-treated patients.[1,20,21]

The postoperative side effects of DBS stimulation of the STN are related to overstimulation of the target structure or current leakage to neighboring structures.[14] Side effects of DBS in the STN include dyskinesia, hypotonia, apraxia of eyelid opening, conjugate ocular deviation, and limbic effects.[9] Likewise, current diffusion to nontargeted areas near the STN induces dysarthria and hypophonia from unintended corticobulbar fiber stimulation, tetanic muscle contraction from corticospinal fiber stimulation, and acute depressive symptoms from substantia nigra stimulation.[9,14]

Finite element models (FEMs) of electric field distribution have significantly contributed to a better understanding of the volume of tissue activated (VTA) surrounding the stimulating electrodes, and have brought new insight when correlating the occurrence of side effects with the position of the activated electrode for each individual situation.[22] Electrode size has an important influence on the occurrence of side effects. Several groups have shown that stimulation of the superior and lateral portion of the STN, i.e., the presumed motor area, correlates with the best clinical efficacy.[23-26] Limiting the VTA to this region improves UPDRS performance.[27]

The models showed that in these patients, complete suppression of tremor was associated most closely with activating an average of 62% of the cerebellothalamic afferent input into VIM ($n = 10$), while persistent paresthesias were associated with activating 35% of the medial lemniscal tract input into Vc thalamus ($n = 12$).

Through computational modeling, Keane and colleagues showed that directional DBS that activates 62% of the cerebellothalamic afferent input into VIM theoretically could result in complete suppression of tremor, while persistent paresthesias were associated with activating 35% of the medial lemniscal tract input into ventral caudal thalamus.[22] Martens and coauthors, using lead design techniques, showed similar results.[28]

DIRECTIONAL DBS CLINICAL PROOF OF CONCEPT

Modern, thin-film microfabrication techniques have made more advanced DBS lead designs with higher resolution of electrodes practically feasible.[29-32] Pollo and colleagues recently provided proof of concept in patients with PD or essential tremor.[33] A total of 13 patients, 11 patients undergoing STN DBS for PD (eight males, three females, age 33–72, median 59 years) and two males undergoing VIM DBS for essential tremor (age 54 and 67 years), at the University Hospital of Bern were included. Monodirectional and omnidirectional simulations were

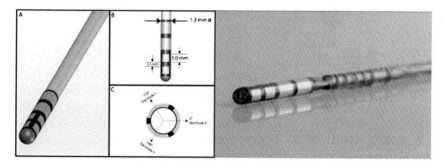

FIGURE 3.1 Schematic of Aleva Neurotherapeutics' directSTN Acute lead and electrode layout (left). Photo of finished device (right). (A) A graphic representation of the distal end of the lead (B) Planar dimensions of the lead demonstrating diameter, electrode height, and separation. (C) An axial view demonstrating the angles that the electrodes are placed.

performed intraoperatively. No device-related or study-related adverse effects were reported during the study period. No complications, such as brain hemorrhage or lesion effect due to insertion or stimulation, were observed during the directional test phase.

A specifically designed DBS lead was used that incorporated a total of eight electrodes consisting of two levels of three-directional electrodes (directSTN Acute, Aleva Neurotherapeutics SA, Lausanne, Switzerland) and two omnidirectional electrodes proximal to the directional contacts. The directional electrodes are each 1×1 mm in dimension, and the longitudinal space between each level is 0.5 mm. The three-directional electrodes give a direction of 0°, 120°, and 240°, respectively (Fig. 3.1).

Preoperative T1- and T2-weighted high-resolution magnetic resonance images (3 Tesla) were coregistered with a stereotactic computer tomography (Leksell frame, Elekta, Sweden) for targeting and planning the implantation trajectories (iPlan, BrainLab, Germany). Intraoperatively, three-trajectory microelectrode recording (FHC, United States) and clinical testing by semimacroelectrode stimulation was performed with the Leadpoint system (Medtronic, MN, United States).

Once the trajectory and site of implantation of the permanent lead had been determined for the first hemisphere operated on (the most symptomatic side), the directional electrode was inserted under fluoroscopic control so that the distal directional ring (contact 0,1,2) was at the Z level of the trajectory that had been chosen for clinical testing and the 0° axis plane of the directSTN lead was directed medially (for STN stimulation) or directed anteriorly (for VIM stimulation).

The proximal end of the directSTN Acute lead was connected to an octopolar extension cable (Model 37081, Medtronic Inc., United States). The extension cable was then connected to a dedicated external neurostimulation cart. This cart was developed in order to pulse any individual directional electrode, or to pulse any combination of two or three electrodes simultaneously. The system features several Osiris Stimulators (Model 504196, Inomed GmbH, Emmendingen, Germany) and includes a custom-made user interface.

The stimulation parameters were current-driven monopolar monophasic pulses, with pulse width 90 µs and frequency 130 Hz. Five different stimulation configurations were tested: each of the three individual directions; the three directions (0°, 120°, 240°) together (omnidirectional stimulation); and a configuration in which two-directional contacts facing the best direction, one above the other, pulse together. Upon completion of the test phase, the directSTN Acute lead was removed and the definitive DBS lead implantation resumed (lead model 3389, Medtronic Inc., United States).

For each patient, a stereotactic postoperative CT scan was performed and coregistered with the preoperative 3D T2-weighted magnetic resonance imaging (iPlan, BrainLab, Germany). Furthermore, the anterior commissure–posterior commissure coordinates of the point for clinical testing were calculated and mapped onto the closest axial slice in the Schaltenbrand atlas templates,[34] and normalized to the intercommissural points. The sequence of stimulation in the three single directions and in the omnidirectional stimulation was determined before the test phase in a randomized fashion, to prevent bias that might arise if an identical sequence was used in all patients. The fifth stimulation configuration (two-directional contacts facing the best direction, one above the other) was performed last, as it required knowledge of the directional contact that gave the best clinical results. The sequence of stimulations was conducted in a double-blinded fashion, unknown to the patient, the neurosurgeon, and the neurologist assessing the patient's reactions. The sequence of directions was known only to the neurologist operating the neurostimulators. All of the patients were operated on by the same surgeon. The same experienced neurologist assessed the intraoperative response of all patients. The patient's motor symptoms were assessed at baseline before stimulation. The total stimulation current was increased in increments of 0.1 mA steps. As the electrical current was increased, the therapeutic effect on the motor symptoms was graded by the neurologist on a four-point scale: no effect, partial effect, very good partial effect, and full effect.

Once the full therapeutic effect was obtained, the neurophysiologist continued to incrementally increase stimulation current until a sustained treatment-limiting side effect arose, such as paresthesia, dysarthria, or focal muscular contraction. These symptoms disappeared as soon as the stimulation turned off, which indicated the upper limit of the TW for stimulation. The current required to obtain a meaningful therapeutic effect (full effect on rigidity or very good partial effect on tremor) which we term the therapeutic current (TC), as well as the side effects encountered, were assessed for the different stimulation configurations. The width of the

TW was defined as the electrical current at which a sustained side effect appeared minus the electrical current at which a meaningful therapeutic benefit was obtained. The impedance through each directional contact was also measured before and after the test phase, as a confirmation that the stimulation did take place as intended.

A three-dimensional FEM of the directional DBS lead was constructed using the COMSOL Multiphysics v4.0 software package (COMSOL Inc., Burlington, MA, United States). The simulation places the lead in a cylinder of diameter 5 cm and height 10 cm. The cylindrical boundary is set to ground while its volume is modeled as an isotropic medium with 0.3 S/m that models the brain tissue resistivity. The model can simulate both constant voltage and constant current stimulation modes.

The model compares the electrical potential around the directional DBS lead for two modes: the omnidirectional mode, in which current is applied to all three-directional electrodes at one level simultaneously, and the directional mode, in which current is applied to only one-directional electrode. A third mode was named "double best," which means turning on two-directional electrodes, one above the other, in the same direction as the best electrode. In the modeling section, this mode is also referred to as 2.5 MM, in order to describe the mode as a 2.5 MM high directional electrode. By solving the model at a given current injection for both cases, an electric potential in the tissue could be determined and the two situations could be compared. Subsequently, the electric potential was superimposed onto the anatomy of the region surrounding the implantation site. This allowed for a comparison of the electrical fields induced in the two cases, i.e., omnidirectional and directional stimulation, to be performed.

Modeling theory also suggests that calculating the VTA is a better indicator of stimulation efficiency in anatomical volumes near the electrode site. Following the method of Buhlmann et al.[35] in which the activating function threshold is derived from a Hodgkin–Huxley model, we computed a VTA by developing a Hessian matrix at each point in the volume surrounding the electrode lead. The maximum absolute eigenvalues of the Hessian matrix were then compared to a voltage strength threshold. Points with eigenvalues greater than the voltage strength threshold were included in the VTA. The voltage strength threshold can be calculated by the method proposed by Rattay. An activation function threshold is defined as $S = I \bullet rs$ where I is the applied current threshold, $rs = 4 \bullet \rho/d$ is the resistivity of the surround tissue with respect to axon diameter, ρ is the resistivity of the axoplasm (70 Ωcm), and d is the diameter of an axon (5.7 μm in this anatomical region). The activation function S can then be compared to previously published values. For example, McIntyre et al.[13] calculated a threshold of ~12 V/cm^2, Martens et al.[28] calculated ~20 V/cm^2, and Buhlmann et al. calculated ~27 V/cm^2.[35] The VTA in Pollo et al.[33] is represented as isolines of threshold values surrounding the lead.

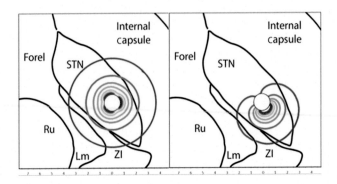

FIGURE 3.2   Axial projection of two stimulation modes using finite element analysis and superposition of electric potential onto anatomy, Plate 54, Hv = −3.5. Left: all three electrodes simultaneously activated with a total applied current of 3 mA (1 mA per contact). Right: posterolateral directional electrode active with an applied current of 1.8 mA, avoiding the internal capsule (IC). Horizontal scale represents the distance from the center of the lead in mm. *Source: Adapted from Schaltenbrand G, Wahren W, Hassler R. Atlas for Stereotaxy of the Human Brain. Chicago: Year Book Medical Publishers; 1977.*

Fig. 3.2 shows the stimulation with the directSTN Acute system in omni-directional and directional modes. The electrical potential is aligned with the anatomy believed to be surrounding the lead during implantation. The isopotential lines are represented with colors, where a darker color means a lower isopotential. The clinically relevant superior and lateral section of the STN has an applied electric potential in both cases, while in the single-directional contact case the internal capsule (IC) is avoided.

Fig. 3.3 shows an analogous comparison of stimulation in the unidirectional and omnidirectional modes superimposed on the anatomy of the VIM, which was the target used for the essential tremor patients. Here, it is apparent that an electric potential directed anteriorly will avoid regions of the sensory thalamus.

The graphs in Fig. 3.4 represent the calculated isolines of the VTA, with a comparison of omnidirectional and directional stimulation modes. Calculations were performed with a stimulation voltage of 1 V on the electrodes, meaning that the current delivered in the omnidirectional mode (three electrodes activated) is three times higher than the current delivered in directional mode. The computation reveals that, when the VTA threshold is set at 12 V/cm^2, a volume of 10.5 mm^3 is activated in omnidirectional mode, whereas a volume of 4.2 mm^3 is activated with a unidirectional electrode.

Finite element modeling was used to simulate and compare the VTA of both one-directional and omnidirectional stimulation. For the models, the total current injected in the omnidirectional simulation was 0.61 mA. As observed in our clinical study, the TC for the one-directional electrode

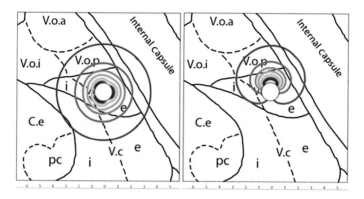

FIGURE 3.3 Anatomical representation in the axial projection of region surrounding the VIM implantation site, Plate 53, Hd = +2. Left: all three electrodes simultaneously activated with a total applied current of 3 mA (1 mA per contact). Right: anterior directional electrode active with an applied current of 1.8 mA, avoiding the sensory thalamus. The horizontal scale represents the distance from the center of the lead in mm. *Source: Adapted from Schaltenbrand G, Wahren W, Hassler R. Atlas for Stereotaxy of the Human Brain. Chicago: Year Book Medical Publishers; 1977.*

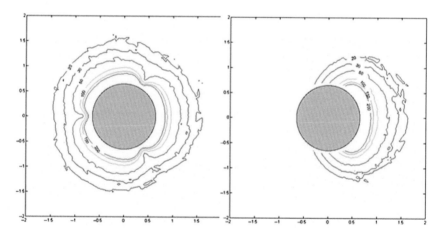

FIGURE 3.4 Transverse view of VTA isolines, when 1 V stimulation is applied. Left: all three electrodes simultaneously activated. Right: one-directional electrode activated. The disk represents a cross-section of the lead. The *x*- and *y*-axis labels represent millimeters from the center of the lead.

stimulation was ~60% of the TC for omnidirectional stimulation. Therefore, for the one-directional electrode stimulation simulations, the total current injected was 0.37 mA (60% of 0.61 mA, the omnidirectional injection current). In order for the total current in the one-directional simulation to match this value, the stimulation level of the one contact needs to be 70% higher, e.g., for a stimulation level of 1 V in the omnidirectional

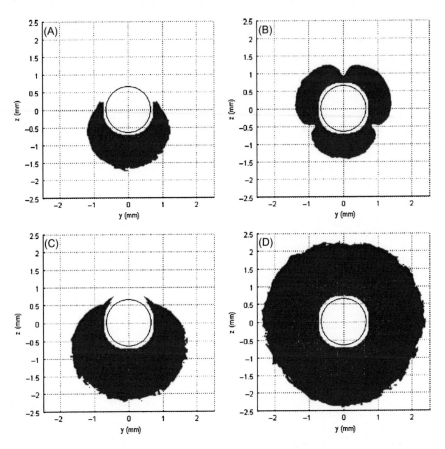

FIGURE 3.5   Top view plots (y–z plane) showing the VTA of the omnidirectional stimulation using all three contacts of one ring on the square ALE lead (plots A and C) compared to the VTA of directional stimulation using only one-directional contact of the same square ALE lead (plots B and D). (A) One contact at 1.6965 V compared to (B) all three contacts at 1 V; and (C) one contact at 5.0895 V compared to (D) all three contacts at 3 V. For the directional simulations (using only one contact), the current injected is equal to 60% of the current injected in the omnidirectional simulation (all three contacts). The activation threshold is 26.66 V/cm^2.

simulation, the level in the one-directional simulation was set to 1.70 V. For the case where 3.00 V were used in the omnidirectional simulation, the corresponding voltage for the one-directional simulation was 5.10 V.

For both one-directional stimulation with 1.70 V and omnidirectional with 1.00 V, the VTA extends into the surrounding tissue approximately 1.5 mm away from the electrode center (see Fig. 3.5A, B). When the stimulation level is three times higher for the omnidirectional (3 V) and the corresponding voltage for one-directional stimulation is 5.10 V, the penetration

FIGURE 3.6   3D image of the VTA when one electrode is turned on.

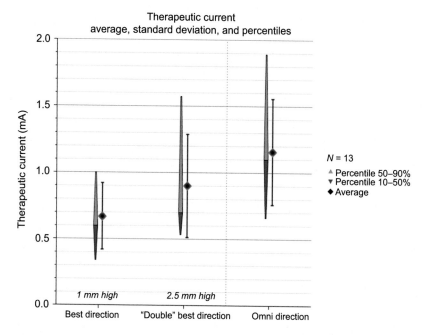

FIGURE 3.7   Therapeutic current generated by 1 MM, 2.5 MM, and omnidirectional electrode configurations.

of VTA into the tissue is between 2 and 2.5 mm, with the VTA of the omnidirectional electrode extending slightly deeper into the tissue (see Fig. 3.5C, D). Based on the FEM simulations, 3D models of the VTA of both one-directional and omnidirectional stimulation were generated (see Fig. 3.6).

As shown in Fig. 3.7, directional stimulation provides a meaningful therapeutic effect with less current when compared to omnidirectional stimulation. The TC was measured for each of the stimulation configurations, in all 13 patients. The average TC in the best direction (best = resulting in the best directional TW) was 0.67 mA (range, 0.3–1.0 mA; see Fig. 3.3, 1 MM directional electrode). The average TC for 1 MM omnidirectional stimulation was 1.17 mA (range, 0.6–1.95 mA). Therefore, the average TC

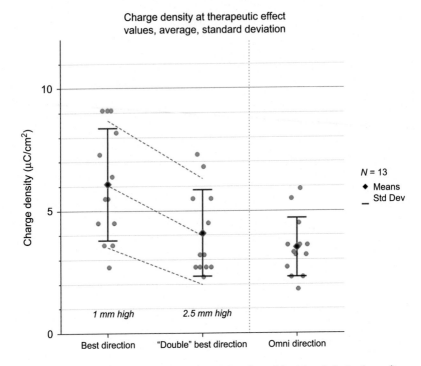

FIGURE 3.8   Charge density for 1 MM, 2.5 MM, and omnidirectional electrode configurations when therapeutic effect was obtained.

in best direction stimulation was approximately 60% of the TC in omnidirectional stimulation. A lower spread of values was also observed for the TC in the best direction stimulation studies. The difference between omnidirectional and best direction TC is statistically significant ($p = 0.002$ with Wilcoxon signed-rank test, $p < 0.001$ with randomization test).

    The charge density ($\mu C/cm^2$) for three electrode configuration (1 MM directional, 2.5 MM directional representing the "double-best" configuration, and 1 MM omnidirectional) was also calculated. As indicated in Fig. 3.8, the highest average charge density ($6.1 \, \mu C/cm^2$) and widest range of charge density ($2.7–9.1 \, \mu C/cm^2$) was observed using 1 MM directional electrodes. By comparison, the 2.5 MM directional electrodes generated average charge density of $4.1 \, \mu C/cm^2$ with a range of $2.3–7.3 \, \mu C/cm^2$ while the 1 MM omnidirectional electrodes generated average charge density of $3.5 \, \mu C/cm^2$ and a range of $1.8–5.9 \, \mu C/cm^2$.

    The charge density was also calculated for each electrode configuration when sustained side effects were observed. As indicated in Fig. 3.9, the highest average charge density ($23.8 \, \mu C/cm^2$) and widest range of charge density ($13.6–30.9 \, \mu C/cm^2$) was observed using 1 MM directional

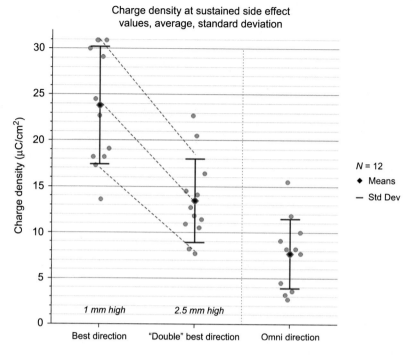

FIGURE 3.9   Charge density for 1 MM, 2.5 MM, and omnidirectional electrode configurations when sustained side effects were observed.

electrodes. By comparison, the 2.5 MM directional electrodes generated average charge density of 13.4 μC/cm² with a range of 7.7–22.7 μC/cm² while the 1 MM omnidirectional electrodes generated average charge density of 7.7 μC/cm² and a range of 2.7–15.5 μC/cm².

In addition to reducing the TC, directional stimulation also widens the TW (see Fig. 3.10). The TW in the best direction (i.e., the one that resulted in the widest directional TW) was 1.93 mA on average (range, 1.0–2.9 mA). The omnidirectional TW average was 1.36 mA (range, 0.15–3.15 mA). The average TW in the best direction is 42% wider than the omnidirectional TW, and with a narrower spread of values. The TW in the best direction (best = resulting in the best directional TW) was larger than omnidirectional TW for 11/12 patients. In one patient with tremor-dominant PD, we found no advantage of directional stimulation over omnidirectional stimulation (omnidirectional TW = 3.15 mA, which was greater than the TW in any of the three individual directions). The difference between omnidirectional and best direction TW is statistically significant ($p = 0.037$ with Wilcoxon signed-rank test, $p = 0.038$ with randomization test).

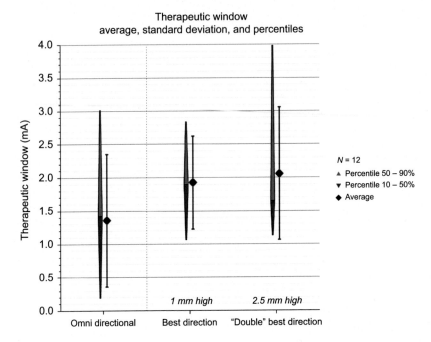

FIGURE 3.10   Therapeutic window generated by 1MM, 2.5MM, and omnidirectional electrode configurations.

The omnidirectional configuration was the first one tested for four patients and was in either second, third, or fourth tested sequence for the other nine patients. Therapeutic effects and side effects were detectable in all five stimulation configurations, but at different electrical current values. A meaningful therapeutic effect was defined as: "full effect" on reduction of rigidity, or "very good partial effect" on reduction of tremor. The first sustained side effect encountered, as current was increased, was either dysarthria, focal muscular contraction, or paresthesias (Fig. 3.11).

One of the directions gave a higher TW than the other two directions for every patient. The best direction (best = resulting in the widest directional TW) varied from patient to patient. The other two single directions were designated as second-best and third-best. Nine of the eleven STN patients had motor side effects (seven dysarthria and two muscular contractions) as their first sustained side effect. Six of these nine patients had the best directional TW in the medial direction, two in the posterolateral and one in the anterolateral direction. The other two STN patients had paresthesia as a first sustained side effect, and their best directional TW was anterolateral. These two patients had a lateral electrophysiological trajectory ≥4mm inside the STN. The two VIM patients had the best direction in the anterior direction, and the third best direction in the

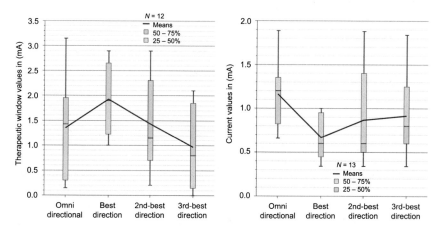

FIGURE 3.11 Box plot representing the width of the therapeutic window (percentiles 0, 25, 75, 100; red line = mean; left) or electrical current producing a meaningful therapeutic effect (percentiles 0, 25, 75, 100; red line = mean; right) for omnidirectional stimulation and for stimulation in each single direction.

posteromedial direction. Both patients had a lateral microrecording trajectory ≥4 mm inside the VIM.

The observed first sustained side effects were correlated with the direction of stimulation.

A representation of TW and current values for omnidirectional and individual directions is shown in Fig. 3.6.

These studies demonstrate the advantage of using one-directional stimulation over omnidirectional stimulation to treat brain disorders. A one-directional stimulation approach achieves a therapeutic effect with lower injection current compared to standard omnidirectional stimulation. Being able to generate an equivalent therapeutic effect at a lower injection current reduces the probability of neural damage. Furthermore, the ability to tune the direction of the stimulation current toward the intended neural target greatly lowers the chance of stimulating off-target neuronal functional areas within the brain, which could trigger unwanted side effects.

There was also a larger TW using one-directional stimulation compared to omnidirectional stimulation. Directional stimulation with an electrode of reduced size, while allowing a specific orientation and reduction of the VTA, provides a new concept of delivering DBS, leading to a more selected activation of the neurons and/or axons surrounding the lead. This enhanced accuracy would be especially desirable in case a DBS lead is not optimally placed, resulting in a reduced intensity of stimulation before the apparition of side effects. Therefore, the ability to direct the stimulation current toward the region of interest enables patient-centric

DBS therapy by allowing the neurosurgeon to tune both the stimulation direction and injection current based on the severity of the patient's neurological disorder and the regions of therapeutic interest.

The posterolateral direction was associated with paresthesias as a first sustained side effect in two of 11 STN patients, which could be explained by stimulation of the medial lemniscus (ML) fibers. In addition, these patients had their best TW in the anterolateral direction, while the posterolateral direction was their worst. Remarkably, the medial direction was never associated with a sustained motor or sensitive side effect at the lowest current threshold.

There was no apparent correlation between the observed best direction TW and the lead location in relation to the STN as defined on postoperative imaging resulting from postoperative computer tomography and preoperative T2-weighted magnetic resonance imaging coregistration. This may be explained by the limited number of patients, but also by the image resolution, which does not provide a well-delineated STN in some cases.

In both VIM patients, posteromedial direction of stimulation was associated with sustained paresthesia. This can be explained by the proximity of the Vc nucleus of the thalamus and of the ML in these directions. Dysarthria could be elicited in the anterior as well as posterolateral direction of stimulation. Both VIM patients had their best TW in the anterior direction, i.e., the direction facing away from the Vc/ML pathways.

The current needed for the generation of meaningful therapeutic effects was remarkably low, less than or equal to 1 mA, in all patients. Intraoperative conditions in terms of tissue reaction to lead insertion (the microlesional effect induced by insertion of the lead and/or surrounding edema) may differ from those seen in a chronic state. For this reason, intraoperative observations may change over time. In order to reduce the risk for an oversized intraoperative TW as well as the risk of a lowered amount of current needed for beneficial effects induced by these particular conditions, the authors excluded patients from our study cohort where a microlesion effect was observed after microrecording and/or microstimulation and before directional stimulation testing.

APPLICATION OF DIRECTIONAL DBS TO OTHER DISEASES

The small volume of targeted areas and close proximity to nontargeted structures makes directional DBS particularly useful in PD and essential tremor treatment. However, several other diseases and disorders that are the focus of omnidirectional DBS treatment studies may be better served by treatment with directional DBS. Benefits would likely be achieved in the global pallidus interus for dystonia or PD. Further benefits may be achieved in other small and complex target regions where a reduced and directional VTA may be desirable.[36] Therefore, highly targeted stimulation fields could optimize DBS not only in currently used targets like STN or VIM, but also in emerging targets and even generate new targets for stimulation.

For example, akinesia and gait disturbances are some of the more debilitating symptoms in patients with PD. One potential DBS target to ameliorate these symptoms is the pedunculopontine nucleus (PPN),[37] which is thought to be involved in the initiation and modulation of gait. More precisely, observations from animal studies have shown that overactive inhibitory influence from the basal ganglia to the PPN contributes to the motor dysfunction in PD and that removing this influence could improve motor function. The PPN is quite small and has two distinct divisions, one containing cholinergic neurons and the other containing glutamatergic neurons. It is almost certainly a case that large, omnidirectional stimulation of the PPN would be fraught with unintended consequences. On the other hand, it is conceivable that modest current delivery within a precise area could be therapeutic.

In phase I trials, DBS stimulation of the fornix/hypothalamus appeared to slow the rate of cognitive decline in six patients with mild Alzheimer's disease.[38] In this study, DBS appeared to drive neural activity in the entorhinal and hippocampal regions. DBS also increased metabolic activity in various cortical regions in these patients. The procedure was well tolerated, however high stimulation settings caused autonomic and cardiovascular side effects. Researchers began with settings commonly used in DBS for PD, 3.5 V, 130 Hz, and pulse width of 90 µs. They observed a dose–response relationship between stimulation and the magnitude of change in the electroencephalography. The authors increased the intensity of stimulation until they encountered adverse effects, usually with stimulation between 6 and 8 V. They then reduced this maximal stimulation by 50% for the chronic implantation and stimulation parameters. It is intriguing to speculate that a directional lead would have permitted higher stimulation intensities along a single lead axis and expanded the TW. Furthermore, as neurons become dysfunctional and die in the progressive course of Alzheimer's disease, directional DBS would allow for higher, focused stimulation and could, perhaps, extend the length of time patients retained memory and cognitive function.

Some of the most exciting work with DBS has been in the treatment of medically refractory psychiatric illnesses. Perhaps the most extensively studied mental health condition for which DBS has been used is treatment-resistant depression. Various target regions have been tried with subcallosal cingulate gyrus, ventral anterior IC and ventral striatum, nucleus accumbens, medial forebrain bundle, inferior thalamic peduncle, and habenula.[39–42] The major limitation to widespread clinical use of DBS in the treatment of depression is a lack of understanding of the neurobiology and neuroanatomy of mental illness. While most of these trials have not included a placebo arm, positive effects have been sustained for years and relapse has occurred when batteries have failed without the patient's knowledge, suggesting a true clinical effect.[43–45] DBS targeting of these disparate structures within brain have led to a wide array of side effects from dysphoria and psychosis to polyuria, tinnitus, and tremor. With the exception of suicide that may or may not be exacerbated by DBS stimulation, each side effect is related to unintended stimulation of nontargeted structures and resolves by reducing stimulation intensity or stopping stimulation altogether.[41] Thus, directional DBS could expand the TW in depression as it has in PD and essential tremor. Furthermore, directional DBS leads would allow additional postsurgical adjustment and refinement of stimulation. This could be useful for targeting neural networks that underlie emotional homeostasis and depression, such as the superolateral branch of the medial forebrain bundle[46] and the nucleus accumbens,[47] respectively.

DBS shows promise for treatment-resistant obsessive-compulsive disorder (OCD). A recent review of OCD DBS trials showed DBS was able to significantly improve scores on the Yale–Brown Obsessive Compulsive Scale.[48] The authors identified 13 stimulation-related adverse effects; 10 of which were transient or reversible with a change in stimulation patterns. Targets included the anterior limb of the IC, ventral capsule/ventral striatum, nucleus accumbens, STN, and inferior thalamic peduncle.[49] As in treatment-resistant depression, progress in OCD DBS is limited by a lack of a clearly defined pathophysiological mechanism for the disorder. Nevertheless, stimulation-associated side effects may be minimized with directional DBS in any small-volume target.

References

1. Benabid AL, Chabardes S, Mitrofanis J, Pollak P. Deep brain stimulation of the subthalamic nucleus for the treatment of Parkinson's disease. *Lancet Neurol.* 2009;8(1):67–81.
2. Dostrovsky JO, Levy R, Wu JP, Hutchison WD, Tasker RR, Lozano AM. Microstimulation-induced inhibition of neuronal firing in human globus pallidus. *J Neurophysiol.* 2000;84(1):570–574.
3. Fox MW, Ahlskog JE, Kelly PJ. Stereotactic ventrolateralis thalamotomy for medically refractory tremor in post-levodopa era Parkinson's disease patients. *J Neurosurg.* 1991;75(5):723–730.
4. Matsumoto K, Asano T, Baba T, Miyamoto T, Ohmoto T. Long-term follow-up results of bilateral thalamotomy for parkinsonism. *Appl Neurophysiol.* 1976;39(3–4):257–260.
5. McIntyre CC, Savasta M, Kerkerian-Le Goff L, Vitek JL. Uncovering the mechanism(s) of action of deep brain stimulation: activation, inhibition, or both. *Clin Neurophysiol.* 2004;115(6):1239–1248.
6. Vaillancourt DE, Sturman MM, Verhagen Metman L, Bakay RA, Corcos DM. Deep brain stimulation of the VIM thalamic nucleus modifies several features of essential tremor. *Neurology.* 2003;61(7):919–925.

7. Esselink RA, de Bie RM, de Haan RJ, et al. Unilateral pallidotomy versus bilateral subthalamic nucleus stimulation in PD: a randomized trial. *Neurology*. 2004;62(2):201–207.
8. Dowling J. Deep brain stimulation: current and emerging indications. *Mo Med*. 2008;105(5):424–428.
9. Krack P, Fraix V, Mendes A, Benabid AL, Pollak P. Postoperative management of subthalamic nucleus stimulation for Parkinson's disease. *Mov Disord*. 2002;17(suppl 3): S188–197.
10. Hariz MI. Complications of deep brain stimulation surgery. *Mov Disord*. 2002;17(suppl 3): S162–166.
11. Temel Y, Kessels A, Tan S, Topdag A, Boon P, Visser-Vandewalle V. Behavioural changes after bilateral subthalamic stimulation in advanced Parkinson disease: a systematic review. *Parkinsonism Relat Disord*. 2006;12(5):265–272.
12. Stefurak T, Mikulis D, Mayberg H, et al. Deep brain stimulation for Parkinson's disease dissociates mood and motor circuits: a functional MRI case study. *Mov Disord*. 2003;18(12):1508–1516.
13. McIntyre CC, Mori S, Sherman DL, Thakor NV, Vitek JL. Electric field and stimulating influence generated by deep brain stimulation of the subthalamic nucleus. *Clin Neurophysiol*. 2004;115(3):589–595.
14. Guehl D, Tison F, Cuny E, et al. Complications and adverse effects of deep brain stimulation in Parkinson's patients. *Expert Rev Neurother*. 2003;3(6):811–819.
15. Gross RE, Krack P, Rodriguez-Oroz MC, Rezai AR, Benabid AL. Electrophysiological mapping for the implantation of deep brain stimulators for Parkinson's disease and tremor. *Mov Disord*. 2006;21(suppl 14):S259–283.
16. Starr PA. Placement of deep brain stimulators into the subthalamic nucleus or Globus pallidus internus: technical approach. *Stereotact Funct Neurosurg*. 2002;79(3–4):118–145.
17. Cuny E, Guehl D, Burbaud P, Gross C, Dousset V, Rougier A. Lack of agreement between direct magnetic resonance imaging and statistical determination of a subthalamic target: the role of electrophysiological guidance. *J Neurosurg*. 2002;97(3):591–597.
18. Schrader B, Hamel W, Weinert D, Mehdorn HM. Documentation of electrode localization. *Mov Disord*. 2002;17(suppl 3):S167–174.
19. Fitzpatrick JM, Konrad PE, Nickele C, Cetinkaya E, Kao C. Accuracy of customized miniature stereotactic platforms. *Stereotact Funct Neurosurg*. 2005;83(1):25–31.
20. Deuschl G, Schade-Brittinger C, Krack P, et al. A randomized trial of deep-brain stimulation for Parkinson's disease. *N Engl J Med*. 2006;355(9):896–908.
21. Weaver FM, Follett K, Stern M, et al. Bilateral deep brain stimulation vs best medical therapy for patients with advanced Parkinson disease: a randomized controlled trial. *JAMA*. 2009;301(1):63–73.
22. Keane M, Deyo S, Abosch A, Bajwa JA, Johnson MD. Improved spatial targeting with directionally segmented deep brain stimulation leads for treating essential tremor. *J Neural Eng*. 2012;9(4):046005.
23. Godinho F, Thobois S, Magnin M, et al. Subthalamic nucleus stimulation in Parkinson's disease: anatomical and electrophysiological localization of active contacts. *J Neurol*. 2006;253(10):1347–1355.
24. Herzog J, Fietzek U, Hamel W, et al. Most effective stimulation site in subthalamic deep brain stimulation for Parkinson's disease. *Mov Disord*. 2004;19(9):1050–1054.
25. Pollo C, Vingerhoets F, Pralong E, et al. Localization of electrodes in the subthalamic nucleus on magnetic resonance imaging. *J Neurosurg*. 2007;106(1):36–44.
26. Rodriguez-Oroz MC, Rodriguez M, Guridi J, et al. The subthalamic nucleus in Parkinson's disease: somatotopic organization and physiological characteristics. *Brain*. 2001;124(Pt 9):1777–1790.
27. Maks CB, Butson CR, Walter BL, Vitek JL, McIntyre CC. Deep brain stimulation activation volumes and their association with neurophysiological mapping and therapeutic outcomes. *J Neurol Neurosurg Psychiatry*. 2009;80(6):659–666.

28. Martens HC, Toader E, Decre MM, et al. Spatial steering of deep brain stimulation volumes using a novel lead design. *Clin Neurophysiol.* 2011;122(3):558–566.

29. Laotaveerungrueng N, Lin CH, McCallum G, et al. 3-D microfabricated electrodes for targeted deep brain stimulation. *Conf Proc IEEE Eng Med Biol Soc.* 2009;2009:6493–6496.

30. Normann RA. Technology insight: future neuroprosthetic therapies for disorders of the nervous system. *Nat Clin Pract Neurol.* 2007;3(8):444–452.

31. Mercanzini A, Colin P, Bensadoun JC, Bertsch A, Renaud P. In vivo electrical impedance spectroscopy of tissue reaction to microelectrode arrays. *IEEE Trans Biomed Eng.* 2009;56(7):1909–1918.

32. Mercanzini A, Reddy ST, Velluto D, et al. Controlled release nanoparticle-embedded coatings reduce the tissue reaction to neuroprostheses. *J Control Release.* 2010;145(3):196–202.

33. Pollo C, Kaelin-Lang A, Oertel MF, et al. Directional deep brain stimulation: an intraoperative double-blind pilot study. *Brain.* 2014;137(Pt 7):2015–2026.

34. Schaltenbrand G, Wahren W, Hassler R. *Atlas for Stereotaxy of the Human Brain.* Year Book Medical Publishers; 1977.

35. Buhlmann J, Hofmann L, Tass PA, Hauptmann C. Modeling of a segmented electrode for desynchronizing deep brain stimulation. *Front Neuroeng.* 2011;4:15.

36. Peppe A, Gasbarra A, Stefani A, et al. Deep brain stimulation of CM/PF of thalamus could be the new elective target for tremor in advanced Parkinson's disease? *Parkinsonism Relat Disord.* 2008;14(6):501–504.

37. Pahapill PA, Lozano AM. The pedunculopontine nucleus and Parkinson's disease. *Brain.* 2000;123(Pt 9):1767–1783.

38. Laxton AW, Tang-Wai DF, McAndrews MP, et al. A phase I trial of deep brain stimulation of memory circuits in Alzheimer's disease. *Ann Neurol.* 2010;68(4):521–534.

39. Hauptman JS, DeSalles AA, Espinoza R, Sedrak M, Ishida W. Potential surgical targets for deep brain stimulation in treatment-resistant depression. *Neurosurg Focus.* 2008;25(1):E3.

40. Rosa MA, Lisanby SH. Somatic treatments for mood disorders. *Neuropsychopharmacology.* 2012;37(1):102–116.

41. Schlaepfer TE, Bewernick BH, Kayser S, Hurlemann R, Coenen VA. Deep brain stimulation of the human reward system for major depression—rationale, outcomes and outlook. *Neuropsychopharmacology.* 2014;39(6):1303–1314.

42. Lozano AM, Mayberg HS, Giacobbe P, Hamani C, Craddock RC, Kennedy SH. Subcallosal cingulate gyrus deep brain stimulation for treatment-resistant depression. *Biol Psychiatry.* 2008;64(6):461–467.

43. Holtzheimer PE, Kelley ME, Gross RE, et al. Subcallosal cingulate deep brain stimulation for treatment-resistant unipolar and bipolar depression. *Arch Gen Psychiatry.* 2012;69(2):150–158.

44. Kennedy SH, Giacobbe P, Rizvi SJ, et al. Deep brain stimulation for treatment-resistant depression: follow-up after 3 to 6 years. *Am J Psychiatry.* 2011;168(5):502–510.

45. Malone Jr. DA, Dougherty DD, Rezai AR, et al. Deep brain stimulation of the ventral capsule/ventral striatum for treatment-resistant depression. *Biol Psychiatry.* 2009;65(4):267–275.

46. Coenen VA, Schlaepfer TE, Maedler B, Panksepp J. Cross-species affective functions of the medial forebrain bundle-implications for the treatment of affective pain and depression in humans. *Neurosci Biobehav Rev.* 2011;35(9):1971–1981.

47. Berton O, Nestler EJ. New approaches to antidepressant drug discovery: beyond monoamines. *Nat Rev Neurosci.* 2006;7(2):137–151.

48. Kisely S, Hall K, Siskind D, Frater J, Olson S, Crompton D. Deep brain stimulation for obsessive-compulsive disorder: a systematic review and meta-analysis. *Psychol Med.* 2014:1–10.

49. de Koning PP, Figee M, van den Munckhof P, Schuurman PR, Denys D. Current status of deep brain stimulation for obsessive-compulsive disorder: a clinical review of different targets. *Curr Psychiatry Rep.* 2011;13(4):274–282.

Waveform Variation in Neuromodulation

J. Arle[1,2,3]

[1]Beth Israel Deaconess Medical Center, Boston, MA, United States;
[2]Mt Auburn Hospital, Cambridge, MA, United States; [3]Harvard Medical
School, Boston, MA, United States

INTRODUCTION

Neuromodulation, whether deep brain stimulation (DBS), spinal cord stimulation (SCS), vagus nerve stimulation (VNS), or some version of peripheral nerve stimulation, is now a widely used approach for treating a number of typically difficult chronic medical conditions such as pain, movement disorders, epilepsy, and a variety of psychiatric problems. Although tremendous advances have been achieved using many of the earliest patterns of electrical stimulation, such as standard

Innovative Neuromodulation.
DOI: http://dx.doi.org/10.1016/B978-0-12-800454-8.00004-5

charge-balanced biphasic square-waves at relatively low frequencies, it has become increasingly apparent in the last decade that other patterns may be more efficacious, more efficient, capture more important salient features of the underlying neural circuitry, or be better able to serve as a useful signal to implement closed-loop paradigms that self-regulate their stimulation moment-to-moment. We explore some aspects of these innovations below, and some of their potential mechanisms of action.

MODIFICATIONS OF TRADITIONAL WAVEFORM PARAMETERS AND SHAPES

Obviously, several of the basic parameters used in any signal can be manipulated outside of typical ranges, especially as technology is developed that accomplishes such changes reliably and without unattainable power requirements. These basic parameters would include frequency, amplitude, and pulsewidth (PW). Some insights have been gained by simply trying different combinations of these basic parameters—e.g., it was appreciated that 60 Hz rather than 130 Hz or higher could achieve equal or better control of dystonia in DBS of the GPi.[1] This finding was driven partly by the simple fact that these patients often were using fairly higher frequencies and PWs to gain benefit and their batteries were draining sooner, requiring more frequent surgeries to replace them. The lower, but still efficacious, frequency allowed for roughly half the amount of power usage and therefore significantly lengthened the time to replacement.

Some attempts to adjust a parameter, however, have been met with problems almost instantly. For example, increasing the amplitude in either VNS or DBS will often merely result in unwanted side effects (vocal paralysis, hoarseness, unwanted muscle contractions or movement, and pain, among others), and side effects may be a boundary on the therapeutic range even when the signal is *within* more typical parameter settings, making the entire process of programming patients still paramount. Nonetheless, advances in just the shape of the stimulus pulse itself have been explored, finding several solutions with a genetic algorithm for wave-shapes that are more energy-efficient, e.g., in monophasic or biphasic modes, than rectangular, exponentially ramping or decaying waveforms.[2] An analysis by Foutz et al.[3] showed that a centered triangular waveshape was more energy-efficient and as efficacious as a traditional rectangular waveshape.

Some variations in typical parameter ranges, however, have been tried using changes of several orders of magnitude. We explore some of those here and also variations in other aspects of the signal such as the temporal characteristics (random, bursting, and paired pulse paradigms), as well as attempts to adjust the stimulus on the fly using information gained by recording (i.e., closed-loop scenarios).

DEEP BRAIN STIMULATION

Since the earliest work with DBS for movement disorders, it has been appreciated that despite exceptionally accurate targeting of the subthalamic nucleus (STN), various nuclei of the thalamus (e.g., ventralis intermedius, or Vim), or the globus pallidum (e.g., pars interna, or GPi), not all patients improved, nor did all patients use the same stimulating patterns or electrodes. Furthermore, it was unclear what changes DBS imparted to the circuitry that bring about the clinical benefit—could it be an increase in regularity of firing downstream, within the nuclear target itself, a more irregular firing, an inhibition of firing, or some other kind of information content that changes? Moreover, were there alterations that worked on longer timescales, receptor up- or downregulation, other protein synthesis changes that regulated transmitter creation, packaging, breakdown, or even more entrenched changes to the DNA or RNA processing itself? Recent work, e.g., has shown that DBS in the STN for Parkinson disease (PD) does alter motor cortex plasticity.[4] If more could be understood about these changes, changes that also run parallel and counter to the changes appreciated with lesioning that had been performed for many years prior to DBS, then perhaps more sophisticated alterations in the DBS signal could take advantage of such knowledge and optimize DBS treatment further. Where optimization of targeting and placement techniques had been achieved, optimization of signal characteristics could be achieved. Furthermore, given that each patient has unique ways in which their disorder has manifested within the neural circuitry, from location to degree, perhaps the signal could be adjusted in real-time or nearly real-time to optimize the signal on a patient-to-patient and moment-to-moment basis.

A few areas of study have made advances in this context. One is to use random or irregular stimulus patterning. Another direction taken is to use sophisticated analysis of recordings to filter changes in the circuitry and match the DBS signal to optimize a particular outcome thought likely to be found in patients with more clinical benefit. Finally, some are examining what is called "coordinated reset" (CR) stimulation, in order to reset synaptic weights endemic within circuitry and thereby desynchronize abnormal synchronized circuitry dynamics.

Random or Irregular Signals in DBS

Brocker et al.[5] point out that efficacy of DBS for PD is sensitive to the stimulation parameters. For example, high-frequency (>100 Hz) is more effective than low-frequency (<100 Hz) stimulation,[6–8] and outcomes are also dependent on the amplitude, polarity, and PW.[9–12] They note, however, that the temporal pattern of stimulation "stands out as a potentially important parameter space that has not been fully explored."

Several groups have begun looking at random or irregular temporal patterns of stimulation in DBS, for movement disorders[5,13,14] and even obsessive-compulsive disorder (OCD).[13] Brocker et al.[5] note that previous studies in tremor suggested that irregular stimulation was not as effective as regular stimulation. However, in re-exploring the underlying nature of the signal to learn what characteristics of the irregular signal were important, they studied several irregular patterns in DBS for PD in a finger-tapping exercise, at both STN and GPi targets (see Fig 4.1 taken from their text) and found three of the four irregular patterns were superior to regular DBS.

Efficacy seemed to be more related to an ability of the signal to lead to more suppression of beta band power than anything else and was not a result of statistical properties of the signal per se.

Karamintziou et al. have examined the relative ability of irregular stimuli in the STN to disrupt synchronization in an MER (microelectrode recording)-based model of PD and OCD pathology in the circuit and found that it was superior to regular stimulation using either 135 or 80 Hz.[13] They tried different combinations of irregularity and bursts in their signals. In a partial contrast, Baker et al.[15] used irregular patterns or regular bursts compared to regular stimulation at 135 and 80 Hz in the GPi treating bradykinesia and found that regular bursts were as effective

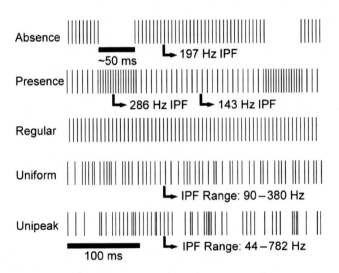

FIGURE 4.1 Exploring boundaries of regularity and irregularity in DBS signals for both tremor and Parkinson disease. Brocker et al.[5] noted that three of the four irregular waveforms they tried for PD were superior to regular stimulation patterns in a finger-tapping exercise. This is from their Figure 1 showing the four irregular patterns they tried (top two and bottom two) and the regular signal in the center.

as regular tonic stimulation but used 40% less current. Other irregular patterns were less effective than regular tonic stimulation, however.

Finally, in a direct comparison of randomized transcranial direct current stimulation (tDCS) with alternating current tACS and regular tDCS to treat tinnitus, the randomized signal resulted in the largest suppressive effect on tinnitus loudness and distress,[16] possibly by better disrupting coordinated activity in auditory cortex.

Closed-Loop Systems Leading to Waveform Adjustment

An active area of neuromodulation research is in the effort to develop closed-loop devices, which typically offer variation from the tonic regular stimulus now used in standard commercially available open-loop systems. Rosin et al.[17] did some of the earliest work in this area when they showed an example of how adaptive stimulation might work in a nonhuman primate model of PD. Two MPTP (1-methyl-4-phenyl-1,2,3,6-tetrahydropyridine) Parkinsonian monkeys were implanted with electrodes recording from regions of GPi and motor cortex providing feedback for adjusting the stimulation, which was in GPi. After assessing several closed-loop paradigms for efficacy versus traditional tonic stimulation, using the motor cortex firing rate changes to drive the timing of a seven-pulse burst in GPi at 130 Hz every 80 ms led to the most significant decrease in bradykinesia. Overall GPi firing rates were reduced and oscillatory activity enhanced, though the number of stimulation pulses overall was significantly reduced as well, making this more energy-efficient. Interestingly, if the activity in GPi was used to drive stimulation in the same way, bradykinesia worsened.

Eventually, realization that beta band power at the stimulating contacts from local field potentials (LFPs), e.g., could be used instead to trigger the DBS stimulus, primarily in STN. Several developments using this information have been tried,[18,19] with results suggesting equivalent or improved motor control in PD patients compared to tonic stimulation but with less than half of the stimulation power requirements, again suggesting that significant improvements in power consumption may be on the near-term horizon. Another recent hybrid development combines the ability to record dopamine release using fast-scan cyclic voltammetry and using the transmitter levels to regulate the amount of stimulation, potentially avoiding overstimulation dyskinesia side effects, as well as reducing power requirements (see Fig. 4.2).[20]

Coordinated Reset

As mentioned above, CR has been tried in the auditory system for tinnitus with some benefit (cf. Ref. [21] for a review). This method is thought

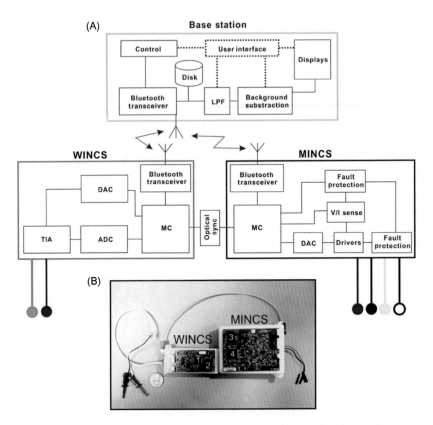

FIGURE 4.2   Schema and picture of the combined WINCS-MINCS device described in Chang et al.[20] toward a reliable useful closed-loop electrochemical feedback system for DBS. WINCS stands for Wireless Instantaneous Neurochemical Concentration Sensing System which allows communication to the MINCS (Mayo Investigational Neuromodulation Control System) using information from fast-scan cyclic voltammetry to inform the DBS output. Communication is through optical fibers. Studies demonstrated stimulation of the median forebrain bundle in rats led to changes in dopamine release in the striatum and levels in near real-time could then feedback to the DBS signaling and autoadjust stimulation to maintain a steady-state level. Such sophisticated devices are continued to be refined and may reach the stage of human trials in the near future. (A) schematic for device, (B) actual device implementation.

to be useful in disorders that involve strong neuronal synchronization, which might include epilepsy, PD, and tinnitus, and attempts to deliver phase-resetting stimuli at different times to different subpopulations involved in abnormal neuronal synchronization.[22,23] It takes advantage of circuits which likely can manifest spike-timing-dependent plasticity leading to a decrease of mean synaptic weights within the target circuitry. In this way, CR stimulation shifts the neuronal network from a pathological attractor with upregulated synchrony and connectivity to a physiological attractor with downregulated synchrony and connectivity.[24–26] It has been described as an "unlearning" or an "antikindling."[27,28]

This technique is also then a modification of traditional tonic stimuli and, again, an innovating neuromodulatory development that has come out of a deeper understanding of the underlying circuitry dynamics. In addition to the work described for tinnitus, some have shown it can be effective in PD and in the STN,[25] and potentially in hippocampus in epilepsy.[29] CR has also itself been modified and other variants explored to some degree. It represents, however, a unique category of waveform variation separate from parameter and shape adjustments and different than using recorded characteristics of the system in real time to make closed-loop adjustments.

SPINAL CORD STIMULATION

While some of the waveform shape, parameter, and timing adjustments described above are also being explored in SCS, two relatively recent developments will be of particular focus here: burst and high frequency (burst and HFS, respectively). Each has now been more thoroughly vetted in clinical trials and reached commercialized levels of support in Europe and the US market. Keep in mind that any of the modifications described in other areas of this chapter could be applied to SCS as well. However, the developments and clinical support for burst and HFS have made them particularly relevant to the discussion at this point in time.

Burst stimulation was hypothesized initially by De Ridder prior to 2007 (cf. Ref. [30] in treating tinnitus on the basis of general thinking about the signal characteristics of pathways reaching auditory cortex, lemniscal and extralemniscal, which preferentially use tonic and burst signaling, respectively). Burst seemed to have more effect than tonic stimulation on cortical neurons. It was tried in the spinal cord with a similar thought process on how medial and lateral pain pathways may use tonic and burst into and after reaching the thalamus. As a burst signal, it is characterized as a signal of five rectangular pulses at 500 Hz with a 1 ms PW, bursting every 25 ms, at 40 Hz (see Fig. 4.3). Part of its uniqueness is the long PW—significantly more than most typical neuromodulation signals. At this point it has been clinically compared to tonic 500 Hz signals (but with the tonic signal using <500 μs PW—cf. Ref. [31]) and is currently being compared to 10 kHz high-frequency stimulation (discussed below). So far, it appears to be either equal or superior to using traditional SCS parameters and is able to salvage patients who have failed traditional SCS (e.g., Refs. [32–35]) (Fig. 4.3 compares burst to tonic).

Interestingly, however, burst stimulation, as used in epidural SCS, does not lead to the typical feeling of vibration-like paresthesias at therapeutic

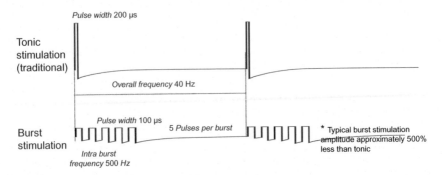

FIGURE 4.3   Rendering of the general "burst" pattern of waveform (see Ref. [30]) investigating tinnitus and then brought to bear on spinal cord stimulation to control pain. Note
that the pulse width of each pulse in a burst is significantly longer than pulses in typical
SCS waveforms (shown above). It remains unclear what aspects of the burst signal are
important for efficacy—intraburst frequency, pulsewidth and amplitudes, varying the burst
pulse amplitudes, overall burst frequency, number of burst pulses per burst, and so forth.
Moreover, it is unclear whether these novel signals act primarily on spinal cord fibers and
circuitry or on higher pain-processing centers.

amplitude levels. Paresthesia-free stimuli seem to be typically better tolerated by patients, already an innovative advance in the field, but it raises
questions about its overall mechanism and how that mechanism could be
further optimized or leveraged.

High-frequency stimulation, specifically using 10 kHz (also known as
HF10), has also become commercialized and has been shown in several
studies to give equal or superior results for pain relief compared to traditional lower-frequency stimulation (cf. Refs. [36–39]). In fact, in a large
randomized controlled trial[39] responders to HF10 outnumbered responders to traditional SCS for back and leg pain by almost 2:1. Again, and
of note, as with burst, patients do not feel paresthesias. Are the mechanisms of eliminating paresthesias the same with burst and HF10? Are the
mechanisms of pain relief the same between burst and HF10? These are
fundamental questions that need to be answered for optimizing these
new waveforms in SCS treatment, but also for developing potentially new
innovations in other areas of neuromodulation as well.

There are a couple of aspects of these two stimulation patterns that
are puzzling. First, if the primary effect of these patterns is inhibitory
or suppressive, and this somehow accounts for preventing paresthesias,
then how can pain be controlled without any neurons being stimulated?
Stimuli only reach the outer 300–500 μm edge of the dorsal columns in the
spinal cord (e.g., Ref. [40]) and there are not significant numbers of pain
fibers in that part of the cord, so it's not as if pain fibers are themselves
directly inhibited, along with the paresthesia-carrying fibers. Second, it
would not make sense that there is stimulation of some fibers which shut

down pain within the spinal cord circuitry, but without stimulation of also the larger lower-threshold paresthesia-carrying fibers at the same time.

A study by Lempka et al.[41] modeling axons and a symmetric rectangular square-wave stimulus at 10 kHz suggested there is no driving of axons within the dorsal columns. Another study by Parker's group recorded compound action potentials superior to the stimulating contacts[42] and suggested there is no signal found using HFS. However, work by our group has modeled axons down to the level of the ionic channel subcomponents across diameters from 5 to 20 µm, as are found in the dorsal columns, and across frequencies from 50 Hz to 10 kHz using a variety of PWs, and shown that with *monophasic* stimuli an interesting phenomenon occurs as frequencies increase above approximately 4–5 kHz (see Fig. 4.4). Because of a combination of the internodal distance in different axon diameters and the consequent activating function related to these different-sized axons, in addition to the channel dynamics at such high

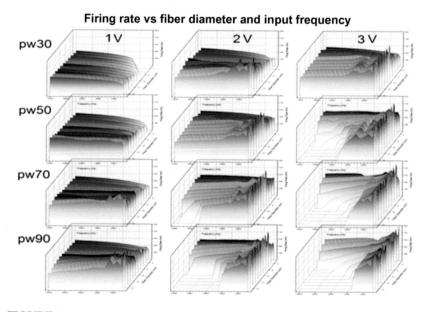

FIGURE 4.4 Composite of graphs showing modeling data across axon diameters (y-axis going into page), frequency of stimulation (up to 10 kHz on far left of each x-axis), and firing rate (z-axes) as amplitudes are increased from 1 to 3 V (columns of panels left to right) and at varying pulse-widths (30, 50, 70, and 90 µs) in rows from top to bottom. Note the main finding that larger fibers (in foreground graphs of each panel waterfall) become blocked and do not generate action potentials by 3 V (typical therapeutic levels), whereas smaller fibers continue to fire. This is a suggested mechanism whereby larger paresthesia-carrying fibers are shut down and the patient feels no stimulation using 10 kHz input. Pain relief is then apparently achieved by the firing of many more medium-sized and smaller fibers.

frequencies, the firing thresholds as related to axon diameter invert—larger axons are suppressed and medium and smaller axons are driven.

This would explain why HF10 leads to paresthesia-free stimulation on the one hand (paresthesia-carrying fibers are larger fibers[43] and would be suppressed), and it would explain why compound action potentials may not be found superiorly, as they would be more desynchronized across many more smaller fibers with smaller amounts of flux overall making the recording of such activity amount to more likely a small rise of background amplitude, which is what was found apparently (Tracy Cameron, personal communication). Pain relief would have to come from the activity of these smaller and some medium fibers. As appreciated from several anatomical studies of the dorsal columns (e.g., Ref. [44]) there are many more fibers between 4 and 9 μm than between 10 and 15 μm and our group has shown in detailed spinal cord circuitry modeling that wide-dynamic range (WDR) cells carrying neuropathic pain signals would be inhibited equally or more effectively by these fibers than if only larger fibers are activated (as in traditional SCS) (see Fig. 4.5).

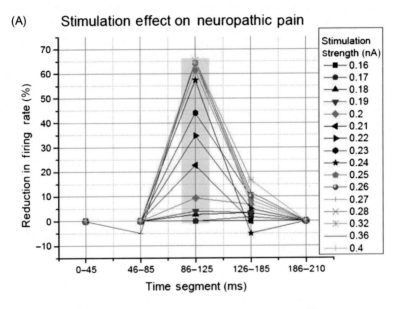

FIGURE 4.5   Spinal cord circuitry models developed by Arle et al.[40] show an amplitude-dependent inhibition in wide-dynamic range (WDR) neurons, when typical (lower-frequency) SCS is used and depends on only a small number of larger fibers in the dorsal columns (A, neuropathic pain; B, acute pain). (C) A similar amplitude-dependent inhibition of the WDR cells can occur when SCS activates only a larger number of medium- and smaller-diameter fibers and blocks the larger fibers.

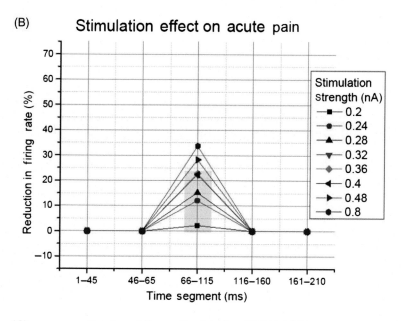

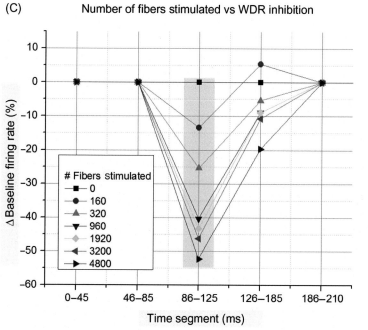

FIGURE 4.5 (Continued)

Finally, it also provides some support for the negative finding by Perruchoud et al.[45] that 5 kHz HFS was no better than placebo stimulation since it appears from the models (and the model parameters used are general estimates, whereas real parameters likely somewhat vary from patient-to-patient and even moment-to-moment) that 5 kHz is still too low to obtain the larger axon diameter suppression reliably. From the modeling, it does seem that somewhere above 7–8 kHz would provide reliable implementation of this phenomenon, and certainly at 10 kHz.

The crux of this explanation for the mechanism of HF10, however, hinges on the use of a monophasic signal in these models and is in stark contrast with the fact that all SCS systems use a charge-balanced biphasic signal. When our group had modeled a symmetric rectangular biphasic signal (as in the Lempka et al. study[41]) we also found no activity being generated. But looking into this situation more deeply it has to be considered that the models are examining a monophasic signal at the axons themselves and it must be asked whether there is any possibility that a symmetric rectangular biphasic source signal at the electrode, in the epidural space, with dura and ionic fluid intervening, could arrive at the cord with a monophasic character. It turns out that this is a complicated question and is also fundamentally different than the DBS picture wherein only the electrode–tissue interface (ETI), with reversible and irreversible faradaic activity, already complicates the signal and requires sophisticated mathematics to describe.

While the ETI creates some degree of pseudocapacitance, the cerebrospinal fluid likely forms an electrical double layer on the inside of the dura, thereby adding a further complicating aspect to understanding the field *at the cord*. In examining this situation, we have explored electrochemical theory using variations of the Randles equation, Gouy–Chapman–Stern theory, the Nernst–Plank–Poisson equations, and the Butler–Volmer equation. While there is likely some increased capacitance from the ETI and electrical double layer, it might be thought to occur equally during both the cathodic and the anodic phases of the biphasic signal, thereby still leading to a symmetric biphasic end result. However, it turns out there are asymmetries in how these effects manifest during the cathodic and the anodic phases, respectively—this effect falls out of the equations themselves and was pointed out in several references obliquely[46,47] and by personal communication (Brian Howell, 2015). Our current estimates suggest that even a 20% asymmetry in the resistivity between anodic and cathodic phases leads to at least a 70% partial half-wave rectification of the original source biphasic signal when measured at the dorsal column. As seen in Fig. 4.6, 70% or more half-wave rectification is enough to account for the diameter inversion threshold effect at high frequency.

Obviously more work needs to be done in understanding the complexities of the signal transformations across the ETI, the dura, and the ionic fluid effects, as well as understanding how suppression and activation

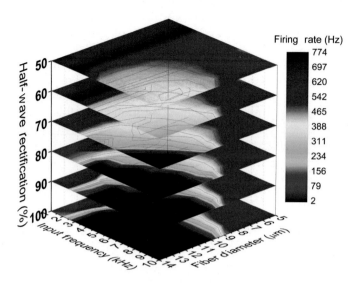

FIGURE 4.6 Composite multilayered set of graphs showing that the axon fiber diameter differential blocking at higher frequencies of stimulation is dependent on some type of monophasic waveform signal reaching the axons, or at least a partially half-wave rectified signal. The z-axis shows the degree of half-wave rectification from 50% to 100% (monophasic), the x-axis the frequency of the signal, and the y-axis the axon diameter. The darkest color shows the least firing, or no firing. Note that even a 70% half-wave rectified signal will inhibit the largest fibers at 10 kHz. How such a somewhat monophasic signal might occur when typical SCS and 10 kHz systems use a balanced biphasic waveform is currently being studied. Various capacitive effects from the ionic fluid of the CSF or membrane properties as a result of ion channel blocking in the axon itself could transform the biphasic signal toward a more monophasic signal, but the mechanisms need to be further elucidated.

within the dorsal columns might truly manifest, but this initial work may be a catalyst in leading the way to that understanding.

OTHER CONSIDERATIONS

Some developments in using neuromodulation to treat epilepsy have broached new territory. In particular, stimulation of the vagus nerve used for many years to treat seizures has now been explored in treating a variety of disorders including depression and heart failure. Because the vagus nerve is involved in so many different organ systems and autonomic control, there is growing interest in understanding how to modulate its fibers in more refined ways. Differential fiber selectivity might be considered in targeting certain axons within particular fascicles of the nerve using a variety of techniques from transmission block to selective activation based potentially on feedback from biomarkers.

In another approach to seizure control, and again different than other attempts to use closed-loop systems, a way of generating signals used to *model* seizures was adapted to *treat* seizures. Zalay and Bardakjian[48] show how sophisticated coupling of cognitive rhythm generators can be linked to generate a very realistic but sophisticated signal as a treatment stimulus to arrest seizures rather than just a seizure-generating network to test other stimulation paradigms. They found that this stimulus, in a closed-loop system for epilepsy, was more effective in stopping seizures than traditional tonic stimulation.

References

1. Alterman RL, Miravite J, Weisz D, Shils JL, Bressman SB, Tagliati M. Sixty hertz pallidal deep brain stimulation for primary torsion dystonia. *Neurology*. 2007;69(7):681–688.
2. Wongsarnpigoon A, Grill WM. Energy-efficient waveform shapes for neural stimulation revealed with genetic algorithm. *J Neural Eng*. 2010;7(4):046009.
3. Foutz TJ, Ackermann Jr DM, Kilgore KL, McIntyre CC. Energy efficient neural stimulation: coupling circuit design and membrane biophysics. *PLoS ONE*. 2012;7(12):e51901.
4. Kim SJ, Udupa K, Ni Z, et al. Effects of subthalamic nucleus stimulation on motor cortex plasticity in Parkinson disease. *Neurology*. 2015;85(5):425–432.
5. Brocker DT, Swan BD, Turner DA, et al. Improved efficacy of temporally non-regular deep brain stimulation in Parkinson's disease. *Exp Neurol*. 2013;239:60–67.
6. Rizzone M, Lanotte M, Bergamasco B, et al. Deep brain stimulation of the subthalamic nucleus in Parkinson's disease: effects of variation in stimulation parameters. *J Neurol Neurosurg Psychiatry*. 2001;71:215–219.
7. Moro E, Esselink RJA, Xie J, Hommel M, Benabid AL, Pollack P. The impact on Parkinson's disease of electrical parameter settings in STN stimulation. *Neurology*. 2002;59:706–713.
8. Kuncel AM, Cooper SE, Wolgamuth BR, et al. Clinical response to varying the stimulus parameters in deep brain stimulation for essential tremor. *Mov Disord*. 2006;21:1920–1928.
9. Kuncel AM, Grill WM. Selection of stimulus parameters for deep brain stimulation. *Clin Neurophysiol*. 2004;115:2431–2441.
10. Kuncel AM, Cooper SE, Wolgamuth BR, Grill WM. Amplitude- and frequency-dependent changes in neuronal regularity parallel changes in tremor with thalamic deep brain stimulation. *IEEE Trans Neural Syst Rehabil Eng*. 2007;15:190–197.
11. Dorval AD, Kuncel AM, Birdno MJ, Turner DA, Grill W. Deep brain stimulation alleviates parkinsonian bradykinesia by regularizing pallidal activity. *J Neurophysiol*. 2010;104:911–921.
12. Birdno MJ, Kuncel AM, Dorval AD, Turner DA, Gross RE, Grill WM. Stimulus features underlying reduced tremor suppression with temporally patterned deep brain stimulation. *J Neurophysiol*. 2012;107:364–383.
13. Karamintziou SD, Deligiannis NG, Piallat B, et al. Dominant efficiency of non-regular patterns of subthalamic nucleus deep brain stimulation for Parkinson's disease and obsessive-compulsive disorder in a data-driven computational model. *J Neural Eng*. 2015;13(1).
14. Birdno MJ, Kuncel AM, Dorval AD, Turner DA, Grill WM. Tremor varies as a function of the temporal regularity of deep brain stimulation. *Neuroreport*. 2008;19(5):599–602.
15. Baker KB, Zhang J, Vitek JL. Pallidal stimulation: effect of pattern and rate on bradykinesia in the non-human primate model of Parkinson's disease. *Exp Neurol*. 2011;231(2):309–313.

16. Vanneste S, Fregni F, De Ridder D. Head-to-head comparison of transcranial random noise stimulation, transcranial AC stimulation, and transcranial DC stimulation for tinnitus. *Front Psychiatry*. 2013;4:1–7.

17. Rosin B, Slovik M, Mitelman R, et al. Closed-loop deep brain stimulation is superior in ameliorating parkinsonism. *Neuron*. 2011;72(2):370–384.

18. Little S, Pogosyan A, Neal S, et al. Adaptive deep brain stimulation in advanced Parkinson disease. *Ann Neurol*. 2013;74(3):449–457.

19. Little S, Beudel M, Zrinzo L, et al. Bilateral adaptive deep brain stimulation is effective in Parkinson's disease. *J Neurol Neurosurg Psychiatry*. 2015;87(7):717–721.

20. Chang SY, Kimble CJ, Kim I, et al. Development of the mayo investigational neuromodulation control system: toward a closed-loop electrochemical feedback system for deep brain stimulation. *J Neurosurg*. 2013;119(6):1556–1565.

21. Williams M, Hauptmann C, Patel N. Acoustic CR neuromodulation therapy for subjective tonal tinnitus: a review of clinical outcomes in an independent audiology practice setting. *Front Neurol*. 2015;6:54.

22. Tass PA. A model of desynchronizing deep brain stimulation with a demand-controlled coordinated reset of neural subpopulations. *Biol Cybern*. 2003;89(2):81–88.

23. Tass PA. Stochastic phase resetting of two coupled phase oscillators stimulated at different times. *Phys Rev E Stat Nonlin Soft Matter Phys*. 2003;67(5 Pt 1).

24. Tass PA, Majtanik M. Long-term anti-kindling effects of desynchronizing brain stimulation: a theoretical study. *Biol Cybern*. 2006;94(1):58–66.

25. Hauptmann C, Tass PA. Therapeutic rewiring by means of desynchronizing brain stimulation. *Biosystems*. 2007;89(1–3):173–181.

26. Popovych OV, Tass PA. Desynchronizing electrical and sensory coordinated reset neuromodulation. *Front Hum Neurosci*. 2012;6:58.

27. Tass PA, Popovych OV. Unlearning tinnitus-related cerebral synchrony with acoustic coordinated reset stimulation: theoretical concept and modelling. *Biol Cybern*. 2012;106(1):27–36.

28. Zeitler M, Tass PA. Augmented brain function by coordinated reset stimulation with slowly varying sequences. *Front Syst Neurosci*. 2015;9:49.

29. Tass PA, Silchenko AN, Hauptmann C, Barnikol UB, Speckmann EJ. Long-lasting desynchronization in rat hippocampal slice induced by coordinated reset stimulation. *Phys Rev E Stat Nonlin Soft Matter Phys*. 2009;80(1 Pt 1):011902.

30. De Ridder D, Vanneste S, van der Loo E, Plazier M, Menovsky T, van de Heyning P. Burst stimulation of the auditory cortex: a new form of neurostimulation for noise-like tinnitus suppression. *J Neurosurg*. 2010;112(6):1289–1294.

31. Schu S, Slotty PJ, Bara G, von Knop M, Edgar D, Vesper J. A prospective, randomised, double-blind, placebo-controlled study to examine the effectiveness of burst spinal cord stimulation patterns for the treatment of failed back surgery syndrome. *Neuromodulation*. 2014;17(5):443–450.

32. De Ridder D, Vanneste S, Plazier M, van der Loo E, Menovsky T. Burst spinal cord stimulation: toward paresthesia-free pain suppression. *Neurosurgery*. 2010;66(5):986–990.

33. De Ridder D, Plazier M, Kamerling N, Menovsky T, Vanneste S. Burst spinal cord stimulation for limb and back pain. *World Neurosurg*. 2013;80(5):642–649.

34. De Ridder D, Lenders MW, De Vos CC, et al. A 2-center comparative study on tonic versus burst spinal cord stimulation: amount of responders and amount of pain suppression. *Clin J Pain*. 2015;31(5):433–437.

35. de Vos CC, Bom MJ, Vanneste S, Lenders MW, de Ridder D. Burst spinal cord stimulation evaluated in patients with failed back surgery syndrome and painful diabetic neuropathy. *Neuromodulation*. 2014;17(2):152–159.

36. Tiede J, Brown L, Gekht G, Vallejo R, Yearwood T, Morgan D. Novel spinal cord stimulation parameters in patients with predominant back pain. *Neuromodulation*. 2013;16(4):370–375.

37. Van Buyten JP, Al-Kaisy A, Smet I, Palmisani S, Smith T. High-frequency spinal cord stimulation for the treatment of chronic back pain patients: results of a prospective multicenter European clinical study. *Neuromodulation*. 2013;16(1):59–65.

38. Al-Kaisy A, Van Buyten JP, Smet I, Palmisani S, Pang D, Smith T. Sustained effectiveness of 10 kHz high-frequency spinal cord stimulation for patients with chronic, low back pain: 24-month results of a prospective multicenter study. *Pain Med*. 2014;15(3):347–354.

39. Kapural L, Yu C, Doust MW, et al. Novel 10-kHz high-frequency therapy (HF10 therapy) is superior to traditional low-frequency spinal cord stimulation for the treatment of chronic back and leg pain: the SENZA-RCT randomized controlled trial. *Anesthesiology*. 2015;123(4):851–860.

40. Arle JE, Carlson KW, Mei L, Shils JL. Modeling effects of scar on patterns of dorsal column stimulation. *Neuromodulation*. 2014;17(4):320–333.

41. Lempka SF, McIntyre CC, Kilgore KL, Machado AG. Computational analysis of kilo-hertz frequency spinal cord stimulation for chronic pain management. *Anesthesiology*. 2015;122(6):1362–1376.

42. Parker JL, Karantonis DM, Single PS, Obradovic M, Cousins MJ. Compound action potentials recorded in the human spinal cord during neurostimulation for pain relief. *Pain*. 2012;153(3):593–601.

43. Ochoa J, Torebjork E. Specific sensations evoked by intraneural microstimulation of single mechanoreceptor units innervating the human hand. *J Physiol*. 1983;342:633–654.

44. Niu J, Ding L, Li JJ, et al. Modality-based organization of ascending somatosensory axons in the direct dorsal column pathway. *J Neurosci*. 2013;33(45):17691–17709.

45. Perruchoud C, Eldabe S, Batterham AM, et al. Analgesic efficacy of high-frequency spinal cord stimulation: a randomized double-blind placebo-controlled study. *Neuromodulation*. 2013;16(4):363–369.

46. Howell B, Grill WM. Evaluation of high-perimeter electrode designs for deep brain stimulation. *J Neural Eng*. 2014;11:046026.

47. Howell B, Naik S, Grill WM. Influences of interpolation error, electrode geometry, and the electrode-tissue interface on models of electric fields produced by deep brain stimulation. *IEEE Trans Biomed Eng*. 2014;61(2):297–307.

48. Zalay OC, Bardakjian BL. Synthesis of high-complexity rhythmic signals for closed-loop electrical neuromodulation. *Neural Netw*. 2013;42:62–73.

NEW MODES OF THERAPY

Ultrasound Neuromodulation

A Chapter for Innovative Neuromodulation

R.F. Dallapiazza, K. Timbie and W.J. Elias

University of Virginia, Charlottesville, VA, United States

Innovative Neuromodulation.
DOI: http://dx.doi.org/10.1016/B978-0-12-800454-8.00005-7 **101**

INTRODUCTION

High-intensity focused ultrasound (HIFU) was originally developed in the 1950s as a neurosurgical tool to create discrete, thermal lesions within the brain.[1,2] However, its widespread adoption was limited by energy dissipation at the skull, which resulted in heating of the scalp and cortical surface. Over the past 15 years, advances in transcranial delivery of ultrasound have rejuvenated an interest in its use among neurosurgeons and neuroscientists.[3–9] Currently, ablative HIFU is being investigated as a treatment for movement disorders, brain tumors, and a wide array of neurological diseases.[10–15]

Acoustic energy has long been known to influence the activity of electrically excitable tissues including cardiac and skeletal muscles,[16] peripheral nerves,[17–25] and the central nervous system. In the central nervous system, high-intensity ultrasound has been used to reversibly inhibit neuronal activity by heating below the temperature threshold for tissue ablation, while low-intensity focused ultrasound (LIFU) has been used to transiently activate and depress neuronal function through nonthermal mechanisms. Although ultrasound-based neuromodulation has been studied for more than half a century, modern studies are emerging which demonstrate the ability to harness acoustic energy for neuromodulation with the exciting potential for noninvasive brain mapping and scientific discovery.

PHYSICS OF ULTRASOUND

Ultrasound can be defined as sound or acoustic pressure waves beyond the range for human hearing (>20 kHz). Ultrasound propagation requires a medium that is ideally a liquid or solid. As an ultrasonic pressure wave travels through a given medium, particles within it may displace and oscillate. The particle's movement within the medium is a reflection of the magnitude of the pressure wave and the elasticity of the medium.[26–28]

Like other waveform energies that follow simple harmonic motion, ultrasound can be characterized by its frequency, wavelength, velocity, amplitude, power, and intensity (Table 5.1 and Fig. 5.1). Similar to electrical resistance, ultrasound waves propagating through media encounter resistance, termed acoustic impedance. Acoustic impedance is largely dependent on the density of the medium. As ultrasound travels from one medium to another, acoustic impedance mismatch results in reflection or absorption of energy at the interface. This is especially important for therapeutic and experimental brain applications of ultrasound since there is a high mismatch between the skull and soft tissues (e.g., scalp and brain).[28]

TABLE 5.1 Common Terminology Used in Ultrasound Neuromodulation

Term	Definition	Units
Frequency	Waves/second	1/s or Hertz (Hz)
Wavelength	Distance between wave peaks	mm
Velocity	Speed of propagation	cm/s
Amplitude	Magnitude of displacement within a medium	Megapascal (MPa)
Power	Rate of energy flow	Watts (W)
Intensity	Power/area	Watts/cm^2
Pulse repetition frequency	Number of pulses in 1 s	kHz
Duty cycle	Percentage of time ultrasound is on during a pulsing protocol	None

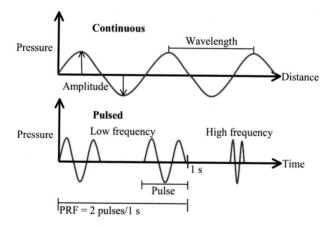

FIGURE 5.1 Continuous versus pulsed ultrasound. Ultrasound can be operated either continuously or in a pulsed fashion, and is defined by various parameters including amplitude, wavelength, frequency, and the pulse repetition frequency (PRF).

The Food and Drug Administration has a long history in regulating the safety of ultrasound used for medical imaging. Current safety measures include thermal index (TI) and mechanical index (MI), which reflect the likelihood of ultrasound causing thermal or biomechanical effects, respectively, in the tissue. The TI is defined as the ratio of the power used to that required to raise the temperature of the tissue by 1°C. The MI, typically used when a patient receives ultrasound contrast agents, provides an estimate of the risk of nonthermal bio effects. MI is defined as the peak negative pressure applied over the square root of the center frequency.[29]

Other safety metrics include various measures of the amount of energy delivered to the tissue, and can be calculated based on the power and frequency of the applied ultrasound. Medical imaging ultrasound typically operates at frequencies between 2 and 20 mega-Hertz (MHz), while ultrasound used in therapeutic and experimental neurological applications is lower in frequency, ranging between 0.2 and 2 MHz.[26–28] Since ultrasound can be delivered in a continuous or pulsed fashion, defining measures of ultrasound intensity becomes complex. The average intensity of an ultrasound protocol is simply defined as the total power delivered divided by the beam area (W/cm^2). Intensity does not provide a measure of the rate of energy accumulation in the tissue, so other intensity-related metrics must be considered. Spatial and temporal peak intensities refer to the instantaneous maximum intensity delivered at any one location or time, respectively (Fig. 5.2). Additionally, spatial average intensity (averaged over the beam area) and the temporal average intensity (averaged over a single pulse repetition period) are sometimes calculated. The pulse average intensity is equivalent to the temporal average intensity over the duty cycle. From these five basic intensity measures, several more standards can be calculated, as shown in Table 5.2.[26–28] Safety metrics are often reported using the spatial peak temporal average intensity, which is an excellent predictor of thermal effects. Current diagnostic ultrasound devices are limited to an MI of 1.9 and spatial peak, temporal average intensity of $720 \, mW/cm^2$.[29,30]

Ultrasound has been classified as either high or low intensity. HIFU is typically used to induce coagulative necrosis and may use power levels that exceed $1000 \, W/cm^2$. Even at low temperatures before tissue ablation, high-intensity ultrasound can induce tissue cavitation. Cavitation

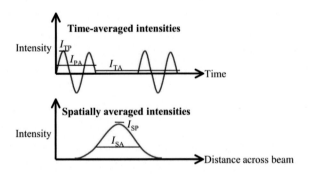

FIGURE 5.2   Ultrasound intensity measurements. Ultrasound safety metrics are often defined in terms of a variety of intensity values. Several intensity measures can be calculated, especially when pulsed ultrasound is applied.

TABLE 5.2 Ultrasound Intensity Metrics

Intensity metric	Abbreviation	Definition
Average intensity	I	Total power/beam area
Spatial peak	I_{SP}	Highest intensity within beam
Temporal peak	I_{TP}	Highest instantaneous intensity
Spatial average	I_{SA}	Average intensity over beam area
Temporal average	I_{TA}	Average intensity over pulse repetition period
Pulse average	I_{PA}	Average intensity over one pulse
Spatial peak temporal average	I_{SPTA}	$I_{SATA}\left(\dfrac{I_{SP}}{I_{SA}}\right)$
Spatial peak pulse average	I_{SPPA}	$\dfrac{I_{SATA}\left(\dfrac{I_{SP}}{I_{SA}}\right)}{duty\,cycle}$
Spatial average pulse average	I_{SAPA}	$\dfrac{I_{SATA}}{duty\,cycle}$
Spatial average temporal average	I_{SATA}	$\dfrac{I_{TA}}{beam\,area}$

occurs when high-intensity ultrasound beams passing through a liquid generate areas of extremely low pressure, which causes low-pressure boiling and produces small gas bubbles in the tissue.[26–28] These bubbles then oscillate in the ultrasonic field. At suitably low intensities, these microbubbles may enter stable cavitation, expanding and contracting in a sustainable, periodic fashion (Fig. 5.3). However, when these microbubbles are subjected to higher intensities, they may collapse violently in a process called inertial cavitation. Inertial cavitation can damage tissue by producing extremely high local temperatures, powerful jet streams and/or high concentrations of free radicals.[26–28] The propensity for microbubble formation and cavitation raises concerns for HIFU ablation and has resulted with the implementation of cavitation monitoring. Theoretically, stable cavitation could be monitored and harnessed for larger therapeutic ablations, but inertial cavitation is dangerous with unpredictable and less-controlled effects. LIFU is more ideally suited for neuromodulation because it utilizes the mechanical and nonthermal properties of ultrasound without the risk of cavitation. Furthermore, the average intensities of LIFU range from 30 to 500 mW/cm² which is well within the Food and Drug Administration (FDA) safety limits.

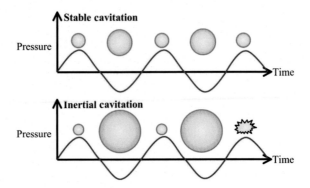

FIGURE 5.3   Stable versus inertial cavitation. Ultrasound can produce and manipulate gas bubbles within tissues. At low power, bubbles oscillate continuously in the ultrasonic field, termed stable cavitation. At higher pressures, bubbles may implode, releasing damaging jet streams and producing high local temperatures and free radicals. This implosion is called inertial cavitation.

HISTORICAL PERSPECTIVE OF ULTRASONIC NEUROMODULATION

Ultrasound has long been known to influence the activity of electrically excitable tissues. In 1929, Harvey published a series of experiments using high-intensity ultrasound to activate cardiac muscle preparations from frogs and turtles.[16] He found that various ultrasound exposures could elicit muscle contractions similar to what was produced by direct electrical stimulation of the tissue.[16] This is one of the first reports describing ultrasound's capability for altering the physiology of living tissue, thus laying the foundation for future investigation in the peripheral and central nervous systems.

During the 1950s, William and Francis Fry from the Bioacoustics Laboratory at the University of Illinois pioneered the application of focused ultrasound (FUS) to the brain.[1,2,31] One of their primary goals was to provide a tool to perform deep brain lesioning for the treatment of movement disorders, a goal they ultimately achieved while in collaboration with neurosurgeon Russell Meyers from the State Hospital of Iowa.[32,33] During early work in the feline brain, they discovered that high-intensity ultrasound could be precisely focused to create reproducible, discrete lesions in the white and gray matter of the brain without damage to the intervening tissue.

After a series of careful observations, the Fry brothers recognized that lower doses of acoustic energy could be used to transiently suppress neuronal function without creating permanent lesions. In an elegant series of experiments, they sonicated the feline lateral geniculate nucleus (LGN) with low doses of high-intensity ultrasound and temporarily suppressed visual-evoked responses in the absence of tissue ablation.[24] This study was among the first to show that nonablative, high-intensity ultrasound could induce reversible changes to intact neural circuits—in essence demonstrating that ultrasonic neuromodulation could be used as a method for brain mapping. Despite the excitement generated by these experiments, the use of FUS posed several difficulties and the mechanisms underlying its bio effects remained poorly understood. Early applications of ultrasound in the brain were limited by energy absorption and reflection by the skull, and required a cranial window to allow unimpeded passage of ultrasound waves. Fry et al. did not closely monitor temperature at the LGN, but histological examination revealed no evidence of tissue damage. It is likely that they empirically determined an acoustic energy dosage that resulted in moderate tissue heating capable of inhibiting neuronal function before neuronal damage. Later studies would confirm that low levels of tissue heating could cause temporary inhibition of neural activity. Using a similar model, Brodkey et al. used radiofrequency stimulation to heat the Edinger–Westphal nucleus in cats. They found that heating this nucleus to 44–49°C produced a reversible dilation of the pupil that returned to baseline size within 20 minutes of heating.[34] Today's premise that low-temperature heating can produce reversible lesions in the brain is based on these studies. More recent thermal dose experiments, however, have proven that even relatively low-temperature heating can result in permanent thermal injury with prolonged exposure. Tissue ablation even occurs ~43°C after continuous exposure for 240 minutes.[35]

The effects of ultrasound have also been studied in the peripheral nervous system. Gavrilov et al. demonstrated that short-duration, nonablative, high-intensity ultrasound applied to the upper extremity could activate peripheral nerves in humans.[21] This activation resulted in a variety of somatic sensations including tactile, thermal, and pain sensations but not tissue damage. They reported that the character of the elicited sensations largely depended on the parameters and localization of the ultrasound application. Further studies varying ultrasound intensity and exposure time preferentially activated small-diameter sensory fibers from feline saphenous nerve preparations.[36,37]

Gavrilov et al. also studied the effects of nonablative high-intensity ultrasound in the auditory system of frogs and humans. In humans, they discovered that transcranial ultrasound could activate the auditory system in human subjects with normal hearing.[22,38] This involved activation of both the auditory hair cells and direct activation of the auditory nerve fibers. Further studies among patients who were completely deaf due to severe cochlear dysfunction demonstrated that nonablative high-intensity ultrasound could elicit an auditory percept.[22,38] In amphibious models, ultrasound was able to evoke auditory brainstem activity even after the labyrinth of the inner ear was destroyed.[25,39] Auditory sensations have also been reported in patients who were undergoing diagnostic, transcranial Doppler ultrasound studies to evaluate clinical cerebrovascular disease involving the vertebral and basilar arteries.[40] These studies suggest that nonablative high-intensity ultrasound can activate the sensory organs of the inner ear and vestibular system as well as the cochlear nerve directly.

Despite early evidence of ultrasound-induced neuromodulation, the previously mentioned studies used higher intensities of ultrasound that could potentially damage tissue. In order to be safe for clinical or diagnostic purposes, ultrasonic neuromodulation protocols using much lower intensities would need to be developed. Currently, several groups are investigating the ability of low-intensity ultrasound to alter neuronal function without thermal effects and the risk of tissue damage.

EXPERIMENTAL CORTICAL NEUROMODULATION

Several studies have investigated transcranial ultrasound delivery to the motor cortex in rodent models. In 2010, Tufail et al. demonstrated that brief ultrasound pulses directed at the somatomotor cortex could elicit local field potentials and multiunit activity in the M1 cortex of lightly anesthetized rats.[41] These experiments utilized ultrasound with a 350 kHz acoustic frequency and 1.5 kHz pulse repetition frequency (PRF) for a total of 100 pulses to induce a variety of somatic movements including forepaw movements, whisker twitches, and tail flicks. Unilateral ultrasound delivery resulted in contraction of the contralateral forelimb triceps, whereas bilateral delivery resulted in contraction of axial musculature and tail flicks.[41] The overall success rate for muscle contraction and limb movement was 92% with a latency of effects of 20 ms. Transcranial ultrasound stimulation of the motor cortex was reproducible over long periods of time when delivered at low repetition rates (0.1–0.25 Hz). However, there was a much higher failure rate when the stimulation frequency was 5 Hz or greater. A variety of acoustic frequencies and intensities were tested, and the authors found that lower frequencies produced more robust electromyography (EMG) activity than higher frequencies.[41] Although various muscle groups were activated with small movements of the ultrasound transducer, the authors were not able to generate a somatic map of the cortex. This is likely because of the small size of the rodent brain and the relatively large size of the acoustic focus.

Two other groups have confirmed these findings with subtle differences in the results. King et al. used a similar experimental model and systematically varied acoustic frequency, acoustic intensity, sonication duration, and depth of anesthesia.[42] They found that low-frequency ultrasound activates motor cortex and elicits movements in rats, increasing the acoustic frequency decreases the probability of activation, and that the depth of anesthesia is just as critical for ultrasound neuromodulation as with other forms of neuromodulation. In addition, they found that the probability of eliciting responses, but not the character of the responses, correlates with pressure amplitude and duration of stimulation, and that continuous waveforms are as effective, or even more so, than pulsed stimulation schemes.[42]

In their subsequent study, King et al. demonstrated a rostral-caudal specificity in the rodent motor cortex stimulated with transcranial ultrasound.[43] They found that rostral midline stimulations were able to stimulate EMG activity in the neck while caudal stimulation resulted in more EMG activity in the tail than the neck.[43] Although a gross representation, this study begins to demonstrate that ultrasound can activate and modulate discrete cortical circuits. The rodent model is limited because of the small cortical size in relation to the size of the pressure wave generated by ultrasound. Larger brain models with more precise ultrasound equipment could allow for improved discrimination.

Younan et al. also replicated the results reported by Tufail et al. in 2013. They used a similar experimental design with an acoustic frequency of 320 kHz (total sonication time of 250 ms, and I_{SPPA} of 17.5 W/cm^2) and were able to elicit motor responses in >60% of trials.[44] The response was highly dependent on depth of anesthesia with more deeply anesthetized animals requiring a greater pressure threshold to activate responses. Although a variety of motor activities were elicited, a conclusive map could not be determined based on small movements of the ultrasound transducer.[44]

Yoo et al. also studied the effects of pulsed ultrasound on the motor cortex using rabbits with craniectomies.[45] In their study, FUS was applied to the motor cortex while EMG activity was recorded from the forepaw during pulsed sonications. Using an acoustic frequency of 690 kHz, a pulse duration of 50 ms, and a PRF of 10 kHz, they induced reliable motor activity in the contralateral forepaw.[45] These results were specific, since moving the transducer as little as 2 mm from the target resulted in no motor activity. Furthermore, fMRI suggested activation of the cortex during sonications. Temperature monitoring with MR thermography showed a temperature change <0.8°C and histological analysis demonstrated no tissue damage. Importantly, this study is one of the first to demonstrate that FUS can be used to elicit fMRI BOLD activations in the brain.[45]

These studies consistently suggest that low-intensity ultrasound can be used to activate neurons in the motor cortex to generate muscle activity and movement (Table 5.3). In general, the ultrasound parameters used in these studies were within the range of reported safety requirements for the FDA. Although various muscle groups were activated individually, there was little evidence that the ultrasound could selectively activate only one muscle group in a targeted fashion, suggesting that the spatial resolution of the ultrasound was too low in the rodent cortex.

TABLE 5.3 Neuromodulation of Somatomotor Cortical Responses

References	Species	Target	Response	Frequency (kHz)	Intensity (W/cm²)
Tufail et al.	Rat	Somatomotor cortex	Tail flick, whisker, and limb contraction	350	36.2 m
Yoo et al.	Rabbit	Somatomotor cortex	Limb contraction	690	6.3
King et al.	Mouse	Somatomotor cortex	Tail flick, neck, and hind limb extension	500	0.1–100
Younan et al.	Rat	Somatomotor cortex	Limb contraction	320	7.5–17.5

NEUROMODULATION OF VISUAL-EVOKED POTENTIALS

Since the first reported reversible suppression of visual-evoked potentials (VEPs) by Fry et al. in 1958, several groups have attempted to test whether low-intensity sonication could affect the transmission of the optic pathways. Adrianov et al. reported reversible suppression of VEP targeting the LGN–optic tract junction with ultrasound intensities ranging from 7 to 63 W/cm^2.[23] Sonication of the LGN resulted in a variety of responses including complete suppression that was fully reversible within minutes, partial suppression, and permanent suppression of the light-evoked response. Electron microscopy identified subtle changes in the optic tract fibers including changes in synaptic vesicle number and increases in mitochondria number.[23] The p30 wave of the VEP response has been reversibly diminished by ~30% by targeting visual cortex in rabbits and corroborated with fMRI measurements.[45]

EXPERIMENTAL NEUROMODULATION OF DEEP CEREBRAL STRUCTURES

Most studies to date have focused on targeting ultrasound to the cerebral cortex; however a few studies have investigated the effects of ultrasound on thalamic targets. One of the principal theoretical advantages of ultrasound neuromodulation compared to transcranial magnetic neuromodulation is that ultrasound can be precisely and discretely focused beyond the cortex into the deep cerebral structures.

Yoo et al. noticed during their studies in rabbits that animals treated with low-intensity ultrasound had shortened anesthesia times. Animals were anesthetized with intraperitoneal ketamine/xylazine injections and allowed to recover either with or without low-intensity ultrasound transmitted to the thalamus.[46] In the group of animals that received thalamic ultrasound treatment, the anesthesia recovery time was significantly shorter than for controls without ultrasound treatment. The authors speculated that low-intensity ultrasound could be influencing anesthesia time by one of two mechanisms. First, pulsed ultrasound could modulate the level of endogenous norepinephrine and thereby overcome the effects of xylazine at alpha-2 adrenergic receptors. Second, ultrasound treatment could aid in reestablishing normal thalamocortical activity that is commonly disrupted during ketamine administration.[46]

It has been suggested that low-intensity thalamic ultrasound could alter seizure activity or treat epilepsy. In a rat model of pentylenetetrazol-induced seizures, bilateral thalamic sonications (690 kHz, 2.6 W/cm^2) resulted in fewer electroencephalography (EEG) spikes and theta peaks compared to control animals.[47] While seizure intensity was lower at day 1, there was no difference by day 2, however, the authors hypothesize that thalamic sonication may have disrupted synchronous cortical activity by disrupting synaptic propagation through the thalamus.[47] Alternatively, ultrasound treatment could have modulated thalamic γ-aminobutyric acid (GABA)ergic activity that is known to be important in some forms of epilepsy.

The effects of thalamic ultrasound on chemical neurotransmission have been measured with microdialysis. Yang et al. demonstrated a 20% reduction in frontal lobe GABA levels but no change in glutamate with thalamic sonications,[48] while Min et al. showed increased levels of both dopamine and serotonin. These results suggest that global changes in neurotransmitter level can be achieved with low-intensity thalamic sonication.

These studies have some limitations. As with cortical sonication, these experiments do not have the spatial resolution to determine which of the thalamic regions are responsible for the observed effects. Despite the exciting promise for precise spatial resolution and targeting of deep cerebral structures that are not afforded by other neuromodulation approaches, studies conducted in rodents have yet to demonstrate these theoretical benefits of neuromodulation with ultrasound.

HIPPOCAMPAL NEUROMODULATION WITH ULTRASOUND

Several studies have investigated the effects of ultrasound in hippocampal preparations from rodents. Rinaldi et al. and Bachtold et al. recorded excitatory postsynaptic potentials from the CA3–CA1 synapse and in the dentate gyrus and studied the effects of ultrasound on response amplitude.[49,50] Rinaldi et al. found that FUS delivered for 2–10 minutes at $80 W/cm^2$ reduced electrically induced synaptic potential amplitudes; and Bachtold found that $40–110 W/cm^2$ of FUS delivered for 5 minutes could reduce presynaptic fiber volley amplitude by 33% and orthodromic population spiking by 25%.[49,50] Temperature changes measured during sonications in each of these studies were minimal (<1.5°C), and were unlikely to be high enough to damage tissue; however it is possible that small changes in tissue temperature could have affected the tissue's response to electrical stimulation.

Taken together, these two studies demonstrate that electrically induced, excitatory potentials can be modulated in well-studied, intact hippocampal circuits. Since there was little temperature change observed during these experiments, it can be concluded that FUS at intensities of $40–110 W/cm^2$ has a mechanical effect on neurons that can either block or enhance their activity.

In the previously considered studies, ultrasound was used to modulate electrically evoked neural activity in the hippocampus. However, ultrasound alone has also been shown to induce neural activity. Tyler et al. used an organotypic hippocampal slice preparation to investigate the role of ultrasound-induced neural activity. In this study, pulsed ultrasound with a central frequency of 440 kHz, pulse average intensity of 2.9 W/cm^2, burst duration of 22.7 μs, PRF of 100 Hz, and 250 total pulses were used to study the effects on neurons and glial cells.[51] Using a series of intracellular, ion-sensitive dyes to Na$^+$ and Ca^{2+} visualized with confocal microscopy, they elegantly demonstrated that pulsed, low-intensity ultrasound could generate Na$^+$ and Ca^{2+} transients in neurons and glia that lasted up to 20 seconds.[51] These transients were reliably reproduced across trials, did not appear to disrupt cellular plasma membranes with chronic stimulation, and were blocked by tetrodotoxin (Na$^+$ channel blocker), cadmium (Ca^{2+} channel blocker), and botulinum toxin (blocks synaptic vesicle release). These results demonstrate that pulsed, low-intensity ultrasound can activate voltage-sensitive ion channels in neurons, which was sufficient to induce SNARE-mediated synaptic vesicle release.[51] Furthermore, ultrasound was found to induce Na$^+$ transients in glial cells that also contain transmembrane ion channels and are important for neurotransmitter uptake and maintenance of extracellular ion concentrations. These results suggest that several transmembrane ion channels (at least voltage-gated Na$^+$ and Ca^{2+} channels) that are known to be critical in the generation and propagation of synaptic transmission are mechanically sensitive to low-intensity ultrasound pulses.

In their study, Tyler et al. report that ultrasound stimulated activity in approximately 30% of exposed neurons per field of view, which indicates that there may be additional factors that mediate neuronal responses.[51] The authors speculate that recent cellular activity could influence the excitability of neurons' response to ultrasound.

Using an intact animal approach, Tufail et al. demonstrated that pulsed low-intensity ultrasound can activate local field potentials in the murine hippocampus.[41] Pulsed ultrasound sequences at an acoustic frequency of 250 kHz, 2.0 kHz PRF, total pulse number of 650, and I_{SPTA} of 84.3 mW/cm^2 were directed along the axis of the hippocampus and local field potentials were recorded from the CA1 region of the hippocampus. Using this scheme, local field potentials were reliably recorded with mean amplitudes of −168 μV and a mean latency of 123 ms.[41] Local field potentials were followed by a short period of after-discharge activity lasting less than 3 seconds. Furthermore, long-term stimulation (30 minutes) using similar sonication parameters (acoustic frequency 350 kHz, I_{SPTA} 36.2 mW/cm^2) was found to induce BDNF expression in the hippocampus of mice exposed to ultrasound compared to unstimulated controls.[41] Taken together these results demonstrate that ultrasound can activate intact circuits in the murine hippocampus and alter transcription of activity-related transcription factors.

CORTICAL NEUROMODULATION IN LARGE ANIMALS AND HUMANS

Few studies have used low-intensity ultrasound for neuromodulation in large animal models or in humans. Deffieux et al. recently reported that antisaccade latencies could be attenuated with ultrasound directed at the frontal eye fields in nonhuman primates (*Macaca mulatta*).[52] In their study, animals were trained to perform an antisaccade visual task, and eye movements were monitored with an infrared eye tracking system. Once the animals were adequately trained, FUS with an acoustic frequency of 320 kHz, pulse duration of 100 ms, and pressure amplitude of 0.6 MPa was delivered to the frontal lobe cortex in the region of the frontal eye field. Control trials were interleaved with trials during which ultrasound was delivered. In both of the animals tested there was an attenuation of ipsilateral antisaccade latency in trials where FUS was delivered compared to control trials.[52] Furthermore, there was no change in contralateral antisaccade latency with or without the use of ultrasound. This study is the first to demonstrate that a complex behavioral task could be affected by transcranial ultrasound in a nonhuman primate brain.[52]

Legon et al. studied the effects of low-intensity, pulsed ultrasound on the human somatosensory cortex.[53] In this study, ultrasound was targeted to the somatosensory cortex, and EEG was used to record cortical activity from median nerve stimulation among a group of human volunteers. Ultrasound was delivered using a 500 kHz acoustic frequency, pulse duration 360 μs, 1 kHz PRF, and total duration of 500 ms. The median nerve somatosensory evoked potential has a well-described waveform with several positive and negative peak potentials that occur with a latency ranging between 20 and 300 ms. Transcranial low-intensity ultrasound was found to significantly decrease the N20–P27 and P27–N33 peak amplitudes compared to sham ultrasound trials.[53] This appeared to have a high degree of spatial resolution, since small movements in the transducer (<5 mm) showed no effects on evoked potential amplitude. Interestingly, despite the decrease in amplitude of evoked potentials, these volunteers had improvements in two-point discrimination during ultrasound trials, demonstrating a physiological effect of ultrasound.[53]

Together these two studies demonstrate that well-defined cortical activity can be modulated transcranially in a large animal model and in humans. This suggests that low-intensity ultrasound could potentially be used for noninvasive cortical mapping. However, both of these studies fail to demonstrate precise mapping of the cortex. Further studies in large animal models are needed to assess whether deep structures such as the basal ganglia or thalamus could be targeted using similar experimental paradigms, and to assess whether this approach can be used for functional brain mapping.

MECHANISMS OF ULTRASONIC NEUROMODULATION

Although neuromodulation with ultrasound has been studied for more than 50 years, the mechanisms of action are poorly understood. In general, they can be classified as thermal and mechanical effects.[54] The pressure wave of high-intensity ultrasound results in frictional energy that is orders of magnitude higher at the focus so the target tissue begins to heat. At very high intensities, ultrasound will induce protein denaturation, cellular fragmentation, coagulative necrosis, and cellular death. Lower intensities, which cause tissue heating without cellular death, can induce ultrastructural changes in synapses including decreases in synaptic vesicle numbers, widening of pre- and postsynaptic junctions, and alterations in the size of postsynaptic densities.[23,30,55,56] Since high-intensity ultrasound can lead to permanent tissue damage, this approach is a less attractive option for studying ultrasound neuromodulation.

Conversely, low-intensity ultrasound does not result in tissue heating and likely exerts its effects through mechanical forces on neurons and glial cells.[54,57] There are several potential mechanisms of mechanical neuromodulation by ultrasound, and it is possible that several of these mechanisms could underlie the physiological effects of low-intensity ultrasound demonstrated in neuronal circuits. First, since ultrasound exerts a mechanical force on neurons, it is possible that these forces alter the fluidity and permeability of the plasma membrane to ions, thus generating neuronal depolarization and action potentials.[54] Second, ultrasound could provide mechanical energy necessary to induce conformational changes in transmembrane receptors and voltage-gated ion channels that could lead to their activation and cellular depolarization.[51] Neurons and glia are rich with voltage-sensitive channels, and there is already evidence that pharmacological antagonists for voltage-gated Na^+ and Ca^{2+} channels can block ultrasound-induced depolarization.[51] However, it remains unknown whether ultrasound alone is sufficient to activate voltage-gated ion channels, or if it exerts its effects through an upstream mediator. Finally, low-intensity ultrasound could induce stable cavitation from molecules and microbubbles of cellular or extracellular gas. This rapid expansion and contraction could disrupt cellular membranes and influence neural excitability.[54,56]

CLINICAL APPLICATIONS OF FUS NEUROMODULATION

Currently, transcranial, MR-guided FUS is being investigated as a treatment for movement disorders (essential tremor and Parkinson's disease) and malignant brain tumors.[10,11,13,15] Transcranial MR-guided FUS has also been used clinically to treat chronic pain and obsessive-compulsive disorder.[12,58] It has also been proposed as a therapy for several other neurological disorders including epilepsy, facial pain, and intracranial hemorrhage.[14,59]

Contemporary MR-guided FUS systems use a phased-array, multielement transducer (Neuro ExAblate, Insightec Ltd.) to deliver HIFU capable of creating a discrete thermal lesion within the brain (diameter <7 mm) without affecting intervening tissues. Current clinical transducers for transcranial treatments operate at a frequency of 0.2, 0.71, or 1 MHz, depending on the indication/application.

Our group first applied FUS technology to the treatment of essential tremor because the symptom of tremor is so readily measured and responsive to a variety of treatments and the ventral intermediate thalamic target is perfectly amenable to test ultrasound neuromodulation.[11] Stereotactic lesioning and deep brain stimulation (DBS) surgery confirm the target with signature electrophysiologic recordings and tremor arrest with high-frequency electrical stimulation. However, since MR-guided FUS treatments do not allow direct brain recording or stimulation of the Vim thalamus, it is difficult to confirm the target prior to a permanent ablation (Fig. 5.4). Current treatment strategies rely on the concept of

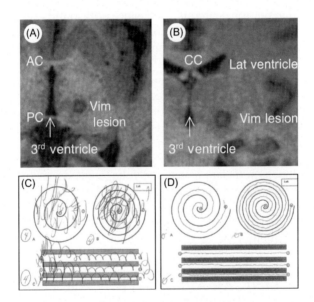

FIGURE 5.4 Vim thalamus ablation with HIFU for essential tremor. (A) Axial and (B) Coronal T1-weighted MRI showing an acute lesion in the Vim thalamus (the third ventricle is indicated by the white arrow; AC, anterior commissure; PC, posterior commissure). (C) Preoperative and (D) Postoperative writing task demonstrating an improvement in writing after FUS thalamotomy.

thermal neuromodulation to aid in confirming the Vim prior to ablation. Thus a series of low-energy sonications that are designed to heat the Vim to 45–50°C are used to temporarily disrupt neural transmission without causing permanent damage.[11] The patient is then assessed for tremor arrest or somatosensory effects.

In a pilot study of 15 essential tremor patients treated with MR-guided FUS thalamotomy, four patients experienced transient paresthesias of the hand, lips, or face during subtherapeutic sonications with peak temperatures ~50°C.[11] This suggested that the ultrasound focus was targeted posteriorly to the ventroposterolateral (sensory) nucleus. In these cases, the acoustic focus was adjusted anteriorly by 1–3 mm to the presumed Vim nucleus with successful tremor suppression. In this study, tremor suppression was seen transiently when peak temperatures of 50°C were reached. Using this thermal neuromodulation approach, Elias et al. were able to selectively target the Vim nucleus and reduce hand tremor by ~75%.[11] However, this method is imperfect. Among the 15 patients who were treated, two had paresthesias of the face or lips, one had paresthesia of the finger, and one patient had painful dysesthesias of the index finger at 1 year follow-up.[11] This finding highlights the need for accurate, reversible, and nondestructive methods for target confirmation during FUS ablations.

FUTURE CLINICAL APPLICATIONS OF FUS NEUROMODULATION

One of the immediate clinical applications for ultrasound neuromodulation is for intraoperative target confirmation and brain mapping during therapeutic, FUS ablations. Pulsed, low-intensity ultrasound could be used to activate, suppress, and essentially map the ventrolateral thalamic nuclear complex in a completely reversible, nondestructive manner prior to therapeutic ablations for tremor treatment since the thalamus has a similar somatotopic arrangement as the cortex.

A second clinical application for ultrasound neuromodulation is noninvasive evaluation of selected targets for therapeutic treatment. Patients with disabling tremor related to multiple sclerosis or posttraumatic tremor are often less responsive to thalamic DBS compared to patients with essential tremor. These patients may undergo invasive brain procedures to evaluate the feasibility and potential efficacy of stimulation, often with mixed results. A noninvasive, reversible means of evaluating thalamic inhibition would be optimal for these patients, which could realistically be achieved with ultrasonic neuromodulation.

A similar principle applies for surgical treatments of psychiatric diseases like severe depression where there is no clear consensus as to the optimal surgical target for effective treatment. Diseases like Tourette's syndrome and obsessive-compulsive disorder could potentially be evaluated with ultrasound neuromodulation for the identification of an optimal target for treatment with any modality, not just FUS.

Finally, ultrasound neuromodulation could be used to study the biology of neurological diseases and any underlying abnormalities in the circuitry. Current FUS applications are largely MR-guided, and MR-based measurements could be combined with neuromodulation as a tool for studying disease. To use Tourette's disease as an example again, low-intensity FUS neuromodulation could be used in combination with functional MRI to study the proposed DBS targets prior to surgery. Baseline patient fMRI could be compared to postneuromodulation fMRI targeting the centrolateral thalamus or limbic area of the globus pallidus. This could conceivably be accomplished with FUS neuromodulation parameters that both activate and suppress neuronal activity.

CONCLUSIONS

Neuromodulation with ultrasound has been studied for more than 50 years, but in many respects, this field is in its infancy compared to direct electrical stimulation and transcranial magnetic stimulation. FUS theoretically offers a noninvasive, deep-penetrating, and spatially well-defined modality to modulate neural activity. Although experimental and clinical studies have demonstrated the capabilities of ultrasound to modulate neural activity, the theoretical benefits of ultrasound neuromodulation have not been fully realized. Further studies are needed to determine precise sonication parameters for neural activation and suppression, and large animal models are needed to demonstrate the highly selective spatial profile offered by ultrasound. Despite these limitations, transcranial FUS neuromodulation has exciting potential to be rapidly translated to clinical use for brain mapping studies and scientific investigations into the nature of neurological disorders.

References

1. Fry WJ, Barnard JW, Fry FJ, Brennan JF. Ultrasonically produced localized selective lesions in the central nervous system. *Am J Phys Med.* 1955;34(3):413–423.
2. Fry WJ, Mosberg Jr. WH, Barnard JW, Fry FJ. Production of focal destructive lesions in the central nervous system with ultrasound. *J Neurosurg.* 1954;11(5):471–478.
3. Aarnio J, Clement GT, Hynynen K. A new ultrasound method for determining the acoustic phase shifts caused by the skull bone. *Ultrasound Med Biol.* 2005;31(6):771–780.
4. Clement GT, Hynynen K. A non-invasive method for focusing ultrasound through the human skull. *Phys Med Biol.* 2002;47(8):1219–1236.
5. Clement GT, Sun J, Giesecke T, Hynynen K. A hemisphere array for non-invasive ultrasound brain therapy and surgery. *Phys Med Biol.* 2000;45(12):3707–3719.

6. Clement GT, White PJ, King RL, McDannold N, Hynynen K. A magnetic resonance imaging-compatible, large-scale array for trans-skull ultrasound surgery and therapy. *J Ultrasound Med.* 2005;24(8):1117–1125.

7. Hynynen K, Freund WR, Cline HE, et al. A clinical, noninvasive, MR imaging-monitored ultrasound surgery method. *Radiographics.* 1996;16(1):185–195.

8. Hynynen K, Jolesz FA. Demonstration of potential noninvasive ultrasound brain therapy through an intact skull. *Ultrasound Med Biol.* 1998;24(2):275–283.

9. Jaaskelainen J. Non-invasive transcranial high intensity focused ultrasound (HIFUS) under MRI thermometry and guidance in the treatment of brain lesions. *Acta Neurochir (Wien).* 2003;88:57–60.

10. Chang WS, Jung HH, Kweon EJ, Zadicario E, Rachmilevitch I, Chang JW. Unilateral magnetic resonance guided focused ultrasound thalamotomy for essential tremor: practices and clinicoradiological outcomes. *J Neurol Neurosurg Psychiatry.* 2015;86(3):257–264.

11. Elias WJ, Huss D, Voss T, et al. A pilot study of focused ultrasound thalamotomy for essential tremor. *N Engl J Med.* 2013;369(7):640–648.

12. Jeanmonod D, Werner B, Morel A, et al. Transcranial magnetic resonance imaging-guided focused ultrasound: noninvasive central lateral thalamotomy for chronic neuropathic pain. *Neurosurg Focus.* 2012;32(1):E1.

13. Lipsman N, Schwartz ML, Huang Y, et al. MR-guided focused ultrasound thalamotomy for essential tremor: a proof-of-concept study. *Lancet.* 2013;12(5):462–468.

14. Monteith S, Sheehan J, Medel R, et al. Potential intracranial applications of magnetic resonance-guided focused ultrasound surgery. *J Neurosurg.* 2013;118(2):215–221.

15. McDannold N, Clement GT, Black P, Jolesz F, Hynynen K. Transcranial magnetic resonance imaging-guided focused ultrasound surgery of brain tumors: initial findings in 3 patients. *Neurosurgery.* 2010;66(2):323–332. discussion 332.

16. Harvey E. The effect of high frequency sound waves on heart muscle and other irritable tissues. *Am J Physiol.* 1929;91:284–290.

17. Colucci V, Strichartz G, Jolesz F, Vykhodtseva N, Hynynen K. Focused ultrasound effects on nerve action potential in vitro. *Ultrasound Med Biol.* 2009;35(10):1737–1747.

18. Foley JL, Little JW, Starr III FL, Frantz C, Vaezy S. Image-guided HIFU neurolysis of peripheral nerves to treat spasticity and pain. *Ultrasound Med Biol.* 2004;30(9):1199–1207.

19. Foley JL, Little JW, Vaezy S. Image-guided high-intensity focused ultrasound for conduction block of peripheral nerves. *Ann Biomed Eng.* 2007;35(1):109–119.

20. Gavrilov LR, Gersuni GV, Ilyinski OB, Tsirulnikov EM, Shchekanov EE. A study of reception with the use of focused ultrasound. I. Effects on the skin and deep receptor structures in man. *Brain Res.* 1977;135(2):265–277.

21. Gavrilov LR, Gersuni GV, Ilyinsky OB, Sirotyuk MG, Tsirulnikov EM, Shchekanov EE. The effect of focused ultrasound on the skin and deep nerve structures of man and animal. *Prog Brain Res.* 1976;43:279–292.

22. Gavrilov LR, Tsirulnikov EM, Davies IA. Application of focused ultrasound for the stimulation of neural structures. *Ultrasound Med Biol.* 1996;22(2):179–192.

23. Adrianov OS, Vykhodtseva NI, Fokin VF, Uranova NA, Avirom VM. [Reversible functional shutdown of the optic tract on exposure to focused ultrasound]. *Biull Eksp Biol Med.* 1984;97(6):760–762.

24. Fry FJ, Ades HW, Fry WJ. Production of reversible changes in the central nervous system by ultrasound. *Science.* 1958;127(3289):83–84.

25. Gavrilov LR, Tsirul'nikov EM, Shchekanov EE. [Responses of the auditory centers of the frog midbrain to labyrinth stimulation by focused ultrasound]. *Fiziol Zh SSSR Im I M Sechenova.* 1975;61(2):213–221.

26. Shung KK, Smith M, Tsui BMW. *Principles of Medical Imaging.* Oxford: Elsevier Science; 1992.

27. Sprawls P. *Physical Principles of Medical Imaging.* Rockville, MD: Aspen; 1987.

28. Szabo T. *Diagnostic Ultrasound Imaging Inside Out.* Amsterdam: Elsevier Academic; 2004.

29. AIUM/NEMA. *Standard for Real-Time Display of Thermal and Mechanical Acoustic Output Indices on Diagnostic Ultrasound Equipment.* Laurel, MD: AIUM Publications; 1992.
30. Dalecki D. Mechanical bioeffects of ultrasound. *Annu Rev Biomed Eng.* 2004;6:229–248.
31. Fry WJ. Intense ultrasound: a new tool for neurological research. *J Ment Sci.* 1954;100(418):85–96.
32. Fry W. Neurosonic surgery. *Trans Am Neurol Assoc.* 1955:86–88. (80th Meeting).
33. Meyers R, Fry WJ, Fry FJ, Dreyer LL, Schultz DF, Noyes RF. Early experiences with ultrasonic irradiation of the pallidofugal and nigral complexes in hyperkinetic and hypertonic disorders. *J Neurosurg.* 1959;16(1):32–54.
34. Brodkey JS, Miyazaki Y, Ervin FR, Mark VH. Reversible heat lesions with radiofrequency current. A method of stereotactic localization. *J Neurosurg.* 1964;21:49–53.
35. Sapareto SA, Dewey WC. Thermal dose determination in cancer therapy. *Int J Radiat Oncol Biol Phys.* 1984;10(6):787–800.
36. Young RR, Henneman E. Functional effects of focused ultrasound on mammalian nerves. *Science.* 1961;134(3489):1521–1522.
37. Young RR, Henneman E. Reversible block of nerve conduction by ultrasound. *Arch Neurol.* 1961;4:83–89.
38. Tsirulnikov EM, Vartanyan IA, Gersuni GV, Rosenblyum AS, Pudov VI, Gavrilov LR. Use of amplitude-modulated focused ultrasound for diagnosis of hearing disorders. *Ultrasound Med Biol.* 1988;14(4):277–285.
39. Vartanian IA, Gavrilov LR, Zharskaia VD, Ratnikova GI, Tsirul'nikov EM. [Stimulating effect of focused ultrasound on auditory fibers of the acoustic nerve in the frog *Rana temporaria*]. *Zh Evol Biokhim Fiziol.* 1981;17(5):512–518.
40. Magee TR, Davies AH. Auditory phenomena during transcranial Doppler insonation of the basilar artery. *J Ultrasound Med.* 1993;12(12):747–750.
41. Tufail Y, Matyushov A, Baldwin N, et al. Transcranial pulsed ultrasound stimulates intact brain circuits. *Neuron.* 2010;66(5):681–694.
42. King RL, Brown JR, Newsome WT, Pauly KB. Effective parameters for ultrasound-induced in vivo neurostimulation. *Ultrasound Med Biol.* 2013;39(2):312–331.
43. King RL, Brown JR, Pauly KB. Localization of ultrasound-induced in vivo neurostimulation in the mouse model. *Ultrasound Med Biol.* 2014;40(7):1512–1522.
44. Younan Y, Deffieux T, Larrat B, Fink M, Tanter M, Aubry JF. Influence of the pressure field distribution in transcranial ultrasonic neurostimulation. *Med Phys.* 2013;40(8):082902.
45. Yoo SS, Bystritsky A, Lee JH, et al. Focused ultrasound modulates region-specific brain activity. *NeuroImage.* 2011;56(3):1267–1275.
46. Yoo SS, Kim H, Min BK, Franck E, Park S. Transcranial focused ultrasound to the thalamus alters anesthesia time in rats. *Neuroreport.* 2011;22(15):783–787.
47. Min BK, Bystritsky A, Jung KI, et al. Focused ultrasound-mediated suppression of chemically-induced acute epileptic EEG activity. *BMC Neurosci.* 2011;12:23.
48. Yang PS, Kim H, Lee W, et al. Transcranial focused ultrasound to the thalamus is associated with reduced extracellular GABA levels in rats. *Neuropsychobiology.* 2012;65(3):153–160.
49. Bachtold MR, Rinaldi PC, Jones JP, Reines F, Price LR. Focused ultrasound modifications of neural circuit activity in a mammalian brain. *Ultrasound Med Biol.* 1998;24(4):557–565.
50. Rinaldi PC, Jones JP, Reines F, Price LR. Modification by focused ultrasound pulses of electrically evoked responses from an in vitro hippocampal preparation. *Brain Res.* 1991;558(1):36–42.
51. Tyler WJ, Tufail Y, Finsterwald M, Tauchmann ML, Olson EJ, Majestic C. Remote excitation of neuronal circuits using low-intensity, low-frequency ultrasound. *PLoS ONE.* 2008;3(10):e3511.
52. Deffieux T, Younan Y, Wattiez N, Tanter M, Pouget P, Aubry JF. Low-intensity focused ultrasound modulates monkey visuomotor behavior. *Curr Biol.* 2013;23(23):2430–2433.

53. Legon W, Sato TF, Opitz A, et al. Transcranial focused ultrasound modulates the activity of primary somatosensory cortex in humans. *Nat Neurosci.* 2014;17(2):322–329.

54. Tyler WJ. Noninvasive neuromodulation with ultrasound? A continuum mechanics hypothesis. *Neuroscientist.* 2011;17(1):25–36.

55. Borrelli MJ, Bailey KI, Dunn F. Early ultrasonic effects upon mammalian CNS structures (chemical synapses). *J Acoust Soc Am.* 1981;69(5):1514–1516.

56. Dinno MA, Dyson M, Young SR, Mortimer AJ, Hart J, Crum LA. The significance of membrane changes in the safe and effective use of therapeutic and diagnostic ultrasound. *Phys Med Biol.* 1989;34(11):1543–1552.

57. Tufail Y, Yoshihiro A, Pati S, Li MM, Tyler WJ. Ultrasonic neuromodulation by brain stimulation with transcranial ultrasound. *Nat Protoc.* 2011;6(9):1453–1470.

58. Jung HH, Kim SJ, Roh D, et al. Bilateral thermal capsulotomy with MR-guided focused ultrasound for patients with treatment-refractory obsessive-compulsive disorder: a proof-of-concept study. *Mol Psychiatry.* 2015;20(10):1205–1211.

59. Monteith SJ, Harnof S, Medel R, et al. Minimally invasive treatment of intracerebral hemorrhage with magnetic resonance-guided focused ultrasound. *J Neurosurg.* 2013;118(5):1035–1045.

Optogenetics

P.S.A. Kalanithi, MD* and D. Purger, PhD

Department of Neurosurgery, Stanford University, Stanford, CA,
United States

*Author P.S.A. Kalanithi has unfortunately passed away since co-authoring this chapter.

Innovative Neuromodulation.
DOI: http://dx.doi.org/10.1016/B978-0-12-800454-8.00006-9

INTRODUCTION

From intraoperative neuromonitoring to white matter tractography-based neuronavigation, modern neurosurgical practice requires exquisite knowledge and, increasingly, manipulation of the neuronal networks involved in health and disease. Focal neuromodulation is evolving beyond its origins in deep brain stimulation (DBS) into new treatment modalities that promise to revolutionize the clinical neurosciences. However, the dream of precise control over neural network function is not limited to neurosurgeons, neurologists, and psychiatrists; in 1979, Francis Crick remarked that "[t]o understand these higher levels of neural activity we would obviously do well to learn as much as possible about the lower levels," going on to suggest that "a method by which all neurons of just one type could be inactivated, leaving the others more or less unaltered" would be required to make advances in basic neuroscience.[55] While electrical manipulation of the nervous system affords the user temporally precise control over neural networks, current electrical methods cannot fulfill Crick's criterion of functional selectivity, as they are not precise enough to target neuronal subpopulations. While pharmacologic and other techniques have shown some selectivity, they operate on long time scales. However, in the laboratory, optical techniques—especially optogenetics—have been remarkably effective, both temporally precise and cell-selective.

Optogenetics is the combination of optical and genetic tools to achieve spatial and temporal control of biological systems. Optogenetic techniques are used in neuroscience to modulate neural circuits with specificity and precision unattainable by traditional methods such as direct electrical stimulation of neuronal populations and pharmacologic activation and inhibition of activity. Optogenetic tools (Fig. 6.1) were developed out of a need to "convert the biological mechanisms underlying neuronal excitability and communication into experimental mechanisms for observing and controlling activity."[1] Some early attempts at driving intracellular events with light used lasers to ablate proteins in signaling pathways (e.g., the Shh receptor Ptc in the Hedgehog signaling pathway of developing *Drosophila* embryos[2]) or to turn them on (e.g., stimulating action potentials via laser irradiation of axon initial segments[3]). Later work began to couple light stimulation with genetic manipulations, such as the targeted expression of *Drosophila* arrestin-2, rhodopsin, and a G-protein subunit in rat hippocampal neurons, light stimulation of which could induce an action potential (i.e., the chARGe strategy[4]); other such early attempts included expression of the ligand-gated ion channels $P2X_2$ and TRPV1 along with versions of their agonists that were chemically modified to be biologically inert, but capable of reactivation after exposure to ultraviolet (UV) laser radiation, such that UV exposure disinhibited the channels, allowing the generation of an action potential.[5,6] These initial efforts, while remarkable for pioneering the coupling of a light stimulus with

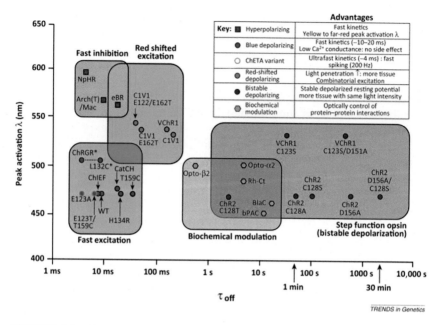

FIGURE 6.1   The variety of optogenetic tools to modulate neural circuit function. *Source: Adapted from Gerits A, Vanduffel W. Optogenetics in primates: a shining future? Trends Genet. 2013; 29: 403–411.*[7]

intracellular phenomena, proved to be unwieldy, as neuronal activity could only be induced very slowly, and targeting specific populations of neurons was difficult. Additionally, insufficient tissue penetration of the electromagnetic radiation stimulus to reach target populations of interest was another limiting factor. Ultimately, the challenges of such systems where the molecular machinery required to sense electromagnetic radiation was distinct from the effector of the desired intracellular event prompted further development of optical tools to remove these barriers.

A way to circumvent the disadvantages of these methods was discovered in a class of light-sensitive ion channels known as microbial opsins. Without the complex sensory organs that characterize higher-order eukaryotes, microbes evolved molecular sensors sensitive to visible light as a way to maintain osmotic balance in seawater and perform other homeostatic functions.[8] Microbial and algal opsins unite the distinct functions of sensing electromagnetic radiation and transducing it into transmembrane ion flux or a signaling cascade in order to effect an intracellular change and thus represented an optimal platform for continued exploration of light-stimulated induction of neuronal activation in the mid-2000s. Despite several current barriers to direct clinical translation, optogenetic techniques seem poised to one day join the neurosurgeon's neuromodulatory toolkit.

OPSINS

Opsins are seven-transmembrane ion channels or G-protein-coupled receptors; they require retinal as a cofactor, a molecule closely related to vitamin A, which absorbs a photon and undergoes isomerization. When retinal is bound to an opsin, its isomerization causes a downstream conformational change in the attached opsin, initiating transmembrane ion movement or a signaling cascade. In ion channel opsins, exposure to light at the characteristic wavelength of maximum absorbance results in a transient peak photocurrent, followed by a lower, stable plateau photocurrent (due to channel desensitization[9]); desensitized channels recover in the dark after a time constant (τ_{off}) unique to each opsin.

The first opsin to be isolated and studied was a proton pump, named bacteriorhodopsin (BR),[10,11] isolated from *Halobacterium halobium*. It responded maximally to green light at 570 nm. For decades, the potential applications of BR for controlling intracellular activity were not appreciated; however, with the advent of early attempts at light-activated neuronal stimulation, renewed interest was directed at the microbial opsins. Nagel et al. soon isolated a similar proton pump from the primitive pigmented eyespot of the algae *Chlamydomonas reinhardtii*, named channelrhodopsin-1 (ChR1), with significant homology to BR especially in the hydrophobic transmembrane core.[12] Shortly thereafter, channelrhodopsin-2 (ChR2) was isolated from *C. reinhardtii*; with a peak absorption at approximately ~460 nm and a time constant of only 18 ms, researchers had finally found an opsin with optimal characteristics for reliably driving neuronal spiking (Fig. 6.2).[9]

Excitatory Opsins

ChR2 was the first opsin to be brought to neuroscience as a single-component optogenetic platform, enabling temporal control of neuronal activity on the millisecond scale.[13] Since it was discovered that retinal cofactor exists in vertebrate tissues in large enough quantities to enable opsin expression as a single component,[14,15] many groups have engineered opsins through codon optimization in order to allow for activation by different wavelengths of light, more consistent expression in mammalian tissues, and alteration of ion conductance properties to modulate the time course of activation. Beginning with the introduction of the H134R mutation into ChR2[16,17] to improve steady-state current size at the expense of temporal precision, much work has been done to enhance excitatory opsin function:

- Endoplasmic reticulum export motifs were added to the ChR2 protein to achieve higher expression and, thus, higher neuronal excitability.[18]

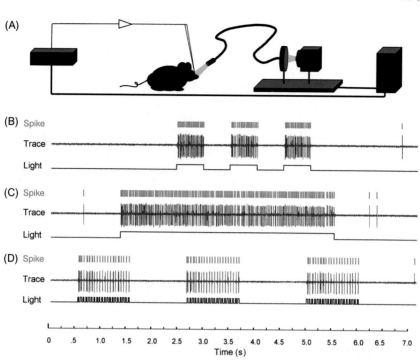

FIGURE 6.2   In vivo channelrhodopsin-2-mediated optogenetic stimulation of layer V cortical output neurons results in a robust and reliable neuronal electrical response. *Source: Adapted from Arenkiel BR et al. In vivo light-induced activation of neural circuitry in transgenic mice expressing channelrhodopsin-2. Neuron. 2007; 54: 205–218.*[19]

- Because the crystal structure of ChR2 had not yet been solved, several changes to the ChR2 amino acid sequence were engineered based on its predicted quaternary structure. A chimeric combination of ChR1 and ChR2, termed ChEF, was generated to decrease photocurrent falloff during persistent light stimulation (33% inactivation vs 77% for ChR2[20]); a further mutation was introduced to yield ChIEF, an opsin with accelerated channel closure to allow for higher-frequency stimulation.[20]
- ChETA[21] further reduced desensitization and introduced the innovation of a destabilized active conformation of retinal, allowing for faster spontaneous reisomerization to the inactive state.
- Step function opsins (SFOs[22]) introduced new mutations in ChR2 to yield bistable activation, realized as prolonged activity after cessation of the light stimulus, up to a time constant of 29 minutes in the advanced stabilized step function opsin (SSFO[23]). SFOs possess the additional characteristic of being able to be inactivated by a pulse of green (542 nm) light, which causes retinal to reisomerize to the

inactive state; as a result, SFOs represented, for the first time, a true "on–off switch" to control neural activation with light.

- Another innovation has been with opsins isolated from different algal species, such as the identification of an opsin from *Volvox carteri* named VChR1; this opsin is activated by red-shifted, or higher-wavelength and lower-energy, light, in contrast with ChR2.[24] When expressed in mammalian cells as a hybrid with *Chlamydomonas* ChR1, the red-shifted chimeric channel (C1V1[23]) allows for combinatorial control of two distinct populations of neurons along with ChR2. Most recently, ReaChR[25] has been engineered as a hybrid of ChIEF[20] and VChR1 to achieve superior plasma membrane expression in mammalian cells and higher photocurrents than other red-shifted ChR2 variants with the added advantage of maximum excitation wavelength 590–630 nm (red light), which is less scattered by tissue and less absorbed by blood and blood vessels, allowing better tissue penetration, even through an intact skull.
- Recently, the crystal structure of ChR2 was solved.[26] This breakthrough will allow for future engineering of opsins to further optimize their optical properties, as it already has for inhibitory opsins (iC1C2[27]; see below in Inhibitory Opsins).

Inhibitory Opsins

The optogenetic toolkit of opsins designed to inhibit neuronal activity is not as extensive as that for excitatory opsins. The first light-sensitive ion pump to prove effective in inhibiting neuronal spiking was NpHR, a chloride channel isolated from the halobacterium *Natronomonas pharaonis*,[28] maximally activated by yellow light at 573–613 nm.

- Later, enhancements to the membrane-trafficking of NpHR yielded the "enhanced" halorhodopsins eNpHR2.0 and eNpHR3.0.[18,29]
- Reminiscent of the bioinformatics work that identified ChR2-like opsins in previously unutilized species (VChR1),[24] proton pumps from other species were identified as potential inhibitory opsins (eBR from *Halobacterium*, Arch from *Halorubrum sodomense*, ArchT from *Halorubrum* strain TP009, and Mac from *Leptosphaeria maculans*, as reviewed in Ref. [30]). Membrane trafficking-enhanced versions (eArch3.0, eArchT3.0, eMac3.0) offer the added benefit of a 3–5-fold increase in photocurrent over the originally isolated opsins.[30]
- Based on the first published crystal structure of a channelrhodopsin, the ChR1–ChR2 chimeric opsin C1C2,[26] a version of C1C2 engineered to conduct chloride ions instead of cations, termed iC1C2, was developed to inhibit neuronal activity with the same blue light activation spectrum of the opsins on which it is based.[27] As a

testament to the efforts of several groups over many years of opsin engineering, altering the kinetics of iC1C2 to resemble the step-function-like properties of SFO has recently resulted in SwiChR, an inhibitory chloride channel that enables stable and reversible (with a pulse of 632-nm red light) neuronal inhibition.[27]

IN VIVO OPTOGENETIC APPLICATIONS

In Vivo Applications

Equally important to the optimization of opsins is the development of delivery technologies to express opsins in vitro and in vivo. Due to high infectivity, low toxicity, and ease of production with standard laboratory materials and equipment, viral delivery systems have been widely used to deliver opsin packages to cells in the dish and in living organisms. Viral expression systems based on lentiviral and adeno-associated vectors have been successfully implemented to stably and reliably express opsins in mammalian neural tissues.[31] In vivo cellular specificity can be achieved by restricting opsin expression to the control of cell type-specific promoters, injecting the virus into specific anatomical sites, or gating light delivery in order to activate opsins in desired anatomical regions.[32] Viral delivery systems, however, have disadvantages; e.g., the transgene payload as well as the promoter sequence used to target specific cell types must necessarily be small in most viral vectors. To overcome these limitations, transgenic, opsin-expressing organisms were developed (as reviewed in Ref. [33]): *Caenorhabditis elegans*, *Drosophila*, zebrafish, rat, and, most prominently, mouse, initially developed by Arenkiel et al. as the Thy1::ChR2 mouse, which stably expresses ChR2 primarily in layer V cortical output neurons.[19] Light stimulation of a desired population of neurons is delivered via optical fiber, encased at its terminal end in a metal ferrule, placed at the pial surface of the exposed brain after stereotactic craniotomy.[19,31,34] Recent clinically and translationally relevant work in mouse models is reviewed below.

Anxiety

Kheirbek et al. used either ChR2 or eNpHR3.0 to activate or inhibit, respectively, hippocampal dentate gyrus granule cells, and found that increasing activity of the ventral dentate gyrus improves performance on the elevated plus maze and open field test (validated assays of conflict anxiety in rodents) without impairing learning, suggesting that anxiety-like behaviors can be optogenetically attenuated.[35]

Obsessive-Compulsive Disorder

In a transgenic mouse model that exhibits compulsive behavior, optogenetic stimulation of the lateral orbitofrontal cortex using ChR2 abolished both stimulus-evoked and spontaneous compulsive grooming behavior, likely by restoring behavioral inhibition provided by the orbitofrontostriatal pathway.[36,37]

Depression

Much work has been done to apply optogenetic principles to mouse models of depression (reviewed in Ref. [38]). Chaudhury et al. used optogenetic stimulation through ChR2 to modulate the ventral tegmental area (VTA)-nucleus accumbens (NA) pathway to induce depression-like behaviors in mice, such as social avoidance, and then suppressed these behaviors by attenuating VTA–NA axis activity using NpHR stimulation.[39]

Addiction

Circuits that underlie reward-seeking behavior, such as the VTA and NA—implicated in addiction—have also been modulated optogenetically (as reviewed in Ref. [40]).

Memory Disorders

Recently, optogenetic techniques have been used to manipulate specific memory engrams, both to elicit, out of context, the behavioral output based on a specific memory,[41] and to generate false memories[42] (reviewed in Ref. [43]). This work carries the intriguing possibility of one day informing our treatments of memory disorders, such as Alzheimer disease and other types of dementia, amnesic disorders, and even posttraumatic stress disorder.

Epilepsy

In a mouse model of temporal lobe epilepsy (the most common variant of epilepsy in adults), optogenetic inhibition using halorhodopsin of excitatory principal cells, or optogenetic activation of a subpopulation of γ-aminobutyric acid (GABA)ergic hippocampal cells, arrested seizure activity rapidly after onset of light stimulation in rodents.[44]

Movement Disorders

One of the only neuromodulatory interventions in the functional neurosurgeon's toolkit today is DBS in treatment of Parkinson disease, in which high-frequency electrical stimulation is delivered to the subthalamic nucleus (STN) via an implanted electrode is highly successful at relieving tremor and other motor dysfunction. However, exactly how DBS functions therapeutically—and specifically which basal ganglia circuits are being activated by electrical stimulation—has historically been an open question. However, systematic optogenetic stimulation of basal ganglia components suggests that direct stimulatory effects on afferent fibers projecting to STN are sufficient to explain the therapeutic effects of DBS.[45] Optogenetic studies have even been useful in testing long-held assumptions about neurobiological structure–function relationships, such as the direct–indirect pathway dichotomy in the basal ganglia,[46,47] lending mechanistic support to current and future therapeutic strategies.

Demyelinating Disorders

Optogenetic technologies have recently been used to reveal that neuronal activity within the premotor circuit can influence oligodendrocyte lineage dynamics to induce differentiation of oligodendrocyte and neural precursors into oligodendrocytes and result in increased thickness of the myelin sheath around corticofugal projection neurons.[48] These cellular changes resulted in increased swing speed of the forelimb correlating to optogenetically stimulated activity,[48] raising the possibility that modulation of motor tract neural activity could one day be exploited for its beneficial effects on motor function in diseases of the motor system or in demyelinating disorders such as multiple sclerosis or the leukodystrophies.

Glioma

It has been suggested that activity-mediated neuron–glia interactions, when dysregulated, could underlie gliomagenesis in pediatric brain tumors.[49] Recent work has revealed that optogenetically induced neuronal activity increases the growth of tumor cells in an orthotopic xenograft model of pediatric high-grade glioma in immunodeficient mice expressing ChR2.[50] Furthermore, proteomic analysis of conditioned medium resulting from optogenetic stimulation of acute cortical slices from mice expressing ChR2 reveals a candidate list of mitogens that might underlie the activity-dependent interaction between neurons and oligodendroglial cells,[50] representing a potentially attractive future therapeutic target for brain cancers.

Disorders of Epigenetic Dysregulation

In a remarkable marriage of optogenetic technologies and epigenetics, Konermann et al. have recently achieved optogenetic control of transcription and chromatin state.[51] This technique, known as LITE, paves the way for intervention at the level of gene expression regulation and promises to be a powerful technique if it can one day be adapted to therapeutic use.

OUTLOOK: NONHUMAN PRIMATES AND HUMAN TISSUE

While optogenetic applications in small animals have yielded new insights into both basic neuroscience as well as diseases of the nervous system, of utmost importance to the eventual translation of these technologies to the clinical realm is their application in nonhuman primates and human tissues. However, several issues prevent direct application of small animal optogenetic techniques to nonhuman primates, including larger brain size, greater importance of safety (i.e., smaller tolerance of vector-related adverse effects), and differing susceptibility to infectious delivery vectors. In 2009, Han et al. were the first group to successfully modulate primate neuronal activity using optogenetics,[52] targeting excitatory neurons of the macaque frontal cortex and demonstrating via electrical recording of surrounding regions that optogenetic activation was limited to the targeted neurons and not upstream afferents as a proof of principle. Since then, optogenetic control over primate behavior has been achieved via both stimulation of excitatory networks (e.g., ChR2-mediated activation of rhesus monkey arcuate sulcus to modulate saccadic motions[53]) and inhibition of activity (e.g., inhibition of monkey superior colliculus neurons via the inhibitory proton pump ArchT, yielding deficits in saccadic eye motion[54]). While current genetic tools preclude the generation of a transgenic line of optogenetically stimulatable primates, Diester et al.[32] have proposed "an optogenetic toolbox" for primates consisting of established opsin/delivery method combinations that conform to the additional necessity to maximize tolerance and safety of opsin expression; until transgenic primates become available, these guidelines serve as "best practices" to guide work through the relatively uncharted territory of higher-order mammalian neuromodulation.

References

1. Miesenböck G, Kevrekidis IG. Optical imaging and control of genetically designated neurons in functioning circuits. *Annu Rev Neurosci.* 2005;28:533–563.
2. Schmucker D, et al. Chromophore-assisted laser inactivation of patched protein switches cell fate in the larval visual system of Drosophila. *Proc Natl Acad Sci USA.* 1994;91:2664–2668.
3. Hirase H, et al. Multiphoton stimulation of neurons. *J Neurobiol.* 2002;51(3):237–247.

4. Zemelman BV, et al. Selective photostimulation of genetically ChARGed neurons. *Neuron*. 2002;33:15–22.
5. Lima SQ, Miesenböck G. Remote control of behavior through genetically targeted photostimulation of neurons. *Cell*. 2005;121:141–152.
6. Zemelman BV, et al. Photochemical gating of heterologous ion channels: remote control over genetically designated populations of neurons. *PNAS*. 2003;100:1352–1357.
7. Gerits A, Vanduffel W. Optogenetics in primates: a shining future? *Trends Genet*. 2013;29:403–411.
8. Stoeckenius W. The rhodopsin-like pigments of halobacteria. *TIBS*. 1985;10:483–486.
9. Nagel G, et al. Channelrhodopsin-2, a directly light-gated cation-selective membrane channel. *PNAS*. 2003;100:13940–13945.
10. Oesterhelt D, Stoeckenius W. Rhodopsin-like protein from the purple membrane of *Halobacterium halobium*. *Nat New Biol*. 1971;233:149–152.
11. Lozier RH, Bogomolni RA, Stoeckenius W. Bacteriorhodopsin: a light-driven proton pump in *Halobacterium halobium*. *Biophys J*. 1975;15:955–962.
12. Nagel G, et al. Channelrhodopsin-1: a light-gated proton channel in green algae. *Science*. 2002;296:2395–2398.
13. Boyden ES, et al. Millisecond-timescale, genetically targeted optical control of neural activity. *Nat Neurosci*. 2005;8:1263–1268.
14. Deisseroth K, et al. Next-generation optical technologies for illuminating genetically targeted brain circuits. *J Neurosci*. 2006;26(41):10380–10386.
15. Zhang F, et al. Channelrhodopsin-2 and optical control of excitable cells. *Nat Methods*. 2006;3(10):785–792.
16. Nagel G, et al. Light activation of channelrhodopsin-2 in excitable cells of *Caenorhabditis elegans* triggers rapid behavioral responses. *Curr Biol*. 2005;15:2279–2284.
17. Gradinaru V, et al. Targeting and readout strategies for fast optical neural control in vitro and in vivo. *J Neurosci*. 2007;27:14231–14238.
18. Gradinaru V, Thompson KR, Deisseroth K. eNpHR: a natronomonas halorhodopsin enhanced for optogenetic applications. *Brain Cell Biol*. 2008;36:129–139.
19. Arenkiel BR, et al. In vivo light-induced activation of neural circuitry in transgenic mice expressing channelrhodopsin-2. *Neuron*. 2007;54:205–218.
20. Lin JY, et al. Characterization of engineered channelrhodopsin variants with improved properties and kinetics. *Biophys J*. 2009;96:1803–1814.
21. Gunaydin La, et al. Ultrafast optogenetic control. *Nat Neurosci*. 2010;13:387–392.
22. Berndt A, et al. Bi-stable neural state switches. *Nat Neurosci*. 2009;12(2):229–234.
23. Yizhar O, et al. Neocortical excitation/inhibition balance in information processing and social dysfunction. *Nature*. 2011;477:171–178.
24. Zhang F, et al. Red-shifted optogenetic excitation: a tool for fast neural control derived from *Volvox carteri*. *Nat Neurosci*. 2008;11(6):631–633.
25. Lin JY, et al. ReaChR: a red-shifted variant of channelrhodopsin enables deep transcranial optogenetic excitation. *Nat Neurosci*. 2013;16:1499–1508.
26. Kato HE, et al. Crystal structure of the channelrhodopsin light-gated cation channel. *Nature*. 2012;482:369–374.
27. Berndt A, et al. Structure-guided transformation of channelrhodopsin into a light-activated chloride channel. *Science*. 2014;344:1509–1511.
28. Zhang F, et al. Multimodal fast optical interrogation of neural circuitry. *Nature*. 2007;446:633–639.
29. Gradinaru V, et al. Molecular and cellular approaches for diversifying and extending optogenetics. *Cell*. 2010;141:154–165.
30. Mattis J, et al. Principles for applying optogenetic tools derived from direct comparative analysis of microbial opsins. *Nat Methods*. 2012;9:159–172.
31. Zhang F, et al. Optogenetic interrogation of neural circuits: technology for probing mammalian brain structures. *Nat Protoc*. 2010;5:439–456.

32. Diester I, et al. An optogenetic toolbox designed for primates. *Nat Neurosci.* 2011;14:387–397.
33. Fenno LE, Yizhar O, Deisseroth K. The development and application of optogenetics. *Annu Rev Neurosci.* 2011;34:389–412.
34. Yizhar O, et al. Optogenetics in neural systems. *Neuron.* 2011;71:9–34.
35. Kheirbek MA, et al. Differential control of learning and anxiety along the dorso-ventral axis of the dentate gyrus. *Neuron.* 2014;77:955–968.
36. Ahmari SE, et al. Repeated cortico-striatal stimulation generates persistent OCD-like behavior. *Science.* 2013;340:1234–1239.
37. Burguiere E, et al. Optogenetic stimulation of lateral orbitofronto-striatal pathway suppresses compulsive behaviors. *Science.* 2013;340:1–15.
38. Albert PR. Light up your life: optogenetics for depression? *J Psychiatry Neurosci.* 2014;39:3–5.
39. Chaudhury D, et al. Rapid regulation of depression-related behaviours by control of midbrain dopamine neurons. *Nature.* 2013;493:532–536.
40. Stuber GD, Britt JP, Bonci A. Optogenetic modulation of neural circuits that underlie reward seeking. *Biol Psychiatry.* 2012;71:1061–1067.
41. Liu X, et al. Optogenetic stimulation of a hippocampal engram activates fear memory recall. *Nature.* 2012;484:381–385.
42. Ramirez S, Tonegawa S, Liu X. Identification and optogenetic manipulation of memory engrams in the hippocampus. *Front Behav Neurosci.* 2013;7:226.
43. Ramirez S, et al. Creating a false memory in the hippocampus. *Science.* 2013;341:387–391.
44. Krook-Magnuson E, et al. On-demand optogenetic control of spontaneous seizures in temporal lobe epilepsy. *Nat Commun.* 2013;4:1376.
45. Gradinaru V, et al. Optical deconstruction of parkinsonian neural circuitry. *Science.* 2009;324(5925):354–359.
46. Kravitz AV, et al. Regulation of parkinsonian motor behaviours by optogenetic control of basal ganglia circuitry. *Nature.* 2010;466(7306):622–626.
47. Freeze BS, et al. Control of basal ganglia output by direct and indirect pathway projection neurons. *J Neurosci.* 2013;33(47):18531–18539.
48. Gibson EM, et al. Neuronal activity promotes oligodendrogenesis and adaptive myelination in the mammalian brain. *Science.* 2014;344:1252304.
49. Monje M, et al. Hedgehog-responsive candidate cell of origin for diffuse intrinsic pontine glioma. *Proc Natl Acad Sci USA.* 2011;108:4453–4458.
50. Venkatesh H, et al. Neuronal activity-regulated secretion of neuroligin-3 promotes glioma growth. In revision.
51. Konermann S, et al. Optical control of mammalian endogenous transcription and epigenetic states. *Nature.* 2013;500:472–476.
52. Han X, et al. Millisecond-timescale optical control of neural dynamics in the nonhuman primate brain. *Neuron.* 2009;62:191–198.
53. Gerits A, et al. Optogenetically induced behavioral and functional network changes in primates. *Curr Biol.* 2012;22:1722–1726.
54. Cavanaugh J, et al. Optogenetic inactivation modifies monkey visuomotor behavior. *Neuron.* 2012;76:901–907.
55. Crick FHC. XI: Thinking about the Brain. *The Brain, A Scientific American Book.* 1979;130–137.

Introduction to Basic Mechanisms of Transcranial Magnetic Stimulation

D. Austin and J. Rothwell

University College London, London, United Kingdom

INTRODUCTION

Although the first demonstration of electrical stimulation of the human brain was reported by Bartholin in 1874,[1] it was more than 100 years later before stimulation parameters were refined sufficiently to allow brain stimulation to be performed in healthy awake volunteers. In the intervening period, attempts to pass electrical current through the skull were restricted by its high electrical resistance, requiring large currents to be applied to scalp electrodes, with intense stimulation of scalp nerves causing considerable discomfort. Electrical stimulation of the human brain was limited to explorations during neurosurgical procedures, with part of the skull removed to expose the brain beneath. In 1980 however, Merton and Morton[2] finally demonstrated that transcranial stimulation was possible using a single brief high-voltage stimulus, and while somewhat uncomfortable the method was used for several years before the introduction of the transcranial magnetic method by Barker and colleagues[3] allowed the high electrical resistance of the skull to be bypassed completely.

TRANSCRANIAL MAGNETIC STIMULATION

The key to the success of transcranial magnetic stimulation (TMS) is that the scalp and skull have negligible impedance to the passage of a magnetic field. TMS produces a time-varying magnetic field that readily penetrates brain tissue and (via Faraday's laws) induces an electrical current over a time course that follows the time differential of the magnetic field.

A typical TMS device consists of a large electrical capacitor charged to a high voltage by a transformer (Fig. 7.1), which is then short-circuited (discharged) through a coiled copper wire. The resultant transient electrical current of up to several thousand amps induces an accompanying perpendicular magnetic field that typically rises to 1–2.5 T within 50–100 μs and then decays more slowly back to zero over the following 1 ms. In a conventional monophasic TMS coil a switch-diode prevents oscillation in coil current, generating a near-monophasic pulse waveform as the current

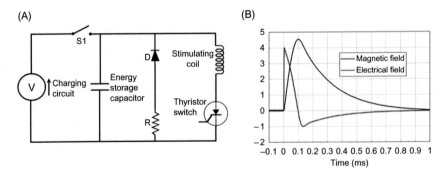

FIGURE 7.1   (A) Simplified circuit diagram of a TMS stimulator. (B) Respective waveform of magnetic and electrical field strength form a TMS pulse—note the electrical field is proportional to the rate of change in the magnetic field. *Source: Adapted from Barker AT, Freeston I. Transcranial magnetic stimulation. Scholarpedia 2007; 2(10): 2936.*[3]

is gradually dissipated during an extremely shallow, low-current second phase of the waveform (Fig. 7.1). For this to be performed safely the switch-diode needs to be turned off precisely when current within the circuit is at zero amps, as otherwise the sudden change in current flow will induce a large-voltage electromotive force with potentially damaging effects.

The original TMS coil design is a single loop of coiled wire, typically around 8–15 cm in diameter and containing approximately 20 turns of wire. Optimal dimensions are considered to be a coil width 60% of its radius and a height 20% of its radius.[4] The current induced in the brain flows in the opposite direction to the current in the coil, and is maximal in an annulus under the windings of the coil. Conventional round coils have poor spatial focality.

More recent designs consist of two round coils sited side by side, with current flowing in opposite directions in each circuit (clockwise vs anti-clockwise) but in the same posterior to anterior (PA) direction at the point where the two coils (and fields) overlap. Each coil is comparatively small (9 cm) compared to the larger circular coils. The induced fields under each loop of the coil summate at the junction, creating greater focality.[5] Use of a ferro-magnetic core within the coil windings can reduce power consumption by the stimulator and consequently decrease coil overheating.[6]

Because the magnetic field falls off rapidly with distance from the coil, it is difficult to stimulate structures deep within the brain. High-intensity stimuli from conventional coils can cause deep stimulation but because the field cannot be focused, they also cause intense stimulation to cortical surface areas. The Hesed coil, or H-coil,[7] is designed to reduce the gradient of intensity between superficial and deep stimulation, creating a more constant level of stimulation in all structures and minimizing the production of poorly tolerated side effects from cortical and surface excitation. It thus affords stimulation of deeper brain structures as a trade-off for reduced focality.

BASIC PRINCIPLES OF NERVE STIMULATION WITH MAGNETIC PULSES

When Barker et al.[8] pioneered transcranial magnetic stimulation (TMS), they were extrapolating an experimental technique that had been previously utilized in research on peripheral nerves.[9] Indeed, they selected the pulse parameters to be optimal for stimulation of large-diameter myelinated axons, inducing short-duration monophasic pulses of electrical current. Maccabee et al.[10] explored in some detail the electrophysiology of magnetic pulse stimulation of long peripheral nerve axons. Axons are activated preferentially at the point where the negative spatial derivative of the electric field along their length is maximal.[11] This causes outward current to flow across the membrane and depolarize the axons. If a straight nerve is aligned along the length of the junction region of a figure-of-eight coil, then the spatial derivative of the induced electric field is maximum at the two points where the windings diverge from each other into their respective circular coils. There is no stimulation in the middle of the junction region where the spatial derivative is smaller. Maccabee et al.[10] confirmed that this was the case in vitro (Fig. 7.2). Using a monophasic

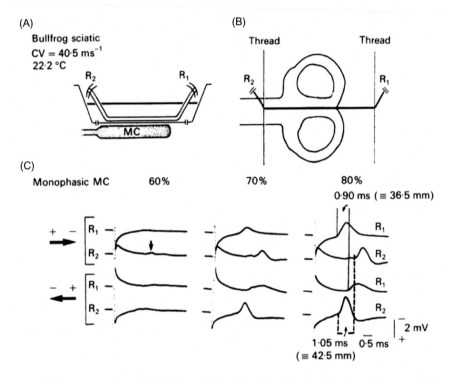

FIGURE 7.2   Maccabee et al.[10] stimulation of peripheral nerves in vitro using magnetic coils. The difference in latencies with opposing directions of stimulation suggest that excitation occurs at the first spatial derivative of the electrical field—the point at which isoelectric lines start to curve away from the straight nerve. The site of activation is thus not directly under the center of the figure-of-eight but at the point(s) where the two loops start to diverge. (A) Shows the experimental arrangement from the side. (B) The same from above. The nerve is immersed in a saline bath resting on a figure-of-eight TMS coil. (C) Shows the responses recorded from two electrodes at each end of the nerve (R1 and R2) at three different intensities of TMS (60%, 70%, and 80% maximum output). The upper two rows show responses evoked with current flowing from right to left; the lower two with the reversed current. Note the difference in onset latencies at R1 and R2 for the two different current directions. It is 0.9 ms for R1 and 1.05 ms for R2. Given the estimated conduction velocity of the nerve, this corresponds to a difference in the site of stimulation using the two different directions of current at 36.5 and 42.5 mm, respectively. In other words, reversing the current in the coil moves the effective stimulation site by around 39 mm, which corresponds to the distance between the two bifurcation points of the coil. *Source: From Maccabee PJ, Amassian VE, Eberle LP, Cracco RQ. Magnetic coil stimulation of straight and bent amphibian and mammalian peripheral nerve in vitro: locus of excitation. J Physiol 1993; 460: 201–219, Fig. 3, p. 208.*

stimulator, if the induced current under the junction region flows from left to right in the figure, stimulation occurs preferentially at the distal (relative to the coil handle) divergence, where the negative spatial derivative is maximum, whereas if the induced current is in the opposite direction, stimulation occurs at the more proximal divergence point.

Changes in spatial derivative of the electric field also occur at points where the nerve bends out of the induced field (rather than the field bending away from the nerve). For example, although no stimulation occurs at the mid-junction region with a straight nerve, it can be induced quite easily if the nerve is bent out of the plane of the induced field at that point. Again the effect is directional: activation occurs if the electric field is aligned so that the bend produces a negative spatial derivative at the bend (i.e., current comes out of the nerve); if the field is in the opposite direction it is ineffective (and will in fact hyperpolarize the membrane at the point) (Fig. 7.3).

The same authors[10] also explored the effect of stimulation with biphasic pulses, in which the peak currents induced in each direction are equal. In this case they found that stimulation occurs preferentially during the reverse phase of the stimulus, rather than on the rising edge as occurs with a monophasic pulse. This is because the reverse phase lasts for longer and hence provides more powerful stimulation than either phase alone. Finally, they also examined the effect of placing resistive barriers around the nerves, simulating the passage of a nerve trunk through the intervertebral foramina. In this case, stimulation occurs preferentially at the foramen.

The conclusion is that the effect of magnetic stimulation on axons is highly directional, and depends critically on the orientation of the induced field with respect to the direction of the axons. The specificity of this interaction is best observed near threshold levels of stimulation, becoming "smeared" at higher intensities of stimulation.

EFFECT OF TMS ON MOTOR CORTEX

The effects of TMS have been studied most extensively on motor cortex. Stimulation here evokes a brief contraction in muscles on the opposite side of the body that can be measured with electromyographic recording techniques. Since each stimulus evokes a measureable response it makes motor cortex the ideal site to investigate the basic mechanisms of TMS. The typical onset latency of electromyography (EMG) responses in intrinsic hand muscles is 20–25 ms (depending on arm length and nerve conduction velocity) and results from activation of rapidly conducting corticospinal fibers from motor cortex that have monosynaptic connections to spinal motoneurons. This descending activity in the spinal cord can be recorded in patients who have had electrodes implanted into the epidural space of the spinal cord for treatment of chronic pain.[12]

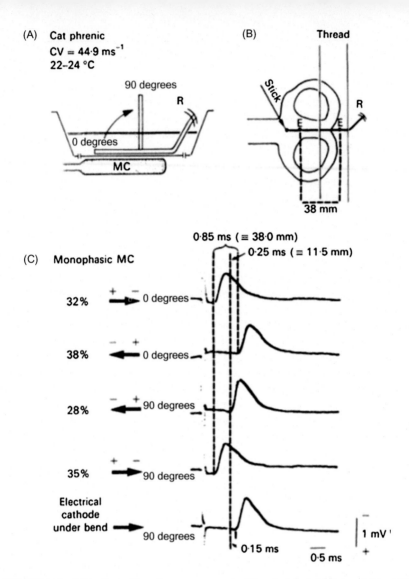

FIGURE 7.3 The effect of bending an axon out of the electric field induced by a TMS pulse. (A) and (B) show the setup as in Fig. 7.2, with the addition that the nerve can be bent upward by 90 degrees from the base of the saline bath. (C) Shows the responses recorded from the electrode (R) on the right of the nerve. With nerve lying flat in the bath (0 degrees) a current induced from left to right of the figure causes activation at a site near the recording electrode (intensity 32%); reversing the current activates the nerve further from the electrode, near the proximal divergence of the figure-of-eight TMS coil (intensity 38%). These two points are indicated in panel (B) as E. When the nerve is bent upward (90 degrees), stimulation with current from right to left (intensity 28%) shifts the point of activation nearer to the recording electrode. The reduction in latency is 0.25 ms which is equivalent to 11.5 mm in this nerve. This latency corresponds to the latency of responses elicited by direct electrical stimulation of the nerve at the bend (bottom trace). The trace one up from the bottom shows that, in contrast, the site of activation with a left-to-right pulse is unchanged, remaining near to the recording electrode at the distal divergence of the TMS coil. *Source: From Maccabee PJ, Amassian VE, Eberle LP, Cracco RQ. Magnetic coil stimulation of straight and bent amphibian and mammalian peripheral nerve in vitro: locus of excitation. J Physiol 1993; 460: 201–219, Fig. 8, p. 213.*

These electrodes are often first implanted with the leads exposed through the skin; several days later, once the integrity of the electrodes has been verified, the leads are reimplanted under the skin and attached to the implanted electrical stimulator. In the intervening "screening" period, it is possible to record the corticospinal activity produced by TMS pulses to motor cortex. Such recordings[13] show that potentials are conducted at around 60 m/second. They also give some insight into how TMS produces EMG activity.

To understand this, it is necessary to review briefly the electrophysiology of direct electrical stimulation of exposed motor cortex in animal experiments. A single brief electrical pulse produces a series of descending volleys, consisting of synchronized action potentials in many individual corticospinal axons. The initial, and lowest threshold, descending volley is termed the D-wave, caused by direct depolarization at the first internode of the corticospinal axon. This volley persists in decorticate animals, consistent with an axonal origin.[14] The D-wave is followed by later volleys, termed I- or indirect waves, which follow at fairly consistent intervals of 1.5 ms. These volleys are absent after decortication, and are therefore thought to reflect synaptic activation of the same corticospinal neurons from other neurons in the cortex. They require higher stimulus intensities than D-waves and increase in number and amplitude the stronger the stimulus becomes. Both EMG and epidural recordings show that the latency of these D-waves shortens slightly with increasing voltage of electrical stimulation—presumably due to deeper penetration of the current and stimulation at more distant nodes on the axon within the subcortical white matter, perhaps even cerebral peduncles or pyramidal decussations with high-intensity stimulation.[15]

Data from epidural recordings in humans are consistent with these findings, at least when the Merton and Morton[2] technique of transcranial electrical stimulation is used. However, there is one important difference with TMS: the lowest-threshold volley (after stimulation of the hand area) is the first I-wave.[16] Later I-waves are recruited at higher stimulus intensities, with the D-wave only appearing at very high intensities. Why does this difference occur if both TMS and transcranial electrical stimulation (TES) produce short-lasting pulses of electrical current in the brain? The lowest-threshold electrical stimulation of the cortex occurs with a surface anode (positive pole). It is thought that this causes current to flow into the apical dendrites of corticospinal pyramidal neurons; it leaves at the axon hillock region or (more likely) the first internode, where the outward current depolarizes the membrane and causes an action potential. Absence of a D-wave with low-intensity TMS means that this is much less likely to happen. It has been proposed that for physical reasons related to the build-up of electrical charge at boundaries between conductive layers of tissue, TMS induces current flow parallel to the surface of the brain with little or no radial component. If the cortex were laid flat and parallel to the scalp, this would mean that current could not flow into and out of vertically oriented pyramidal neurons. Instead, "horizontal" current flow parallel to the surface would tend to activate intracortical elements that synaptically activate corticospinal discharges.

However, the cortical surface is not flat, but highly curved, so this simple explanation seems unlikely to account for all of the differences. Modeling studies (see "Models" below) are underway to try to calculate in detail the distribution of currents induced in the cortex and their relationship with the various types of cortical neurons.

I-WAVES

Models to describe the production of I-waves are considered below. Here we describe some of the main experimental properties of the waves that must be accounted for by the models. The initial animal experiments of Patton and Amassian[14] showed that I-waves persisted after large thalamic lesions, suggesting that they did not depend on activation of thalamocortical fibers. But this leaves many other sources of possible synaptic inputs still unexplored. Cooling of the surface of the cortex caused late I-waves to disappear before early I-waves, consistent with late I-waves reflecting input to more distal dendrites. In humans, the EMG response produced by a given intensity of TMS is always larger if applied during a voluntary contraction of the muscle than at rest. Most of the increase in amplitude is due to the fact that contraction increases the excitability of spinal motoneurons, making them easier to discharge by the descending corticospinal volleys. However, during strong contractions, epidural recordings[17] also show that the amplitude of I-waves also increases, consistent with the idea that cortical excitability has also increased, making it easier for I-wave synaptic input to discharge corticospinal neurons. All I-waves are affected in the same way, but the D-wave is unchanged, consistent with its being a response initiated at the first internode of the axon.

Early and late I-waves in contrast have different sensitivity to GABA-A,[18] with later I-waves being suppressed by benzodiazepines while D- and early I-waves are relatively unaffected. These I-waves are also suppressed by a preceding subthreshold conditioning pulse in the short-interval intracortical inhibition (SICI) paradigm (short-interval intracortical inhibition).[19] Finally, modulation of cortical excitability through excitatory forms of repetitive TMS (rTMS)[20] tends to increase late I-waves, whereas inhibitory forms suppress them.[21,22]

Taken together the data suggest that although all I-waves are produced by excitatory synaptic inputs to corticospinal neurons, the synapses responsible for later I-waves are more easily modulated by GABAergic and other inputs. This could be due, e.g., to the early I-wave inputs being located on different parts of the dendritic tree or cell body than the late I-wave inputs.

I-wave inputs are also differentially sensitive to the direction of the current induced by TMS over M1.[23] TMS that induces a monophasic current pulse from PA perpendicular to the line of the central sulcus evokes the lowest-threshold EMG responses in hand muscles. Computer modeling of the distribution of the electric field induced by TMS indicate that this is because stimulation perpendicular to a gyrus induces a larger electrical field at the crown of the gyrus than stimulus oriented parallel to the gyrus.[24] Thus we might expect monophasic stimulus pulses to favor PA current. However, we would also expect that the reverse current (anterior-posterior, AP) should be equally effective, since it too is aligned perpendicular to the gyrus. But this is not the case; the threshold for AP stimulation is higher than for PA stimulation, and the onset latency of the evoked motor evoked potentials (MEPs) is often 1–2 ms longer.[25]

In fact, epidural recordings[23] show that while PA stimulation evokes early (I1-waves), AP stimulation tends only to evoke later I-waves, with I1-wave recruitment only occurring at suprathreshold intensities. The most likely reason for the difference is that TMS activates neural structures (presumably axons) that have a specific orientation with respect to the magnetic pulse. It would be very similar to the bent axon illustrated in Fig. 7.3; activation at the bend occurs much more easily when the induced current is aligned to exit the nerve at the bend. Stimulation in the opposite direction tends to cause hyperpolarization and the threshold is much higher.

But this simple concept is still not quite sufficient to explain the difference between PA and AP stimulation, since not only is the threshold of AP stimulation higher than for PA pulses, the latency of the effect is longer. One possible explanation is that AP stimulation must be stimulating another set of fibers that themselves are specifically oriented for activation by AP current. If correct, the conclusion is that within M1 there are two sets of axons preferentially aligned to be stimulated by PA or by AP current.

TMS OF MOTOR CORTEX EXCITES INHIBITORY AS WELL AS EXCITATORY NEURONS: PAIRED PULSE EVIDENCE

Generation of MEPs and I-waves might be seen as indicating that TMS activates only excitatory inputs to the corticospinal system. Of course, there are multiple other neural types that could well be activated by the induced current pulses. Detecting activity of these elements requires more complex methods, such as the paired pulse protocol.

A subthreshold stimulus, too small in itself to produce an MEP even in preactivated muscle (i.e., subactive threshold), will supress a suprathreshold stimulus that follows it by 1–6 ms and facilitate one following 10–15 ms later.[26] These phenomena are termed SICI and facilitation (ICF), respectively. This subthreshold condition stimulus does not itself initiate discharges in corticospinal axons and therefore its effect should be restricted to the cerebral cortex. Epidural recordings[19] have shown that effect of SICI on MEPs is mediated through an effect on I-waves, since these are suppressed while D-waves generally are not, suggesting that the subthreshold conditioning stimulus is acting presynaptically to the pyramidal neuron. Indeed, the suppression is selective for later I-waves, with little or no effect on the first I-wave (I1). Consistent with this, SICI appears to be more effective if the test MEP is evoked with an AP-directed current pulse. AP-evoked MEPs consist of a larger proportion of late I-wave activity and should therefore be more sensitive to SICI. Interestingly, the orientation of the (subthreshold) conditioning pulse has no effect on the depth of SICI, suggesting that the inhibitory neurons have no preferred alignment within cortex. A large number of pharmacological studies suggest that SICI is mediated by a GABA-Aergic connection. For example, SICI of late I-waves in epidural recordings is facilitated by GABA-A agonists.[18] Paradoxically, paired pulse stimulation at a facilitatory interstimulus interval (ICF) produced facilitation of MEPs with no recordable change in I-wave amplitude or quantity,[27] possibly due to an increase in asynchronous low-level activity, which is masked by I-waves on epidural recording.

Intracortical inhibition can be produced through direct stimulation of exposed cortex using electrodes up to 1 cm apart, but not at larger distances,[28] suggesting that SICI interneuron circuits are located within M1. ICI is not however demonstrated with a TES test stimulus[26]—potentially because presynaptic inhibition taking place at level of dendrites/cortex may have a limited impact on TES activation of descending axons with white matter.

While SICI is a relatively well understood interaction, much less is known about the inhibitory interaction between two stimuli at longer intervals. This requires higher-intensity conditioning stimuli that are usually 120% or 130% above resting motor threshold. Such stimuli suppress the response to a test stimulus for 100–200 ms, a phenomenon termed long-interval intracortical inhibition (LICI).[29] The mechanism is complex since the first stimulus evokes corticospinal activity that can change the excitability of spinal circuits as well as evoke activity within motor cortex. LICI, like SICI, is usually studied in the resting state. Studies of spinal excitability using H-reflex and F-wave testing suggest that spinal inhibition occurs over the first 50–100 ms. Recordings of descending activity evoked by the test stimulus show that suppression of late I-waves continues for longer.[30] Thus the later part LICI is usually presumed to be primarily of cortical origin. Pharmacological studies suggest it may be a GABA-B form of inhibition[31] representing a different set of inhibitory connections than are activated in SICI.

MODELS

Various network models have attempted to account for the properties of single and paired pulse testing of motor cortex. They have to reproduce two main physiological features described above: the periodicity of I-waves (at approximately 600 Hz) and the sensitivity of late I-waves to excitatory and inhibitory interactions. Periodicity can result either from intrinsic properties of a single cell type, or from feedback activity in a reverberating circuit. The latter solution was proposed by Di Lazzaro,[34] who suggested that the basic "canonical" model of the cortical circuit[35] could oscillate at high frequency after a TMS pulse. In this model, excitatory interneurons in cortical layers II and III synapse on pyramidal neurons in layer V, which have axon collaterals that reciprocally excite the layer II/III neurons. Both sets of neurons are also reciprocally connected to GABAergic inhibitory neurons.

In this model, D-waves result from direct activation of the axon of the layer V pyramidal neuron. I1 waves result from activation of layer II/III neurons that monosynaptically excite layer V neurons. Layer II/III neurons also excite GABAergic interneurons that evoke an inhibitory postsynaptic potential in layer V cells immediately after the monosynaptic excitation that abruptly terminates its action. Later I-waves result from reverberating activity in the connection between layers II/III and V, which is consistent with the known interval between I-wave populations of approximately 1.5 ms.[36] Since this time interval is shorter than the known refractory period of individual excitatory and inhibitory interneurons, the MEP must represent the net output of parallel neuronal networks activating in synchrony. In this scheme, SICI is caused by facilitation of the GABA interneurons, which results in more extensive inhibition of layer V neurons after the I1-wave, and greater feedback suppression of layer II/III neurons. The result is that I1 waves in response to the test pulse are unaffected, whereas later I-waves are suppressed.

A variation on this basic hypothesis was suggested by Phillips[37] who proposed that layer V neurons might have intrinsic oscillatory properties that resulted in repetitive volleys of I-waves without requiring additional triggering from cortical neurons. The problem with this suggestion is that it does not readily explain why SICI preferentially affects later I-waves, since all I-waves are essentially produced by the same mechanism.

The model of Di Lazzaro assumes that repetitive firing of pyramidal neurons is caused by repeated excitatory/inhibitory inputs at I-wave frequency. A key feature is that cortical interneurons fire repetitively at the same rate as pyramidal neurons. A second class of model was proposed by Esser[38] and by Rusu and Ziemann.[33] In this model, only pyramidal neurons fire at high frequency; cortical interneurons do not. Instead, the cortical circuitry generates strong excitatory input to pyramidal neurons that fire repetitively at a frequency determined by their refractory period. This is consistent with experimental studies that show that pyramidal neurons that receive very strong depolarization can generate activity at a maximum of about 600 Hz for short periods. Both models are similar in essence but differ in details of the physiological properties of pyramidal neurons and the interconnections within cortex. In addition, Esser et al.[38] include a cortico-thalamic circuit.

In detail, the recent model of Rusu et al.[33] postulates a simple feed-forward architecture with connections between layer II/III neurons and layer V pyramidal neurons, with a more detailed morphology of the layer V cytoarchitecture (Fig. 7.4). In concordance with earlier models it

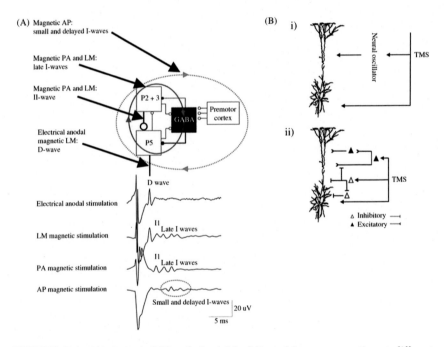

FIGURE 7.4 (A) Canonical (Douglas) model of D- and I-wave generation at different points of the same neuronal circuit by different forms of TMS. (B) Alternative model with separate I-waves generated by distinct inhibitory and excitatory circuits. *Source: From (A) Di Lazzaro V, Ziemann U. Modelling of I waves in human motor cortex. The contribution of transcranial magnetic stimulation in the functional evaluation of microcircuits in human motor cortex. Front Neural Circuits. 2013;7(18):1–9*[32] *with permission. (B) Rusu CV, Murakami M, Ziemann U, Triesch J. A model of TMS-induced I-waves in motor cortex. Brain Stimulation 2014; 7: 401–414, Fig. 14, p. 411.*[33]

postulates that the D-wave originates from direct axonal depolarization of layer V pyramidal neurons, with depolarization focused on the region distal to the axonal hillock where the neuronal axis curves within the generated electrical field. As in the Di Lazzaro model, I-waves are then generated through synaptic inputs on to layer V neurons from cells in layer II/III. However in the Rusu model, the layer II/III cells have synapses on proximal dendrites as well as on distal dendrites in superficial cortical layers. I1 waves originate from the initial excitation of inputs to the proximal dendrites. Excitation to the distal dendrites arrives later at the cell body and prolongs the depolarization so that the pyramidal neurons fire repetitively. The input to distal dendrites is more affected by inhibitory inputs. This explains the preferential suppression of late I-waves in SICI.[19] It is important to note that inputs to layer V neurons within motor cortex originate not just from neurons within primary motor cortex but also from premotor and supplementary motor cortex and somatosensory cortex. Transcranial electrical stimulation of these secondary areas is indeed capable of generating I-waves, an effect which seems nonetheless dependent on M1 neurons as the effect is abolished by ablation of M1.[39]

SYNAPTIC PLASTICITY

One of the most important discoveries in synaptic physiology of the past 50 years is long-term potentiation - LTP (and depression (LTD), discovered some years later). Repeated patterns of activity can change the effectiveness of synaptic connections for hours, days, or longer. In animal experiments, such changes are induced in two different ways: repetitive activation of the presynaptic input (e.g., 100 Hz for 10 seconds) or repeated inputs that are carefully timed to precede/follow the discharge of the postsynaptic neuron (spike-timing-dependent plasticity, STDP). In the first method the usual rule is that the high-frequency stimulation produces facilitation at the synapse, whereas low-frequency depresses the synapse. In the second method, the usual rule is that if the input precedes the postsynaptic action potential then the synapse will strengthen, whereas the opposite occurs if the presynaptic input follows the postsynaptic action potential. These rules, however, are only approximate guides, with many exceptions possible.

With the development of TMS there has been much interest in trying to replicate some of these effects in the human brain. Thus rTMS of motor cortex can lead to aftereffects on excitability such that the MEP evoked by a standard single TMS pulse may be larger or smaller than at baseline for the 30–60 minutes after application of rTMS. Recordings of descending corticospinal activity show[40] that in almost all cases, the later I-waves are more affected by these interventions than the I1- or D-waves, and pharmacological studies[41] suggest they depend on activity of N-methyl-D-aspartate (NMDA) receptors. The effects are relatively short-lasting compared with those reported in animal preparations. However, it is important to bear in mind that much of the basic animal work on Long Term Potentiation (LTP)/Long Term Depression (LTD) is performed in slice preparations from the hippocampus of dead animals. Far fewer studies have been performed on neocortex, and even fewer in awake animals. In the latter, it is difficult to induce reliable LTP/LTD. Such studies might be a much better model for plasticity studies in the human brain.

Work in humans has also replicated the paired presynaptic/postsynaptic approach to generating synaptic plasticity (Spike-Timing-Dependent Plasticity - STDP). A widely employed protocol is paired associative stimulation,[42] where a peripheral (median) nerve electrical stimulus is paired with TMS to motor cortex. If the stimuli are timed such that the peripheral stimulus reaches the cortex just prior to the TMS pulse, a facilitatory effect is observed. With a slightly later peripheral nerve stimulus, calculated to reach cortex just after the TMS pulse, there is an inhibitory effect.

There are many other variations on these protocols, from theta burst stimulation[43] to quadrupulse stimulation,[44] with subtly different effects from each type. Nevertheless, the problem with all of them is that the aftereffects are extremely variable both between and within individuals. Several factors are known to contribute to this variability. Age, sex, physical fitness, genetics, and brain anatomy contribute to interindividual differences; time of day, circulating hormones, drug levels, and brain state contribute to both intra- and interindividual differences. Present efforts are now concentrated on trying to reduce variability by controlling some of these factors but, nonetheless, TMS has firmly established itself as one of the innovative means of achieving therapeutic neuromodulation.

References

1. Bartholow R. Experimental investigations into the functions of the human brain. *Am J Med Sci*. 1874;66:305–313.
2. Merton PA, Morton HB. Stimulation of the cerebral cortex in the intact human subject. *Nature*. 1980;285(5762):227.
3. Barker AT, Freeston I. Transcranial magnetic stimulation. *Scholarpedia*. 2007;2(10):2936.
4. Mouchawar GA, Nyenhuis JA, Bourland JD, Geddes LA. Guidelines for energy efficient coils: coils designed for magnetic stimulation of the motor cortex. *J Clin Neurophysiol*. 1991;10:353–362.
5. Ueno S, Tashiro T, Harada K. Localized stimulation of neural tissues in the brain by means of a paired configuration of time-varying magnetic fields. *J Appl Phys*. 1988;64:5862–5864.
6. Epstein CM, Davey KR. Iron-core coils for transcranial magnetic stimulation. *J Clin Neurophysiol*. 2002;19(4):376–381.
7. Roth Y, Zangen A, Hallett M. A coil design for transcranial magnetic stimulation of deep brain regions. *J Clin Neurophysiol*. 2002;19(4):361–370.
8. Barker AT, Jalious R, Freeston IL. Non-invasive magnetic stimulation of human motor cortex. *Lancet*. 1985;1(8437):1106–1107.

9. Polson MJ, Barker AT, Freeston IL. Stimulation of nerve trunks with time-varying magnetic fields. *Med Biol Eng Comput.* 1982;20(2):243–244.

10. Maccabee PJ, Amassian VE, Eberle LP, Cracco RQ. Magnetic coil stimulation of straight and bent amphibian and mammalian peripheral nerve in vitro: locus of excitation. *J Physiol.* 1993;460:201–219.

11. Roth BJ. Mechanisms for electrical stimulation of excitable tissue. *Crit Rev Bioeng.* 1994;22(3–4):253–305.

12. Di Lazzaro V, Oliviero A, Profice P, et al. Comparison of descending volleys evoked by transcranial magnetic and electric stimulation in conscious humans. *Electroencephalogr Clin Neurophysiol.* 1998;109:397–401.

13. Boyd SG, Rothwell JC, Cowan JM, et al. A method of monitoring function in corticospinal pathways during scoliosis surgery with a note on motor conduction velocities. *J Neurol Neurosurg Psychiatry.* 1986;49(3):251–257.

14. Patton HD, Amassian VE. Single and multiple-unit analysis of cortical stage of pyramidal tract activation. *J Neurophysiol.* 1954;17(4):345–363.

15. Rothwell J, Burke D, Hicks R, Stephen J, Woodforth I, Crawford M. Transcranial electrical stimulation of the motor cortex in man: further evidence for the site of activation. *J Physiol.* 1994;481(1):243–250.

16. Di Lazzaro V, Oliviero A, Pilato F, et al. The physiological basis of transcranial motor cortex stimulation in conscious humans. *Clin Neurophysiol.* 2004;115:255–266.

17. Di Lazzaro V, Restuccia D, et al. Effects of voluntary contraction on descending volleys evoked by transcranial stimulation in conscious humans. *J Physiol.* 1998;508:625–633.

18. Di Lazzaro V, Oliviero A, Meglio M, et al. Direct demonstration of the effect of lorazepam on the excitability of the human motor cortex. *Clin Neurophysiol.* 2000;111(5):794–799.

19. Di Lazzaro V, Restuccia D, Oliviero A, et al. Magnetic transcranial stimulation at intensities below active motor threshold activates intracortical inhibitory circuits. *Exp Brain Res.* 1998;119:265–268.

20. Di Lazzaro V, Pilato F, Dileone M, et al. The physiological basis of the effects of intermittent theta-burst stimulation of the human motor cortex. *J Physiol.* 2008;586:3871–3879.

21. Di Lazzaro V, Pilato F, Dileone M, et al. Low-frequency repetitive transcranial magnetic stimulation suppresses specific excitatory circuits in the human motor cortex. *J Physiol.* 2008;586(18):4481–4487.

22. Di Lazzaro V, Ziemann U, Lemon RN. State of the art: physiology of transcranial motor cortex stimulation. *Brain Stimulation.* 2008;1(4):345–362.

23. Sakai K, Ugawa Y, Terao Y, Hanajima R, Furubayashi T, Kanazawa I. Preferential activation of different I waves by transcranial magnetic stimulation with a figure-of-eight-shaped coil. *Exp Brain Res.* 1997;113(1):24–32.

24. Opitz A, Windhoff M, Heidemann RM, Turner R, Thielscher A. How the brain tissue shapes the electric field induced by transcranial magnetic stimulation. *Neuroimage.* 2011;58(3):849–859.

25. Day BL, Dressler D, Maertens de Noordhout A, et al. Electric and magnetic stimulation of human motor cortex: surface EMG and single motor unit responses. *J Physiol.* 1989;412:449–473.

26. Kujirai T, Caramia MD, Rothwell JC, et al. Corticocortical inhibition in human motor cortex. *J Physiol.* 1993;471:501–519.

27. Di Lazzaro V, Pilato F, Oliviero A, et al. Origin of facilitation of motor-evoked potentials after paired magnetic stimulation: direct recording of epidural activity in conscious humans. *J Neurophysiol.* 2006;96(4):1765–1771.

28. Ashby P, Reynolds C, Wennberg R, Lozano AM, Rothwell JC. On the focal nature of inhibition and facilitation in the human motor cortex. *Clin Neurophysiol.* 1999;110(3):550–555.

29. Valls-Sole J, Pascual-Leone A, Wassermann EM, Hallett M. Human motor evoked responses to paired transcranial magnetic stimuli. *Electroencephalogr Clin Neurophysiol.* 1992;85(6):355–364.

II. NEW MODES OF THERAPY

30. Chen R, Lozano AM, Ashby P. Mechanism of the silent period following transcranial magnetic stimulation: evidence from epidural recordings. *Exp Brain Res.* 1999;128(4):539–542.
31. McDonnell MN, Orekhov Y, Ziemann U. The role of GABAB receptors in intracortical inhibition in the human motor cortex. *Exp Brain Res.* 2006;173(1):86–93.
32. Di Lazzaro V, Ziemann U. Modelling of I waves in human motor cortex. The contribution of transcranial magnetic stimulation in the functional evaluation of microcircuits in human motor cortex. *Front Neural Circuits.* 2013;7(18):1–9.
33. Rusu CV, Murakami M, Ziemann U, Triesch J. A model of TMS-induced I-waves in motor cortex. *Brain Stimulation.* 2014;7:401–414.
34. Di Lazzaro V, Profice P, Ranieri F, et al. Origin and modulation. *Brain Stimulation.* 2012;5(4):5512–5525.
35. Douglas RJ, Martin KA, Whitteridge D. A canonical microcircuit for neocortex. *Neural Comput.* 1989;1:480–488.
36. Thomson AM, West DC, Wang Y, Bannister AP. Synaptic connections and small circuits involving excitatory and inhibitory neurons in layers 2–5 of adult rat and cat neocortex: triple intracellular recordings and biocytin labelling in vitro. *Cereb Cortex.* 2002;12:936–953.
37. Phillips CG. Epicortical electrical mapping of motor areas in primates. *Ciba Found Symp.* 1987;132:5–20.
38. Esser SK, Hill SL, Tononi G. Modeling the effects of transcranial magnetic stimulation on cortical circuits. *J Neurophysiol.* 2005;94(1):622–639.
39. Patton HD, Amassian VE. The pyramidal tract: its excitation and functions. 2nd ed. Field J, editor. *Handbook of Physiology-Neurophysiology*, 1960. Washington, DC: American Physiological Society; 1960:837–861.
40. Di Lazzaro V, Profice P, Pilato F, Dileone M, Oliviero A, Ziemann U. The effects of motor cortex rTMS on corticospinal descending activity. *Clin Neurophysiol.* 2010;121(4):464–473.
41. Hoogendam JM, Ramakers GM, Di Lazzaro V. Physiology of repetitive transcranial magnetic stimulation of the human brain. *Brain Stimulation.* 2010;3(2):95–118.
42. Steffan K, Kunesh G, Cohen LG, Benecke R, Classen J. Induction of plasticity in the human motor cortex by paired associative stimulation. *Brain.* 2000;123:573–584.
43. Huang YZ, Edwards MJ, Rounis E, Bhatia KP, Rothwell JC. Theta burst stimulation of the human motor cortex. *Neuron.* 2005;45(2):201–206.
44. Hamada M, Hanajima R, Terao Y, et al. Quadro-pulse stimulation is more effective than paired-pulse stimulation for plasticity induction of the human motor cortex. *Clin Neurophysiol.* 2007;118(12):2672–2682.

8

Transcranial Direct Current Stimulation: From Historical Foundations to Future Directions

F. Fregni[1] and T. Wagner[2]

[1]Harvard Medical School, Boston, MA, United States;
[2]Highland Instruments, Harvard Medical School, and MIT,
Cambridge, MA, United States

Innovative Neuromodulation.
DOI: http://dx.doi.org/10.1016/B978-0-12-800454-8.00008-2

HISTORY

The use of electricity to influence the nervous system predates the invention of the battery by nearly 2000 years. In AD 43 in ancient Greece, a physician, named Scribonious Largus, began experimenting with electrical currents to treat various physiological ailments, such as headaches and gouty arthritis, by applying electric torpedo fish to patients' scalps to relieve headaches or to arthritic joints to relieve pain.[1] Others physicians, such as Pedanius Dioscorides,[2] Charles Le Roy,[3] and Duchenne de Boulogne[4] explored various applications of electromagnetic energy to provide stimulation, but it was Luigi Galvani who ultimately began laying the foundations for modern electrical stimulation in the 18th century.

Galvani demonstrated that muscle that was obtained from a frog could be made to contract if a zinc electrode that was attached to the muscle and a copper electrode on the nerve that innervated the muscle were brought in contact.[5] Galvani incorrectly concluded that the contractions were the result of "animal electricity" or, more specifically, the wire that was attached to the muscle releasing "animal electricity" to return through the closed circuit that was formed by the zinc and copper path through the nerve.[6] In 1793, the Italian physicist Alessandro Volta proposed that the electrical stimulus that mediated the contraction was attributed to the dissimilar electrical properties at the metal–tissue saline interface.[7] Subsequently, in 1800, Volta showed that the voltage difference, due to the unbalanced half-cell potentials of the zinc–saline and copper–saline interfaces, excited the neuromuscular preparation.[5] Then, in 1804, Galvani's nephew, Giovanni Aldini, used voltaic cells to evaluate the use of weak transcranial direct current (DC) to treat individuals who were suffering from depression-like syndromes.[8,9] This work on noninvasive stimulation was largely ignored for over 100 years, although it was one of the first potential therapeutic applications of transcranial direct current stimulation (tDCS).

In the 1960s, researchers began reexamining the effects of weak DC currents on the brain in various animal studies. Bindman reported that currents with magnitudes as low as $0.25\,\mu A/mm^2$, applied to exposed pia via surface electrodes ($3\,\mu A$ from a 12-mm^2 saline cup on the exposed pia surface), could influence spontaneous activity and evoked response of neurons for hours, after several minutes of stimulation in rat preparations.[10,11] Purpura and McMurtry showed similar effects in animal preparations for currents magnitudes as low as $20\,\mu A/mm^2$ from cortical surface electrodes.[12] Furthermore, researchers demonstrated that current polarity (orientation), relative to a neural fiber, was a key factor in determining whether the neural targets were facilitated or suppressed (i.e., whether the spontaneous activity increased or declined and whether the magnitudes of evoked potentials rose or fell following stimulation).

Such studies from the 1960s[10–13] showed that surface-positive cortical polarization (anode placement) excites the cortex and that the opposite effect is seen with surface-negative polarization (cathodal placement). Landau et al. observed that the surface effects could be reversed by placing the stimulation source in deeper locations, such that the current density orientations are reversed relative to the stimulated neurons compared with the surface electrode locations.[13] In an ex vivo neural preparation, Terzuolo and Bullock noted that the change in neural firing frequency due to weak DC currents could be modulated, based on the relative current to neural fiber orientations.[14] Overall, these researchers showed that currents, at magnitudes that were much lower than those necessary to initiate an action potential, could still alter levels of neural excitability and that the direction of modulation (i.e., inhibition or facilitation) was affected by the relative neural fiber-to-current orientation. These studies led physicians to examine the efficacy of weak transcranial DC currents for the treatment of depression,[15–18] but due to inconsistencies in treatment protocols and clinical outcomes, the use of transcranial DC stimulation was largely abandoned until the late 1990s since when its use has greatly expanded.

TECHNICAL ASPECTS

During tDCS, a low-amplitude current is applied to the cortex transcranially via electrodes that are fixed to the scalp surface (see Fig. 8.1A). In their simplest form, tDCS stimulation units are DC sources (batteries) that are placed in series, with scalp electrodes and potentiometers (variable resistors) to adjust the constant current (Fig. 8.1B), although in commercial practice, systems usually rely on more complex circuitry to ensure safety and reliability. tDCS electrodes can be simple saline-soaked cotton pads or specifically designed conductive patches and range in size, depending on the application (from ~1 to 35 cm^2; see "Applied Dose (Dose at the tDCS Source)" section).

For stimulation, tDCS implements DCs for a fixed period across a range of intensities and durations, depending on the application (e.g., ~0.5–2 mA applied for minutes in single or multiple sessions for several days; see "Applied Dose (Dose at the tDCS Source)" section). Whereas DCs are fundamental to tDCS, various applied current waveforms have been implemented for other transcranial electrical stimulation (TES) methods, including balanced stepped signals (cranial electrical stimulation), low-frequency sinusoidal signals (transcranial alternating current stimulation), and randomized signals (transcranial random noise stimulation); although these techniques are used in TES, this section focuses on tDCS.

tDCS can be characterized by the *applied stimulation dose* at the stimulation source, based on the total current, electrode size/shape and position,

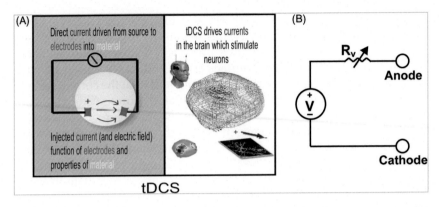

FIGURE 8.1   (A) Transcranial Direct Current Stimulation (tDCS) currents are influenced by the tDCS electrodes (e.g., geometry and location) and electromagnetic properties (e.g., impedance properties) of the stimulated tissue. Partially adapted from Refs. [19,20]. (B) A tDCS device in its most simple form is a battery and a variable resistor (i.e., potentiometer). Partially adapted from Refs. [19,20].

and time of application; but, the *effective dose of stimulation* (at the site of activation [e.g., cortical targets]) is influenced by the anatomic characteristics of the subject who is undergoing stimulation, the properties of the tissues in the head, and the direction of the current relative to the stimulated neural targets. The applied dose can be definitively characterized relatively easily. However, the accuracy of the effective dose of stimulation at the target site depends on the quality of the analysis and patient-specific information that are used to calculate the dose; as technological resources become more readily available, the quality of these data will continue to improve.

To intuitively understand transcranially injected cortical currents and the importance of the parameters that are used to determine the active and effective dose of stimulation, we present a simple resistor model of a head system with a 7 × 5-cm anode above M1 and a 7 × 5-cm cathode above the contralateral orbit that is receiving tDCS. (Please note that this overly simple model, based on a basic multisphere model that was developed from the MRI scan of a 38-year-old male, is provided to facilitate an understanding of the effects of tissues on current intensities and current directions, whereas more complicated issues are addressed below.)

To calculate the resistance of the tissue, we assume that currents can flow parallel to the surface of the tissue or axially through the tissue and that the tissue resistance can be estimated as rectangular resistors (resistance = length/[area × σ]) (see Fig. 8.2). The length of the parallel tissue resistors was determined by assuming that the current flowed along the shortest distance from the anode to cathode. Thus, for a parallel skin resistor, the resistor length would be 6 cm (the circumferential distance from M1 to the contralateral orbit along the scalp of a 38-year-old male). We

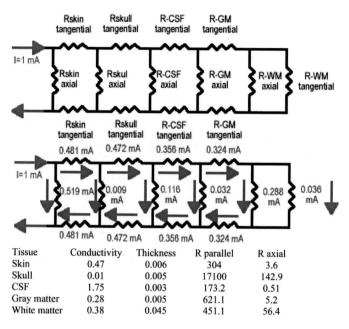

Tissue	Conductivity	Thickness	R parallel	R axial
Skin	0.47	0.006	304	3.6
Skull	0.01	0.005	17100	142.9
CSF	1.75	0.003	173.2	0.51
Gray matter	0.28	0.005	621.1	5.2
White matter	0.38	0.045	451.1	56.4

FIGURE 8.2   Simplified tDCS circuit model of currents injected in the human brain. From Ref. [21].

assumed that the current flowed uniformly from electrode to electrode, and thus, the area could be determined from the thickness of the tissue region and the dimension of the electrode, assumed to be normal to the current flow (determined by the shortest distance). For the skin, the area of the parallel resistor would be 7 × 0.6 cm, which is the cross-length of the electrode on the skin and the thickness of the skin. For simplicity, the circumferential length was considered to be 6 cm for each tissue. With regard to axial resistance, the electrode area was used as the resistor area, and the thickness of the tissue was considered to be the resistor length. For white matter, the distance from electrode to electrode was estimated to be 6.5 cm.

The values in the model are tabulated and displayed in Fig. 8.2 (with the solved currents and resistor values). With the circuit as solved in Fig. 8.2, the tangential current magnitude in the cortex is 31.6 μA, and the axial current magnitude is 0.324 mA. Using the areas of the resistors to determine the current densities of each current component, the axial and tangential current densities in the cortex are 0.093 and 0.090 A/m², respectively. These values have the same order of magnitude as the current densities that were recorded by Bindman in the animal experiments reviewed above[10,11] that were performed to alter neural excitability levels (and similar magnitudes as the values in the finite element model tDCS models reviewed below).

Although the simplified resistor model above is not appropriate to guide stimulation decisions, it has been provided to highlight the importance of the relative source characteristics, electromagnetic tissue properties of the head, and anatomic tissue distribution in influencing the magnitude and orientation of the stimulating cortical current density. To examine complicated aspects of current flow in the targeted tissue, one generally relies on sophisticated biophysical models of electromagnetic fields.[20] In turn, electromagnetic field distributions have been used to predict the cellular mechanism of activation,[22,23] location,[20,24] focality,[25–27] depth of penetration,[28,29] and degree of stimulation.[20,30] The field distributions can also be used to perform a quantitative analysis of the safety parameters[20,31,32] and the technological potential of brain stimulation.[20]

Although electromagnetic models provide information about stimulating field distributions, they are merely one source of information in validating the technical aspects of brain stimulation. Phantom studies, animal-based field recordings, human-based field recordings, and imaging studies are additional points of reference in analyzing the fundamental aspects of brain stimulation.[19,33–42]

PARAMETERS OF STIMULATION

Applied Dose (Dose at the tDCS Source)

In clinical practice, the applied "dose" of a tDCS session is determined by the following factors: (1) the size and location of the electrodes, (2) the current intensity, (3) the duration of the sessions, and (4) the total number of sessions (and the interval between them). Note that the effective dose at the site of stimulation is not equivalent to the applied dose (see "Effective Dose (Dose at Site of Activation)" section).

1. Size/shape/position—tDCS electrodes usually measure 25–35 cm^2 (5 × 5 to 5 × 7 cm^2). In two-electrode systems, larger electrodes render the stimulus less focal; conversely, smaller electrodes increase the focality of the stimulus;[43,44] although it can make the effects of stimulation more variable. In addition, the enhanced focality from smaller electrodes often comes at the expense of current penetration, especially with atypically small electrodes,[20] and can necessitate higher source current densities (which can be painful or result in scalp irritation) to reach cortical targets.
2. Electric current intensity—The first modern tDCS studies used low current intensities in the range of 0.5 mA,[45,46] whereas more current tDCS studies and clinical trials apply higher doses (1–2 mA).[47] For electrodes between 25 and 35 cm^2, the applied current density is 0.4–0.8 A/m^2. Electric currents below 0.5 mA do not seem to have

neuromodulatory effects with typical electrode sizes (i.e., 25–35 cm^2), especially when applied for short periods[46]; in turn, current doses of 1.5–2 mA are often perceived by the subject (with typical electrode sizes), and doses that exceed 2 mA might be painful or uncomfortable to participants.

Although currents higher than 2 mA (given traditional electrode sizes) are potentially safe according to animal studies; it has not been formally tested. Higher electric source currents are associated with greater current densities at a fixed target point in the brain. However, it is unknown whether higher doses are associated with an increased impact on neuroplasticity. Some studies have reported greater cognitive improvement with higher current doses,[48,49] whereas recent meta-analyses have failed to demonstrate any intensity-dependent effects of tDCS in cognitive tDCS studies[50] and in clinical trials of tDCS for depression.[51]

3. Duration of the tDCS session—A tDCS session last from 5 to 35 minutes, but the maximum "safe" period for which tDCS can be applied and the optimal time for clinical efficacy have not been established. For practical purposes, tDCS sessions that exceed 30 minutes are undesirable in cognitive studies (because longer stimulation periods can increase fatigue and compromise performance in cognitive tasks) and clinical trials, in which patients should return to receive tDCS for several consecutive days.

4. Total number of and interval between sessions—Neuropsychological studies, in which tDCS is usually applied two or three times (anodal, cathodal, and sham sessions), are designed to address mechanistic questions and typically do not evaluate the cumulative effects of tDCS. Thus, such studies usually implement a 2–7-day interval between tDCS sessions.

In contrast, clinical trials aim to determine the cumulative effects of tDCS; thus, tDCS is applied once or twice daily for several days, usually excluding weekends (for a review, see Ref. [52]). For instance, most clinical studies on major depression[53–55] have applied tDCS once per day for 10–15 days. Conversely, the largest randomized clinical trial that administered tDCS for schizophrenia performed two sessions per day for five consecutive days.[56] Further studies are warranted to determine the optimal interval between tDCS sessions and to examine how long the effects of tDCS persist after several tDCS sessions.

Effective Dose (Dose at Site of Activation)

The effective dose of stimulation can help one understand the unique response of an individual patient and help establish patient-specific dosing regimens (however, complete knowledge of the effective dose is not necessary to apply tDCS effectively in the clinic just as an incomplete understanding of the fundamental pharmacological biochemistry does not preclude one from establishing dosing guidelines of drug therapies). The effective dose at the target site of stimulation is influenced by the patient head anatomy, patient tissue characteristics, and neural distribution at the target site, in addition to the criteria above on the characteristics of the applied dose of stimulation (i.e., at the stimulation source).

1. Patient anatomy: The shape of the head (and the distribution of the various individual tissues below the scalp) influences the distribution of the stimulation current. As demonstrated above with the simple resistor model, the relative shape of the head and stimulating electrode montage are key in determining the shape and distribution of the resistive network along which the stimulating currents flow (i.e., the magnitude of a resistor depends directly on its geometry, and the relative distribution of multiple resistors determines the total resistance of the resistor circuit that makes up the head and brain).

2. Tissue characteristics: The electromagnetic properties of the tissues (i.e., tissue conductivities) influence and constrain the stimulating electromagnetic fields in them. As demonstrated above with the simple resistor model, tissue conductivities govern the magnitude of the resistance of the resistive network along which the stimulating currents flow (i.e., the magnitude of a resistor depends directly on its conductivity and electromagnetic boundary conditions, which constrain the current flow between tissue layers of dissimilar tissue conductivities).

3. Neural distribution: Since the early animal studies of DC fields in neural activity,[10–13] it has been known that the relative distribution of electromagnetic fields to the orientation of the neural cell influences the neural response. Ultimately, the integration of cortical neural distribution models (and potentially tractography for methods that penetrate deep enough) and electromagnetic field distribution models through neural response models could guide patient-specific dosing recommendations.

With improved computational resources, computational models now include more realistic geometries[25,32,57–62] and tissue properties,[24,36,63] all of which can be used to predict the effective dose of stimulation more effectively. Similarly, phantom models, animal models, and neural preparation studies are means for studying the effective dose of stimulation. Ultimately, these fundamental studies can increase our understanding of the effective dose of stimulation and tailor stimulation to individual patients.

SAFETY

With typical current levels and experimental protocols, the side effects of tDCS are mild, benign, and short-lived. In a recent systematic review,[64] data from tDCS studies were reviewed through 2010. Of 172 articles, 56% discussed adverse effects and 63% reported at least one adverse effect. Notably, when assessed systematically, the rates of common adverse effects did not differ between the active and sham arms of the studies. These effects included itching (39.3% vs 32.9%, respectively), tingling (22.2% vs 18.3%), headache (14.8% vs 16.2%), burning sensation (8.7% vs 10%), and discomfort (10.4% vs 13.4%). However, most studies did not systematically evaluate adverse effects. There have been no phase I studies published using tDCS.

Although there are no data that correlate the presence of local adverse effects with the total amount of charge that was delivered in this systematic review, clinically, high current intensities (>2 mA with typical electrode sizes [≥25 cm^2], i.e., with higher applied current densities) are associated with more adverse effects. Also, electrolyte solutions with lower NaCl concentrations (15 mM) appear to be more comfortable during tDCS than those with higher NaCl concentrations (220 mM). Dundas et al.[65] recommended solutions with relatively low NaCl concentrations, in the range 15–140 mM, within which tDCS is more likely to be perceived as comfortable, requires low voltage, and still allows good conduction of current.

Although commonly ignored, tDCS-induced erythema (skin reddening) is an adverse effect that is significantly more frequent in active versus sham groups.[66] This condition is likely attributed to an increase in blood flow in dermal vessels that accompanies the current application. Although this effect is generally benign, it might compromise the blinding of the study in randomized, sham-controlled trials[66] and thus should be minimized. On rare occasions, tDCS causes skin burns[67] but only when standard procedures regarding tDCS application (such as correct preparation of the skin, humidification of sponges with saline, and limit of voltage/current above maximum impedance) are not followed.[68,69] Thus, the safety of tDCS is ensured only with the appropriate tDCS equipment, accessories, and protocols.

Studies have not found any significant abnormal changes in electroencephalographic activity[70] or heart rate variability.[71–73] The threshold for adverse effects was suggested in a safety study in rats,[74] in which the charge density that was necessary to induce brain damage was found to be at least 100 times higher than that in tDCS trials. Because skin discomfort and pain are induced with currents that are 2–3 times higher than those in most tDCS experiments, it is highly unlikely that the safety threshold would ever be reached in human tDCS studies.

tDCS is considered to be safe—the (battery-driven) tDCS device is bio-medically secure, delivering low-dose current with subthreshold effects in cortical excitability, and no major or serious adverse effects of tDCS have been reported. Nevertheless, such findings do not guarantee that tDCS is "universally safe" and thus can be "allowed" to be used loosely. There are no data regarding tDCS use beyond the common limits in experimental settings regarding current intensity, session duration, and the interval between sessions. Given the ease in both developing and applying tDCS devices, there are potential risks in the use of tDCS using adapted, non-commercial devices and/or applying tDCS without proper supervision and regulatory approval. Furthermore, it is possible that tDCS enhances activity in a particular area of the brain at the expense of declining activity in another region. For instance, a recent trial has shown that tDCS induces antidepressant effects, but it also prevents the acquisition of implicit learning during a probabilistic classification learning task, possibly by decreasing the activity in parts of the brain that mediate implicit memory learning.[75] In this context, application of the incorrect stimulation parameters for several days might have undesired consequences, leading to maladaptive plasticity.

In summary, although potentially safe, tDCS is a relatively novel technique, necessitating longer-term follow-up studies to fully determine its clinical safety.

CLINICAL APPLICATION

One of the basic effects of tDCS is to modulate cortical excitability.[20,44,46,76,77] tDCS has been examined as a therapeutic intervention in many clinical disorders, including depression, chronic pain, stroke, and Parkinson disease (PD).[78–86] After stroke, daily sessions of tDCS improve upper limb function (effect size [ES = 0.49, 95% CI = 0.18–0.81]).[87] At the 3-month follow-up, tDCS increased scores on activities of daily living (MD 11.13 Barthel Index points; 95% CI 2.89–19).[88] A meta-analysis demonstrated that in patients with mild-to-moderate stroke impairments (ES = 0.37), various tDCS techniques—with or without adjunct physical therapy—improved motor function (ES = 0.45).[89] Anodal tDCS over perilesional areas improves language function, but the effect persisted only when tDCS was coupled with language training.[90,91] More research is required to determine the efficacy of tDCS for practical language rehabilitation (anodal/cathodal/dual), primarily by examining the stability of the improvement over clinically significant periods.[88]

For example, administering cathodal stimulation over the injured cortex, Monti et al.[92] reported that although tDCS in aphasia elicited a gain in speech performance of approximately 25%, this effect was transient.[92]

There has been considerable interest in treating depression with asymmetrical application of tDCS to the frontal lobes (typically with the anodal electrode over the left dorsolateral prefrontal cortex (DLPFC) and the cathode over the right supraorbital cortex). The most recent meta-analysis, incorporating all randomized controlled trials (RCTs) to date, found that active tDCS was more effective than a sham stimulation comparator.[93] However, based on the limited number of RCTs that exist ($n = 7$), the evidence for the antidepressant efficacy of tDCS can not be considered conclusive, for which further trials are required. Earlier meta-analyses reported mixed findings, likely due to the heterogeneity in the evidence base.[51,94] The concurrent antidepressant drug treatment may interfere with tDCS effects and explain some of the variability in its effects.

As monotherapy, tDCS effected a 63% response rate, with remission rates more than doubling versus sham control.[51] In other reviews of tDCS and depression, the odds ratio (OR) for a favorable symptom response was 1.63 (95% CI = 1.26–2.12), and the OR for remission was 2.50 (95% CI = 1.26–2.49).[93] When an acute course of tDCS was followed by weekly to biweekly maintenance tDCS sessions, the cumulative probability of avoiding relapse was 83.7% at 3 months and 51.1% at 6 months.[95] Five sessions of anodal stimulation induced a beneficial effect in major depressive disorder and bipolar depressive disorder, examined separately, that persists at 1 week and 1 month in both groups.[96]

In schizophrenic patients who were refractory to medication, cathodal tDCS over the left temporoparietal junction, coupled with anodal tDCS over the left DLPFC, reduced auditory verbal hallucinations by 31%, lasting for up to 3 months. Also, the general severity of illness improved on the positive and negative syndrome scale (ES = 0.98, 95% CI = 0.22–1.73).[56]

In studies of the effects of tDCS on pain sensitivity in healthy subjects, anodal stimulation increases the pain threshold and improves tolerance compared with sham stimulation.[97] Cathodal stimulation reduces the sensitivity to Aδ-fiber-mediated cold sensations and C-fiber-mediated warm sensations versus baseline, whereas Aß-fiber-mediated somatosensory inputs are less affected.[98] In patients who undergo total knee arthroplasty, tDCS reduces opioid consumption and pain levels.[99]

In treating chronic pain, regardless of etiology, the ES of tDCS ranges from −2.29 (95% CI = −3.5 to −1.08)[100] to −0.86 (95% CI = −1.54 to −0.19).[101] Although a prespecified subgroup analysis in a meta-analysis of distinct types of chronic pain indicated that tDCS was superior than sham (ES − 0.59, 95% CI = −1.10 to −0.08),[102] a subsequent meta-analysis failed to detect the superiority of tDCS over sham in reducing pain,[103] possibly due to heterogeneity. The analgesic effects of tDCS, combined with a technique of visual illusion, were better for all pain subtypes, whereas tDCS alone only improved continuous and paroxysmal pain.[104] Also, tDCS, combined with visual illusion, improves neuropathic pain in spinal cord injury patients, who experienced a 50% mean decrease in symptoms.[85] In episodic migraine without aura, anodal preventive treatment reduces the frequency of migraine attacks, days with migraine, attack duration, and intake of acute medication. These benefits persisted for an average of 4.8 weeks after the end of treatment.[105] In chronic migraine, the anodal effect on the primary motor cortex induces a delayed response.[81] Recent evidence also suggests the potential of tDCS in treating phantom limb pain.[106,107]

Although the effects of tDCS on pain vary, the benefits in chronic pain are promising and justify the use of tDCS in treating pain in select patient populations. Overall, studies of anodal stimulation have demonstrated at least a moderate effect. Two excitability-enhancing (anodal) tDCS techniques have analgesic effects—one with the anode over the primary motor cortex, with a mean ES of 9.59%,[108–110] and the other with the anode over the DLPFC, with a mean ES of 15.79%.[111] Typically, the analgesic effects are cumulative, with most clinical trials providing stimulation on five consecutive days (with some extending over 10 days).

This area of research is plagued by several problems, such as the heterogeneity of the studies, which makes specific comparisons difficult; the lack of systematic intention-to-treat designs; and the high dropout rates. New placebo-controlled studies on tDCS for the treatment of pain that include systematic follow-up per the Initiative on Methods, Measurement, and Pain Assessment in Clinical Trials are required.[112]

A recent meta-analysis examined the use of frontal lobe tDCS (and rTMS [repetitive transcranial magnetic stimulation]) to reduce craving substance dependence and highly palatable food.[113] rTMS and tDCS over the DLPFC had an SE of 0.48 (95% CI = 0.316–0.636), with no significant difference between treatments. In the management of tinnitus, anodal tDCS reduces the intensity of symptoms, with an SE of 0.77 (95% CI = 0.23–1.31).[114] Anodal tDCS over premotor areas also improves sleep and fatigue symptoms in patients with postpolio syndrome.[115]

FUTURE DIRECTIONS

Future Studies With tDCS

These 15 years of research with tDCS have confirmed that tDCS induces significant neurophysiological and clinical effects. Effects are robust in some of the clinical conditions tested. Based on these results, we recommend the following future studies:

1. *Replication of clinical studies*: it is critical that initial clinical trials are replicated independently by other laboratories. These results are important to validate tDCS use for a future clinical application.

For most of the clinical applications, there is a lack of independent replications of tDCS findings.

2. *Larger sample size clinical studies*: accordingly, future clinical trials testing initial pilot and preliminary findings with a more robust sample sizes are also necessary for future development of tDCS. These clinical trials need to also test clinical functional outcomes.

3. *Combined treatments*: given the initial results of combined treatment effects; further testing of tDCS with other behavioral therapies and pharmacological approaches would be useful for enhancing tDCS clinical effects.

4. *Use of neurophysiological outcomes*: the use of neurophysiological outcomes is important to predict responders and also to adjust parameters of tDCS. Further research in this area is needed.

Future Technologies

The past decade has witnessed a rapid increase in the application of neurostimulation methods to treat various diseases, such as chronic pain and PD.[20,108,116–118] Current stimulation techniques attempt to balance invasiveness and efficacy, wherein the most effective methods require surgical procedures to implant stimulation devices in the nervous system.[20,116] Thus, the most widely used stimulation tools are invasive, such as deep brain stimulation.[116,119–121] These techniques rely on implanted devices that stimulate brain tissue by injecting electrical currents directly into the tissue. Although the stimulating electrode and targeted tissues influence the final stimulating current density distributions, the major limiting factor is not the technology or physics of the stimulation but the potential for surgical complications.[122–124] These invasive methods are most effective due to their focality, ability to stimulate deeper locations, and ability to precisely target neural tissue. However, because of their associated costs and risks, the therapeutic need for noninvasive options is enormous.

Noninvasive methods, such as tDCS, have been developed to provide stimulation without the risks that accompany surgical stimulation methods.[20] These techniques are notable for their online (i.e., during stimulation) and offline effects, in which the therapeutic activity continues past the period of stimulation if the appropriate stimulation parameters are applied over multiple sessions on consecutive days.[49,118,125–138] tDCS takes advantage of electromagnetic principles to inject currents into cortical tissue. However, these principles limit the focality, penetration, and targeting control of the stimulating currents, translating into limited therapeutic efficacy compared with invasive modalities.[20,63,139–141]

Methods for improving or replacing conventional tDCS have been explored, such as high-definition tDCS (HD-tDCS),[142] which uses multiple electrodes to localize the fields, and electrosonic stimulation, which combines independently controlled electromagnetic and ultrasonic fields. In electrosonic stimulation, the combined fields are believed to focus and boost neurostimulation currents via tuned electromechanical coupling in neural tissue. Electrosonic stimulation, with DC fields coupled to ultrasound, has shown superiority to tDCS and transcranial ultrasound (provided individually) in preclinical studies, and electrosonic stimulation has demonstrated clinical and statistical effectiveness in both Parkinson disease and chronic pain conditions.[143,144]

CONCLUSION

tDCS is a technique that has considerable potential in examining and altering brain function. As we raise our understanding of tDCS methods and their supporting technologies, the limitations that are associated with them will be overcome, leading to improved tDCS technologies and possibly entirely new noninvasive methodologies that can selectively provide controlled cortical and deep brain stimulation.

References

1. Largus S. *De compositionibus medicamentorum*. Paris: Wechel; 1529.
2. Kellaway P. The part played by electric fish in the early history of bioelectricity and electrotherapy. *Bull Hist Med*. 1946;20(2):112–137.
3. Pascual-Leone A, Wagner T. A brief summary of the history of noninvasive brain stimulation (supplement to noninvasive human brain stimulation). *Annu Rev Biomed Eng*. 2007;9:s1–7.
4. Duchenne de Boulogne G. L'Electrisation Localisee; 1855.
5. Randall D, Burggren W, et al. *Animal Physiology*. New York, W.H: Freeman and Company; 1997.
6. Piccolino M. Luigi Galvani and animal electricity: two centuries after the foundation of electrophysiology. *Trends Neurosci*. 1997;20(10):443–448.
7. Galvani L, Valli E, et al. Aloysi Galvani abhandlung über die kräfte der thierischen elektrizität auf die bewegung der muskeln. Prag J.G. Calve; 1793.
8. Aldini G. De animali electricitate dissertationes duae. Bologna; 1794.
9. Aldini G. *Essai theorique et experimental sur le galvanisme*. Paris: Fournier; 1804.
10. Bindman LJ, Lippold OC, et al. Long-lasting changes in the level of the electrical activity of the cerebral cortex produced bypolarizing currents. *Nature*. 1962;196:584–585.
11. Bindman LJ, Lippold OC, et al. Comparison of the effects on electrocortical activity of general body cooling of the surface of the brain. *Electroencephalogr Clin Neurophysiol*. 1963;15:238–245.
12. Purpura D, McMurtry J. Intracellular activities and evoked potential changes during polarization of motor cortex. *J Neurophysiol*. 1965;28:166–185.
13. Landau WM, Bishop GH, et al. Analysis of the form and distribution of evoked cortical potentials under the influence of polarizing currents. *J Neurophysiol*. 1964;27:788–813.
14. Terzuolo CA, Bullock TH. Measurement of imposed voltage gradient adequate to modulate neuronal firing. *Proc Natl Acad Sci USA*. 1956;42(9):687–694.
15. Sheffield LJ, Mowbray RM. The effect of polarization on normal subjects. *Br J Psychiatry*. 1968;114:225–232.

16. Hall KM, Hicks RA, et al. The effects of low level DC scalp positive and negative current on the performance of various tasks. *Br J Psychiatry*. 1970;117:689–691.

17. Lippold OC, Redfearn JW. Mental changes resulting from the passage of small direct currents through the human brain. *Br J Psychiatry*. 1964;110:768–772.

18. Lolas F. Brain polarization: behavioral and therapeutic effects. *Br J Psychiatry*. 1976;12(1):1977.

19. Wagner T, Rushmore J, et al. Biophysical foundations underlying TMS: setting the stage for an effective use of neurostimulation in the cognitive neurosciences. *Cortex*. 2009;45(9):1025–1034.

20. Wagner T, Valero-Cabre A, et al. Noninvasive human brain stimulation. *Annu Rev Biomed Eng*. 2007;9:527–565.

21. Wagner T. *Non Invasive Brain Stimulation: Modeling and Experimental Analysis of Transcranial Magnetic Stimulation and Transcranial DC Stimulation as a Modality for Neuropathology Treatment*. MIT/Harvard Medical School; 2006.

22. Roth B, Basser P. A model of stimulation of a nerve fiber by electromagnetic induction. *IEEE Trans Biomed Eng*. 1990;37:588–597.

23. Nagarajan S, Durand DM, et al. Effects of induced electric fields on finite neuronal structures: a simulation study. *IEEE Trans Biomed Eng*. 1993;40(11):1175–1188.

24. De Lucia M, Parker GJ, et al. Diffusion tensor MRI-based estimation of the influence of brain tissue anisotropy on the effects of transcranial magnetic stimulation. *Neuroimage*. 2007;36(4):1159–1170.

25. Toschi N, Welt T, et al. Transcranial magnetic stimulation in heterogeneous brain tissue: clinical impact on focality, reproducibility and true sham stimulation. *J Psychiatr Res*. 2008;43(3):255–264.

26. Ueno S, Tashiro T, et al. Localised stimulation of neural tissues in the brain by means of a paired configuration of time-varying magnetic fields. *J Appl Phys*. 1988;64:5862–5864.

27. Cohen D, Cuffin BN. Developing a more focal magnetic stimulator. Part 1: some basic principles. *J Clin Neurophysiol*. 1991;8:102–111.

28. Zangen A, Roth Y, et al. Transcranial magnetic stimulation of deep brain regions: evidence for efficacy of the H-coil. *Clin Neurophysiol*. 2005;116(4):775–779.

29. Heller L, Hulsteyn DBV. Brain stimulation using electromagnetic sources: theoretical aspects. *Biophys J*. 1992;63:129–138.

30. Bohning DE, Pecheny AP, et al. Mapping transcranial magnetic stimulation (TMS) fields in vivo with MRI. *Neuroreport*. 1997;8(11):2535–2538.

31. McCreery D, Agnew W. Neuronal and axonal injury during functional electrical stimulation; a review of the possible mechanisms. *Annual International Conference of the IEEE Engineering in Medicine and Biology Society*. IEEE; 1990.

32. McCreery D, Agnew W, et al. Charge density and charge per phase as cofactors in neural injury induced by electrical stimulation. *IEEE Trans Biomed Eng*. 1990;37(10): 996–1001.

33. Tay G. Measurement of current density distribution induced in vivo during magnetic stimulation. PhD, Marquette University; 1992.

34. Tay GCM, Battocletti J, Sances Jr. A, Swiontek T. Mapping of current densities induced in vivo during magnetic stimulation. *Annual International Conference of the IEEE Engineering in Medicine and Biology Society*. IEEE; 1991.

35. Tay GCM, Battocletti J, Sances Jr. A, Swiontek T, Kurakami C. Measurement of magnetically induced current density in saline and in vivo. *Engineering in Medicine and Biology Society, 1989. Images of the Twenty-First Century. Proceedings of the Annual International Conference of the IEEE*. 1989;4:1167–1168.

36. Wagner TA, Zahn M, et al. Three-dimensional head model simulation of transcranial magnetic stimulation. *IEEE Trans Biomed Eng*. 2004;51(9):1586–1598.

37. Yunokuchi K, Cohen D. Developing a more focal magnetic stimulator. Part 2: fabricating coils and measuring induced current distributions. *J Clin Neurophysiol*. 1991;8(1):112–120.

38. Yunokuchi K, Koyoshi R, et al. Estimation of focus of electric field in an inhomogenous medium exposed by pulsed magnetic field. *IEEE First Joint BMES/EMBS Conference Serving Humanity and Advancing Technology.* Atlanta, GA, USA: IEEE; 1999.

39. Cohen LG, Roth BJ, et al. Effects of coil design on delivery of focal magnetic stimulation. Technical considerations. *Electroenceph Clin Neurophysiol.* 1989;75:350–357.

40. Joy ML, Lebedev VP, et al. Imaging of current density and current pathways in rabbit brain during transcranial electrostimulation. *IEEE Trans Biomed Eng.* 1999;46(9):1139–1149.

41. Lisanby S. Intercerebral measurements of rTMS and ECS induced voltage in vivo. *Biol Psychiatry.* 1998;43:100s.

42. Maccabee PJ, Eberle L, et al. Spatial distribution of the electric field induced in volume by round and figure '8' magnetic coils: relevance to activation of sensory nerve fibers. *Electroenceph Clin Neurophysiol.* 1990;76:131–141.

43. Parazzini M, Fiocchi S, et al. Transcranial direct current stimulation: estimation of the electric field and of the current density in an anatomical human head model. *IEEE Trans Biomed Eng.* 2011;58(6).

44. Nitsche MA, Doemkes S, et al. Shaping the effects of transcranial direct current stimulation of the human motor cortex. *J Neurophysiol.* 2007;97(4):3109–3117.

45. Priori A, Berardelli A, et al. Polarization of the human motor cortex through the scalp. *Neuroreport.* 1998;9(10):2257–2260.

46. Nitsche MA, Paulus W. Excitability changes induced in the human motor cortex by weak transcranial direct current stimulation. *J Physiol.* 2000;527(Pt 3):633–639.

47. Brunoni AR, Amadera J, et al. A systematic review on reporting and assessment of adverse effects associated with transcranial direct current stimulation. *Int J Neuropsychopharmacol.* 2011;14(8):1133–1145.

48. Iyer MB, Mattu U, et al. Safety and cognitive effect of frontal DC brain polarization in healthy individuals. *Neurology.* 2005;64(5):872–875.

49. Boggio PS, Ferrucci R, et al. Effects of transcranial direct current stimulation on working memory in patients with Parkinson's disease. *J Neurol Sci.* 2006;249(1):31–38.

50. Jacobson L, Koslowsky M, et al. tDCS polarity effects in motor and cognitive domains: a meta-analytical review. *Exp Brain Res.* 2012;216(1):1–10.

51. Berlim MT, Van den Eynde F, et al. Clinical utility of transcranial direct current stimulation (tDCS) for treating major depression: a systematic review and meta-analysis of randomized, double-blind and sham-controlled trials. *J Psychiatr Res.* 2013;47(1):1–7.

52. Kuo MF, Paulus W, et al. Therapeutic effects of non-invasive brain stimulation with direct currents (tDCS) in neuropsychiatric diseases. *Neuroimage.* 2013;85(Pt 3).

53. Shiozawa P, Fregni F, et al. Transcranial direct current stimulation for major depression: an updated systematic review and meta-analysis. *Int J Neuropsychopharmacol.* 2014:1–10.

54. Brunoni AR, Valiengo L, et al. The sertraline versus electrical current therapy for treating depression clinical study: results from a factorial, randomized, controlled trial. *JAMA Psychiatry.* 2013;70(4):383–391.

55. Loo CK, Alonzo A, et al. Transcranial direct current stimulation for depression: 3-week, randomised, sham-controlled trial. *Br J Psychiatry.* 2012;200(1):52–59.

56. Brunelin J, Mondino M, et al. Examining transcranial direct-current stimulation (tDCS) as a treatment for hallucinations in schizophrenia. *Am J Psychiatry.* 2012;169(7):719–724.

57. Sadleir RJ, Vannorsdall TD, et al. Transcranial direct current stimulation (tDCS) in a realistic head model. *Neuroimage.* 2010;51(4):1310–1318.

58. Salvador R, Mekonnen A, et al. Modeling the electric field induced in a high resolution realistic head model during transcranial current stimulation. *Conf Proc IEEE Eng Med Biol Soc.* 2010:2073–2076.

59. Datta A, Bansal V, et al. Gyriprecise head model of transcranial DC stimulation: Improved spatial focality using a ring electrode versus conventional rectangular pad. *Brain Stimul.* 2009;2(4):201–207.

60. Datta A, Elwassif M, et al. Transcranial current stimulation focality using disc and ring electrode configurations: FEM analysis. *J Neural Eng*. 2008;5(2):163–174.

61. Lu M, Ueno S, et al. Calculating the activating function in the human brain by transcranial magnetic stimulation. *IEEE Trans Mag*. 2008;44(6):1438–1441.

62. Nadeem M, Thorlin T, et al. Computation of electric and magnetic stimulation in human head using the 3-D impedance method. *IEEE Trans Biomed Eng*. 2003;50(7):900–907.

63. Miranda PC, Hallett M, et al. The electric field induced in the brain by magnetic stimulation: a 3-D finite-element analysis of the effect of tissue heterogeneity and anisotropy. *IEEE Trans Biomed Eng*. 2003;50(9):1074–1085.

64. Brunoni AR, Amadera J, et al. A systematic review on reporting and assessment of adverse effects associated with transcranial direct current stimulation. *Int J Neuropsychopharmacol*. 2011:1–13.

65. Dundas JE, Thickbroom GW, et al. Perception of comfort during transcranial DC stimulation: effect of NaCl solution concentration applied to sponge electrodes. *Clin Neurophysiol*. 2007;118(5):1166–1170.

66. O'Connell NE, Cossar J, et al. Rethinking clinical trials of transcranial direct current stimulation: participant and assessor blinding is inadequate at intensities of 2mA. *PLoS ONE*. 2012;7(10):e47514.

67. Palm U, Keeser D, et al. Transcranial direct current stimulation in a patient with therapy-resistant major depression. *World J Biol Psychiatry*. 2009;10(4 Pt 2):632–635.

68. Brunoni AR, Nitsche MA, et al. Clinical research with transcranial direct current stimulation (tDCS): challenges and future directions. *Brain Stimul*. 2012;5(3):175–195.

69. Nitsche MA, Cohen LG, et al. Transcranial direct current stimulation: state of the art 2008. *Brain Stimul*. 2008;1(3):206–223.

70. Tadini L, El-Nazer R, et al. Cognitive, mood, and electroencephalographic effects of non-invasive cortical stimulation with weak electrical currents. *J ECT*. 2011;27(2):134–140.

71. Sampaio LA, Fraguas R, et al. A systematic review of non-invasive brain stimulation therapies and cardiovascular risk: implications for the treatment of major depressive disorder. *Front Psychiatry*. 2012;3:87.

72. Brunoni AR, Kemp AH, et al. Heart rate variability is a trait marker of major depressive disorder: evidence from the sertraline vs. electric current therapy to treat depression clinical study. *Int J Neuropsychopharmacol*. 2013;16(9):1937–1949.

73. Clancy JA, Johnson R, et al. Anodal transcranial direct current stimulation (tDCS) over the motor cortex increases sympathetic nerve activity. *Brain Stimul*. 2014;7(1):97–104.

74. Liebetanz D, Koch R, et al. Safety limits of cathodal transcranial direct current stimulation in rats. *Clin Neurophysiol*. 2009;120(6):1161–1167.

75. Brunoni AR, Zanao TA, et al. Bifrontal tDCS prevents implicit learning acquisition in antidepressant-free patients with major depressive disorder. *Prog Neuropsychopharmacol Biol Psychiatry*. 2012;43C:146–150.

76. Dieckhofer A, Waberski TD, et al. Transcranial direct current stimulation applied over the somatosensory cortex – differential effect on low and high frequency SEPs. *Clin Neurophysiol*. 2006;117(10):2221–2227.

77. Fregni F, Boggio PS, et al. Anodal transcranial direct current stimulation of prefrontal cortex enhances working memory. *Exp Brain Res*. 2005;166(1):23–30.

78. Riberto M, Alfieri FM, et al. Efficacy of transcranial direct current stimulation coupled with a multidisciplinary rehabilitation program for the treatment of fibromyalgia. *Open Rheumatol J*. 2011;5:45–50.

79. Borckardt JJ, Bikson M, et al. A pilot study of the tolerability and effects of high-definition transcranial direct current stimulation (HD-tDCS) on pain perception. *J Pain*. 2012;13(2):112–120.

80. Borckardt JJ, Romagnuolo J, et al. Feasibility, safety, and effectiveness of transcranial direct current stimulation for decreasing post-ERCP pain: a randomized, sham-controlled, pilot study. *Gastrointest Endosc*. 2011;73(6):1158–1164.

81. Dasilva AF, Mendonca ME, et al. tDCS-induced analgesia and electrical fields in pain-related neural networks in chronic migraine. *Headache*. 2012;52(8):1283–1295.

82. Antal A, Paulus W. A case of refractory orofacial pain treated by transcranial direct current stimulation applied over hand motor area in combination with NMDA agonist drug intake. *Brain Stimul*. 2011;4(2):117–121.

83. Hansen N, Obermann M, et al. Modulation of human trigeminal and extracranial nociceptive processing by transcranial direct current stimulation of the motor cortex. *Cephalalgia*. 2011;31(6):661–670.

84. Knotkova H, Rosedale M, et al. Using transcranial direct current stimulation to treat depression in HIV-infected persons: the outcomes of a feasibility study. *Front Psychiatry*. 2012;3:59.

85. Kumru H, Soler D, et al. The effects of transcranial direct current stimulation with visual illusion in neuropathic pain due to spinal cord injury: an evoked potentials and quantitative thermal testing study. *Eur J Pain*. 2013;17(1):55–66.

86. Lindenberg R, Renga V, et al. Bihemispheric brain stimulation facilitates motor recovery in chronic stroke patients. *Neurology*. 2010;75(24):2176–2184.

87. Butler AJ, Shuster M, et al. A meta-analysis of the efficacy of anodal transcranial direct current stimulation for upper limb motor recovery in stroke survivors. *J Hand Ther*. 2013;26(2):162–170. quiz 171.

88. Elsner B, Kugler J, et al. Transcranial direct current stimulation (tDCS) for improving function and activities of daily living in patients after stroke. *Cochrane Database Syst Rev*. 2013;11 CD009645.

89. Marquez J, van Vliet P, et al. Transcranial direct current stimulation (tDCS): does it have merit in stroke rehabilitation? A systematic review. *Int J Stroke*. 2013;10(3).

90. Marangolo P, Fiori V, et al. Something to talk about: enhancement of linguistic cohesion through tDCS in chronic non fluent aphasia. *Neuropsychologia*. 2014;53:246–256.

91. Monti A, Ferrucci R, et al. Transcranial direct current stimulation (tDCS) and language. *J Neurol Neurosurg Psychiatry*. 2013;84(8):832–842.

92. Monti A, Cogiamanian F, et al. Improved naming after transcranial direct current stimulation in aphasia. *J Neurol Neurosurg Psychiatry*. 2008;79(4):451–453.

93. Shiozawa P, Fregni F, et al. Transcranial direct current stimulation for major depression: an updated systematic review and meta-analysis. *Int J Neuropsychopharmacol*. 2014;17(9):1443–1452.

94. Kalu UG, Sexton CE, et al. Transcranial direct current stimulation in the treatment of major depression: a meta-analysis. *Psychol Med*. 2012;42(9):1791–1800.

95. Martin DM, Alonzo A, et al. Continuation transcranial direct current stimulation for the prevention of relapse in major depression. *J Affect Disord*. 2013;144(3):274–278.

96. Brunoni AR, Ferrucci R, et al. Transcranial direct current stimulation (tDCS) in unipolar vs. bipolar depressive disorder. *Prog Neuropsychopharmacol Biol Psychiatry*. 2011;35(1):96–101.

97. Zandieh A, Parhizgar SE, et al. Modulation of cold pain perception by transcranial direct current stimulation in healthy individuals. *Neuromodulation*. 2013;16(4):345–348. discussion 348.

98. Grundmann L, Rolke R, et al. Effects of transcranial direct current stimulation of the primary sensory cortex on somatosensory perception. *Brain Stimul*. 2011;4(4):253–260.

99. Borckardt JJ, Reeves ST, et al. Transcranial direct current stimulation (tDCS) reduces postsurgical opioid consumption in total knee arthroplasty (TKA). *Clin J Pain*. 2013;29(11):925–928.

100. Luedtke K, Rushton A, et al. Transcranial direct current stimulation for the reduction of clinical and experimentally induced pain: a systematic review and meta-analysis. *Clin J Pain*. 2012;28(5):452–461.

101. Zaghi S, Thiele B, et al. Assessment and treatment of pain with non-invasive cortical stimulation. *Restor Neurol Neurosci*. 2011;29(6):439–451.

102. O'Connell NE, Wand BM, et al. Non-invasive brain stimulation techniques for chronic pain. A report of a Cochrane systematic review and meta-analysis. *Eur J Phys Rehabil Med*. 2011;47(2):309–326.

103. O'Connell NE, Wand BM, et al. Non-invasive brain stimulation techniques for chronic pain. *Cochrane Database Syst Rev*. 2014;4:CD008208.

104. Soler MD, Kumru H, et al. Effectiveness of transcranial direct current stimulation and visual illusion on neuropathic pain in spinal cord injury. *Brain*. 2010;133(9):2565–2577.

105. Vigano A, D'Elia TS, et al. Transcranial direct current stimulation (tDCS) of the visual cortex: a proof-of-concept study based on interictal electrophysiological abnormalities in migraine. *J Headache Pain*. 2013;14(1):23.

106. Bolognini N, Olgiati E, et al. Motor and parietal cortex stimulation for phantom limb pain and sensations. *Pain*. 2013;154(8):1274–1280.

107. Bolognini N, Spandri V, et al. Long-term analgesic effects of transcranial direct current stimulation of the motor cortex on phantom limb and stump pain: a case report. *J Pain Symptom Manage*. 2013;46(4):e1–4.

108. Fenton BW, Palmieri PA, et al. A preliminary study of transcranial direct current stimulation for the treatment of refractory chronic pelvic pain. *Brain Stimul*. 2009;2(2):103–107.

109. Fregni F, Gimenes R, et al. A randomized, sham-controlled, proof of principle study of transcranial direct current stimulation for the treatment of pain in fibromyalgia. *Arthritis Rheum*. 2006;54(12):3988–3998.

110. Knotkova H, Portenoy RK, et al. Transcranial direct current stimulation (tDCS) relieved itching in a patient with chronic neuropathic pain. *Clin J Pain*. 2013;29(7):621–622.

111. Vaseghi B, Zoghi M, et al. Does anodal transcranial direct current stimulation modulate sensory perception and pain? A meta-analysis study. *Clin Neurophysiol*. 2014;125(9):1847–1858.

112. Dworkin RH, Turk DC, et al. Core outcome measures for chronic pain clinical trials: IMMPACT recommendations. *Pain*. 2005;113(1–2):9–19.

113. Jansen JM, Daams JG, et al. Effects of non-invasive neurostimulation on craving: a meta-analysis. *Neurosci Biobehav Rev*. 2013;37(10 Pt 2):2472–2480.

114. Song JJ, Vanneste S, et al. Transcranial direct current stimulation in tinnitus patients: a systemic review and meta-analysis. *ScientificWorldJournal*. 2012;2012:427941.

115. Acler M, Bocci T, et al. Transcranial direct current stimulation (tDCS) for sleep disturbances and fatigue in patients with post-polio syndrome. *Restor Neurol Neurosci*. 2013;31(5):661–668.

116. Perlmutter JS, Mink JW. Deep brain stimulation. *Annu Rev Neurosci*. 2006.

117. Villamar MF, Wivatvongvana P, et al. Focal modulation of the primary motor cortex in fibromyalgia using 4x1-ring high-definition transcranial direct current stimulation (HD-tDCS): immediate and delayed analgesic effects of cathodal and anodal stimulation. *J Pain*. 2013;14(4):371–383.

118. Fregni F, Boggio PS, et al. A sham-controlled, phase II trial of transcranial direct current stimulation for the treatment of central pain in traumatic spinal cord injury. *Pain*. 2006;122(1–2):197–209.

119. Tehovnik EJ. Electrical stimulation of neural tissue to evoke behavioral responses. *J Neurosci Methods*. 1996;65(1):1–17.

120. Yeomans JS. *Principles of Brain Stimulation*. London: Oxford University Press; 1990.

121. McIntyre CC, Mori S, et al. Electric field and stimulating influence generated by deep brain stimulation of the subthalamic nucleus. *Clin Neurophysiol*. 2004;115(3):589–595.

122. Ranck Jr. JB. Extracellular stimulation. *Electr Stimul Res Tech*. Academic Press; 1981:1–36.

123. Butson CR, McIntyre CC. Role of electrode design on the volume of tissue activated during deep brain stimulation. *J Neural Eng*. 2006;3(1):1–8.

124. Grill WM. Effects of tissue electrical properties on neural excitation. *18th Annual International Conference of the IEEE Engineering in Medicine and Biology Society*. Amsterdam: IEEE; 1996.

125. Boggio PS, Rigonatti SP, et al. A randomized, double-blind clinical trial on the efficacy of cortical direct current stimulation for the treatment of major depression. *Int J Neuropsychopharmacol*. 2007:1–6.
126. Williams JA, Imamura M, et al. Updates on the use of non-invasive brain stimulation in physical and rehabilitation medicine. *J Rehabil Med*. 2009;41(5):305–311.
127. Wu AD, Fregni F, et al. Noninvasive brain stimulation for Parkinson's disease and dystonia. *Neurotherapeutics*. 2008;5(2):345–361.
128. Cardoso EF, Fregni F, et al. rTMS treatment for depression in Parkinson's disease increases BOLD responses in the left prefrontal cortex. *Int J Neuropsychopharmacol*. 2008;11(2):173–183.
129. Fregni F, Boggio PS, et al. Transcranial direct current stimulation of the unaffected hemisphere in stroke patients. *Neuroreport*. 2005;16(14):1551–1555.
130. Fregni F, Boggio PS, et al. Noninvasive cortical stimulation with transcranial direct current stimulation in Parkinson's disease. *Mov Disord*. 2006;21(10):1693–1702.
131. Fregni F, Freedman S, et al. Recent advances in the treatment of chronic pain with non-invasive brain stimulation techniques. *Lancet Neurol*. 2007;6(2):188–191.
132. Fregni F, Pascual-Leone A. Technology insight: noninvasive brain stimulation in neurology-perspectives on the therapeutic potential of rTMS and tDCS. *Nat Clin Pract Neurol*. 2007;3(7):383–393.
133. Fregni F, Santos CM, et al. Repetitive transcranial magnetic stimulation is as effective as fluoxetine in the treatment of depression in patients with Parkinson's disease. *J Neurol Neurosurg Psychiatry*. 2004;75(8):1171–1174.
134. Fregni F, Thome-Souza S, et al. Antiepileptic effects of repetitive TMS in patients with cortical malformations: an EEG and clinical study. *Stereotact Func Neurosurg*. 2004;83(2–3):57–62.
135. Jensen MP, Hakimian S, et al. New insights into neuromodulatory approaches for the treatment of pain. *J Pain*. 2008;9(3):193–199.
136. Mansur CG, Fregni F, et al. A sham-stimulation controlled trial of rTMS of the unaffected hemisphere on hand motor function after stroke. *Neurology*. 2004;64(4).
137. Martin PI, Naeser MA, et al. Transcranial magnetic stimulation as a complementary treatment for aphasia. *Semin Speech Lang*. 2004;25(2):181–191.
138. Boggio PS, Fregni F, et al. Effect of repetitive TMS and fluoxetine on cognitive function in patients with Parkinson's disease and concurrent depression. *Mov Disord*. 2005;20(9):1178–1184.
139. Wagner T, Fregni F, et al. Transcranial magnetic stimulation and stroke: a computer-based human model study. *Neuroimage*. 2006;30(3):857–870.
140. Wagner T, Fregni F, et al. Transcranial direct current stimulation: a computer-based human model study. *Neuroimage*. 2007;35(3):1113–1124.
141. Miranda PC, Lomarev M, et al. Modeling the current distribution during transcranial direct current stimulation. *Clin Neurophysiol*. 2006;117(7):1623–1629.
142. Edwards D, Cortes M, et al. Physiological and modeling evidence for focal transcranial electrical brain stimulation in humans: a basis for high-definition tDCS. *Neuroimage*. 2013;74:266–275.
143. Doruk D, Luque L, et al. Electrosonic stimulation as adjunctive therapy to dopaminergic treatments in Parkinson's disease. 5th International Symposium on Neuromodulation, Sao Paulo, Brazil.5.7 (1855). L'Electrisation Localisee; 2013.
144. Moreno-Duarte I, Diaz-Cruz C, et al. Effects of electrosonic stimulation on the perception of chronic pain due to osteoarthritis of the knee. 5th International Symposium on Neuromodulation, Sao Paulo, Brazil; 2013.

Viral Vectors and Other Modulatory Biologics

B.J. Mader and N.M. Boulis

Emory University, Atlanta, GA, United States

Innovative Neuromodulation.
DOI: http://dx.doi.org/10.1016/B978-0-12-800454-8.00009-4

INTRODUCTION

Neurological pathologies characterized by impaired neuronal function or neurodegeneration can either be caused by inherited genetic alterations or appear sporadically. The factors that eventually lead to nervous system pathologies have extremely diverse origins that include both local and global alterations to neural metabolism, development, functionality, and viability. Modern medical interventions and surgical practices have yet to provide effective therapeutic benefit for many of these neuropathologies. Gene therapy aims to treat disease processes through gene expression within functionally impaired cells or tissue with the goals of providing normal functionality, relieving disease symptoms, and halting disease progression. Gene-based neuromodulatory techniques can successfully introduce or alter gene function within a specific population of cells and networks leading to exogenous control of neural excitation or inhibition. This approach is in contrast to therapies that protect and support neuronal cells that may be at risk in many types of early-stage neurodegeneration. State-of-the-art therapies, such as viral-mediated neuromodulation, are currently being engineered and for the treatment of Parkinson's disease and forms of chronic pain, which may eventually provide superior benefit to the present-day treatment options across the spectrum of neurological disorders.

Gene therapy was first conceived as a promising method to combat disease as early as 1970.[1] This mode of therapy is achieved by delivery of exogenous genetic material to either increase gene expression or inhibit dysfunctional gene expression. This therapeutic development gave great hope for the potential of correcting genetic diseases, with many being evaluated at the preclinical and clinical levels. However, most neurological diseases are due to sporadic or unknown mechanisms. Thus, more generalized approaches are needed. It is the goal of viral-based neuromodulatory therapeutics to improve on current treatment options for pathologies, including movement disorders, chronic pain, psychiatric disease, and epilepsy.

In conventional small-molecule pharmacology it is accepted that dosage, distribution, and kinetics play an essential role in safety and efficacy. As such, therapies designed for gene-based neuromodulation must also adhere to these principles. Manipulating genetic material at the cellular level is a relatively simple process. However, in clinical applications these manipulations are much less precise when tissue and systemic complexities contribute to the overall outcome of gene-based therapies. A major difference between viral-mediated therapeutics and classical small-molecule therapeutics is the potential ability of the virus to persist within tissue and express the therapeutic molecule over an extended period of time. Viral-based gene therapy utilizes a recombinant virus that contains one or more trans-genes intended to express a therapeutic product. Viral vector-mediated delivery of molecular therapeutics is a clever usage of viruses, exploiting their naturally evolved mechanisms of infection for therapeutic benefit. Eukaryotic viral vectors currently being used are derived from many both pathogenic and innocuous viruses, including adenoviruses (Ads), adeno-associated viruses (AAVs), lentiviruses (LVs) (retroviruses), and herpes simplex viruses (HSVs). These modified viral constructs can support transgene inserts in a range of sizes in both RNA and DNA forms.[2]

Many of the therapeutic viral constructs originate from human pathological viruses. Therefore, safety concerns are paramount during viral-mediated therapeutic development. Removing viral genetic material from vectors to prevent viral replication is a logical safety measure to prevent viral expansion in host tissue and limit the unintended spread of the virus and transgene expression. However, it is necessary to retain certain viral sequences to allow vector packaging and infection. Limiting transgene expression to the target cell type, tissue, or organ is another method to improve vector safety. Accuracy of targeting and expression can be improved by interchanging natural or synthetically produced capsid proteins and gene promoters. For example using the inherent neurotropism of neurotoxin peptides in combination with viral constructs could provide a way to target vectors to neurons efficiently.[3,4] Different capsids may also permit safer delivery routes. The capsid proteins of AAV9 are particularly good at crossing the blood–brain barrier and transfecting neuronal cells, whereas other AAV serotypes cannot cross the blood–brain barrier.[5,6] Viral constructs intended for use in the central nervous system (CNS) would likely have the ability to cross the blood–brain barrier so that therapies could be administered by way of peripheral injections, which are much less invasive than direct injections to the CNS. However peripheral administration of viral vectors through intravenous injection causes expression in off-target tissue with limited expression in the CNS.[7]

There are other hurdles that lie beyond targeting the correct cells. For example, multiple administrations of viral vector will likely prove to be less than effective because antibodies are created against the virus capsid and will likely be blocked from cell entry after vector readministration.[8] Furthermore, previous exposure by a patient to wild-type virus could result in the production of antibodies that prevent efficient delivery to target cells. To circumvent these particular immune issues researchers must explore serotype alternatives through capsid protein modification along with possible use of nonhuman-associated viral constructs.[9–11]

An additional concern of therapeutic viral vector development is the potential risk of insertional mutagenesis caused by integration of the vector into the host genome, resulting in an unintended deleterious loss or gain of function. Insertional mutagenesis can produce tumorigenic effects as seen in a clinical trial treating X-linked severe combined immuno-deficiency.[12,13] Vector-induced host immune response can cause adverse effects and must also be taken into consideration when characterizing viral vectors for therapeutic interventions.[14] In addition to the risk of an immune response against the vector, overexpression of therapeutic genes may result in a deleterious immune response as well.

The overall goal of gene-based neuromodulation is to identify the optimal vector and trans-gene combination that can partially or completely correct neurological dysfunction. This chapter is intended to give an in-depth look at the most up-to-date knowledge of vector-mediated gene-based neuromodulation. First we will discuss characterizations of commonly used viral and nonviral constructs which efficiently introduce therapeutic gene expression in neurological disease-associated cells and tissue. Next we will explore the applications of these vector-based neuromodulation strategies that have advanced to clinical trials as well as relevant preclinical studies that could soon progress into early-phase clinical testing.

VIRAL VECTORS

There are a variety of viral vectors currently being used in preclinical research as well as clinical trials. The predominant viral vector systems that have been used in the nervous system are: (1) Ad, (2) AAV, (3) HSV, and (4) LV (lentivirus, from the retroviral family). These vectors are summarized in Fig. 9.1. The ideal gene therapy vector will selectively target the cell type or tissue of interest, express the transgene at an appropriate level, have minimal off-target effects, and evade the immune system for extended therapeutic expression.

Viral vectors can be targeted to specific tissues by specific capsid or envelope proteins. These proteins define the virus's "serotype." Within the AAV population of viruses, e.g., there are over 100 known serotypes, creating the potential for differential targeting via serotype choice. Researchers commonly create vectors to harness the most attractive aspects of the natural viral tropism and promoter activity.[15] Vectors have been engineered that increase vector potency, cell specificity, and further reduce side effects.[16,17]

An additional technical improvement for viral vector efficacy is the use of pharmaceuticals to regulate gene expression, allowing the transgene to be turned on and off at will. Drugs commonly used as a molecular on/off switch include tetracycline, rapamycin, ecdysone, and progesterone. In some cases, one may wish to control the polarity of a neuron, to cause or prevent it from firing. This need has led to the creation of

Vector	Specifications	Application in the CNS
Adeno-associated virus (AAV) 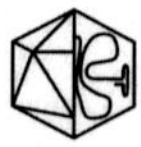 ~20 nm	Genome: ssDNA Capacity: ~4.7 kb (~ 2.2 kb with scAAV, ~8 kb with dual vectors) Forms circular and linear episomes; integrates with very low frequency Shown to infect neurons, astrocytes, glial and ependymal cells	Used extensively in clinical trials, including Parkinson's, Alzheimer's, Batten, and Canavan diseases Preliminary studies suggest AAV vectors could also be used to treat mucopolysaccharidoses (MPS), spinocerebellar ataxia, amyotrophic lateral sclerosis (ALS), epilepsy, and Huntington's disease
Retrovirus: human immunodeficiency virus (HIV) 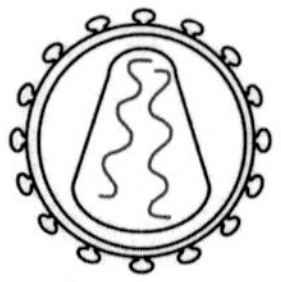 ~100 nm	Genome: ssRNA Capacity: ~ 8 kb NIL vectors form linear and circular episomes; integration is low. Other HIV vectors integrate with high efficiency Shown to infect neurons and astroglial cells	Used in clinical trials for treatment of Parkinson's and Alzheimer's diseases Vectors are being developed for use with Huntington's and lysosomal storage diseases
Adenovirus 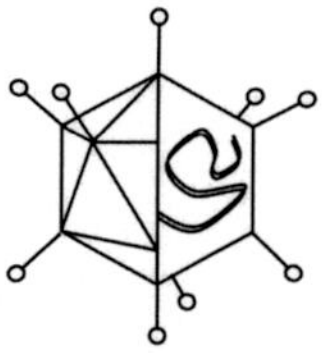 ~70 – 100 nm	Genome: dsDNA Capacity: ~36 kb Maintained as linear episomes; integration is minimal even with extensive homology to genome Shown to infect neural, astroglial, and human glioma cells	Not in clinical use for gene therapy in the CNS due primarily to vector toxicity Has been used for oncolytic potential as an anticancer agent
Herpesvirus: herpes simplex virus-1 (HSV-1) 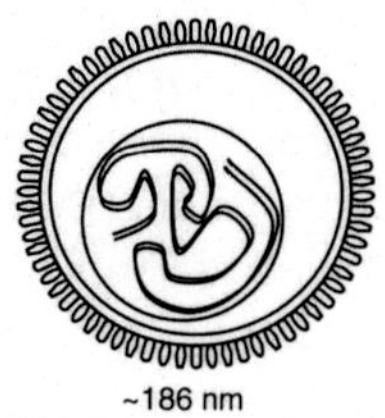 ~186 nm	Genome: dsDNA Capacity: ~150 kb Genome circularizes upon entering nucleus and is maintained episomally; integration is minimal Shown to infect neurons	Not in clinical use for gene therapy in the CNS due to problems with vector toxicity and production Vectors are being developed for use with Parkinson's disease Has also been developed for anticancer therapy

FIGURE 9.1   Common viral vector constructs used in gene therapy.

viral-mediated expression of cell receptors (designer receptors exclusively activated by designer drugs, or DREADDs) or ligand-gated ion channels that can be controlled by small-molecule agonists.[18,19] These exogenously expressed receptors and ion channels can be controlled by specific small-molecule activators that enable researchers to precisely control inhibitory or excitatory synaptic transmission which could be applied ubiquitously to potentially any brain pathway. In a similar fashion, the field of optogenetics uses viral vectors to express rhodopsins that can be activated to induce neuromodulatory alteration. Proteins used in optogenetic studies are light-sensitive and can be controlled with specific wavelengths of light. A more detailed description of optogenetics and DREADDs can be found in their own chapters within this book.

Recently, viral vectors have been used in applications that require the inhibition of gene expression using RNA interference (RNAi).[20] This methodology was developed using scientific knowledge of the naturally occurring gene-silencing mechanism performed by micro-RNA which induce degradation of mRNA at the posttranscriptional level. Synthetically produced RNA used for inhibition is termed small interfering RNA (siRNA). Similar to gene expression, RNAi-mediated gene inhibition can also be regulated by pharmacological molecular switches.[20,21] siRNA has shown particular therapeutic promise in preclinical models of ALS and Alzheimer disease.[22,23] Although relatively new, RNAi technology is a promising strategy to develop potential therapies in diseases where gene alterations may result in deleterious gains of function.

ADENOVIRUS

Wild-type Ad virus is known to cause pathologies in humans including conjunctivitis, pharyngitis, and respiratory ailments.[24,25] As a vector for gene delivery, Ad was attractive for many reasons, including: its high efficiency of transduction in a multitude of cell types; lack of chromosomal integration; high titer production capability; and finally accurate targeting ability by capsid modification. However, these vectors, in early years, had a transgene capacity that is relatively small (~8.3 kb) when compared to other vector systems such as HSV and LV[26] and transgene expression was transient. Current work seeks to reduce vector toxicity and extend the length of transgene expression. Fig. 9.2 provides a detailed map of Ad (as well as the other common viral vectors) and the modifications that are made to this vector system. Ultimately, the main setback to therapeutic use of Ad vectors is due to the severe host immune responses it evokes, which subsequently led to a patient's death in a clinical trial using Ad.[27,28]

Constant adaptation of these vectors has led to their characterization in terms of first-, second-, or third-generation Ad vector systems. The first generation of Ad vectors had genes removed that coded for viral proteins involved in early gene expression, replication, and packaging. Effective CNS transduction using Ad virus was exciting given that it could provide stable treatment for chronic pathologies affecting CNS. Early Ad vectors demonstrated residual viral toxicity indicating the need for further modifications to increase their safety profile.[29,30] This toxicity was attributed

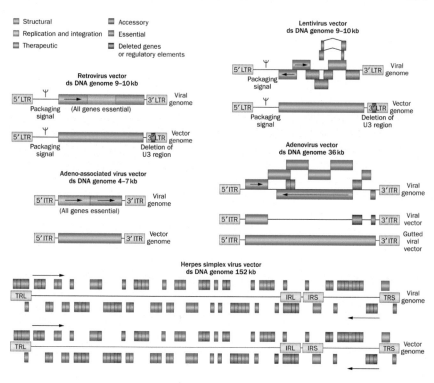

FIGURE 9.2 Diagrams of the genomes of various viral vectors used in gene therapy approaches. Each diagram depicts the genome of the virus along with that of the corresponding viral vector, showing viral structural genes, viral genes involved in replication, and genes essential or nonessential (accessory) for virus replication or growth. Viral genes that are transcribed in the 5′ to 3′ direction (rightward arrow) are depicted above the viral genome, and those transcribed in the opposite direction (leftward arrow) are depicted below the genome. Genes or regulatory elements deleted from viral vectors are shown in red and common locations for introduction of the therapeutic gene in the vector genome are depicted in green. HSV, herpes simplex virus; ds, double-stranded; ITR, inverted terminal repeat; IRL, inverted repeat long; IRS, inverted repeat short; LTR, long terminal repeat; TRS, terminal repeat short.

to a robust immune response, which also was implicated in decreased gene expression within 2 months that correlated with the disappearance of Ad DNA.

Second-generation vector design required the additional removal of viral genes making the vector safer as well as expanding the transgene capacity to ~14 kb.[31] Unfortunately, while much of the viral genome was deleted there remained unresolved toxicity as a result of inflammation and host immune response.[32] Further subsequent removal of endogenous viral genetic material has led to the production of third-generation vectors commonly referred to as either "gutless" or "helper-dependent" Ad, and improved their transgene capacity to ~36 kb. These third-generation Ad vectors were unable to replicate without helper virus or a complementary cell line that express viral genes required for replication.[8] In contrast to earlier Ad generations, and their short-lived transgene expression, the use of a more advanced gutless Ad vector provided evidence of expression detected for 2 years within the CNS after administration.[33] Ad vectors can express genes in neuronal cells and control their activity, regardless of which neuronal pathway they are part of. For example, in neurons the ion-channel Kir2.1 contributes to stabilizing the neuronal resting potential below the threshold of activation of voltage-gated sodium channels. When Kir2.1 is exogenously expressed in the rat spinal cord using an Ad vector construct, neuromuscular function was inhibited in the absence of neuron death.[34] This approach may be useful for treating diseases caused by aberrant neurotransmission, such as dystonia. If specific network synaptic activity can be either inhibited or activated then this methodology could be developed into powerful therapies for a wide range of neurological diseases.

While much research has been done employing Ad as a vector for gene delivery, its frequency of use has been on the decline in deference to other seemingly safer and more effective viral vector systems. Although not ideal for neuromodulatory clinical application, the ease of production and high level of transgene expression when using Ad renders it useful as an effective proof-of-concept tool for robust, short-term gene expression in preclinical studies.

ADENO-ASSOCIATED VIRUS

The majority of viral vectors currently being in development for therapeutic use are derived from AAV.[35] The AAV virion capsid is about 20 nm and is the smallest of the vectors discussed in this chapter. The AAV genome is ~4.7 kb of ssDNA and the capsid can package up to ~4.9 kb, limiting the size of potential transgene. This limitation is considered a major setback to this vector system. Similar to the development of other vector systems, recombinant AAV vectors had 95% of the viral genome removed.[36] These vectors have been shown to transduce both dividing and nondividing cells, making it very amenable to CNS transduction. A very attractive characteristic of AAV is that it is not associated with any human disease process, thus decreasing the potential safety concerns relating to host immune response and other vector-mediated toxicity (as seen with the use of Ad and other vectors). Although, AAVs are not known to be associated with disease pathology and do not exhibit adverse effects, there is evidence that AAV antibodies are found within human populations.[37] A clinical phase I trial using AAV2 to deliver a transgene to the CNS for the treatment of Canavan disease showed no "overt" signs of inflammation within the CNS. Additionally, AAV2 neutralizing antibody was found in only 3 out of 10 patients within the cerebrospinal fluid.[38] This study was the first to use a viral vector for the treatment of a neurodegenerative disorder, and reported critical safety data showing muted immune responses in human subjects. This safety trial has paved the way for the development and use of this vector type in other CNS pathologies. Additional benefits to using these vectors include their inability to replicate or integrate into host genome without helper viruses or plasmids providing the genes essential for viral replication. AAVs naturally contain ssDNA but can be engineered to deliver dsDNA for quicker transgene expression, though this cuts the packaging size by half.[39,40]

Targeting specificity in AAV transduction is regulated by the proteins of the capsid. The capsid controls viral binding to the cell surface. AAV2 preferentially binds heparin sulfate proteoglycans as its primary receptor,[41] while AAV 1, 4, 5, and 6 bind sialic acid,[42] AAV8 binds laminin, and AAV9 binds N-linked galactose.[43] Fig. 9.3 illustrates the major factors affecting tropism, transduction, and transgene expression of the AAV, but also applies to other vectors as well. Over 100 different specific AAV serotypes have been identified to date, with serotype 2 being the most widely studied.[44] The therapeutic potential of AAV is highlighted by the approval of AAV1, 2, 5, 9, and AAVRh10 by the US Food and Drug Administration for use in multiple clinical trials (www.clinicaltrials.gov).

Many studies report that AAVs exhibit a predominant neuronal tropism and biodistribution in the rodent CNS, particularly in the brain. While there are a wide variety of choices in the AAV toolkit, it is imperative to state that an optimal AAV serotype does not exist for general application within the nervous system. There appears to be significant variability in AAV distribution and expression levels after introduction to the nervous system.[35] AAV2 has a strong neuronal tropism when injected intraparenchymally because of its propensity to bind heparan sulfate proteoglycan present in the extracellular matrix.[44] Furthermore, binding of the vector to heparin sulfate proteoglycan limits viral spread to surrounding tissue. AAV2 is also reported to be effective in transducing both neuronal and glial cell populations in the hippocampus of nonhuman primates after multiple direct injections.[45] While AAV2 is known to transduce neuronal and other CNS populations, it may be an inferior AAV choice when compared to other serotypes. AAV5 has been reported to more effectively transduce the CNS and give a higher level of expression.[46] AAV9 could be particularly beneficial in delivering CNS-centered therapies because AAV9 can be administered peripherally as it has been shown to cross the blood–brain barrier.[7,47] Intrathecal administration of AAV9 provides a superior method for widespread biodistribution of the vector when compared to intravenous injection.[7,48,49] While these are just a few examples of serotype-specific transduction patterns using AAV, there

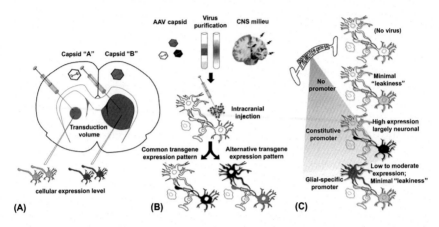

FIGURE 9.3   Major factors affecting tropism, transduction, and transgene expression properties of AAV. (A) Encapsidation of different AAV serotypes can dramatically alter both overall tissue transduction volume and specific cellular transduction and transgene expression. (B) Neurons are the primary targets of most AAV serotypes after intracranial viral delivery to nonpathological CNS tissue. However, some AAV serotypes, cruder purification strategies, and/or a pathological CNS milieu can result in a shift of transgene expression to nonneuronal cells. (C) Promoter selection can dramatically affect transgene expression patterns. While the AAV terminal repeat (TR) can itself contribute to minimal transgene expression, some constitutive promoters, such as the hybrid chicken beta-actin (CBA) promoter lead to very high levels of primarily neuronal transgene expression. Use of a cell-specific promoter, such as the astrocyte-specific GFAP promoter can result in low to moderate transgene expression in these cells. However, cell-specific expression requires transduction of the cell of interest, and some "leaky" expression can occur in other cell types (presumably due to TR-directed promoter activity).

is a rapidly growing body of knowledge regarding serotype specificity. A complete detailed review of AAV vectors was written by Asokan et al.[50]

Although not extensively covered in this chapter, differences in expression can also be affected by differences in vector purity and promoter. As with all types of gene vector systems, the expression of endogenous host promoter activity in the specific tissue of interest must be confirmed if long-term gene therapeutic expression is to be achieved.

AAV has shown particular utility in transducing a variety of cells in the CNS including neurons, glia, astrocytes, and ependymal cells. The seemingly endless combination of capsid proteins and promoter sequences available to assess specific neuronal tropism and expression characteristics provides translational research the flexibility that may eventually create extremely accurate and exclusive vector targeting of many neural pathways for future therapeutic development. Clinical trials, including studies involving Parkinson and Alzheimer disease, have used AAV vector systems as their viral vector of choice because AAV is considered safe and provides long-term gene expression.

HERPES SIMPLEX VIRUS

HSV is a naturally neurotropic virus known to target and infect many types of neurons, such as sensory neurons of the peripheral nervous system. Peripheral neuron infectivity makes HSV a particularly attractive vector for gene therapy applications within the nervous system. Modifications to the wild-type HSV are necessary in order to increase its safety profile as a potential therapeutic vector,[51] and like other vector systems nearly 80 viral genes have been removed for the production of safe therapeutic vectors.[35] An inherent advantage of HSV is its remarkably large transgene capacity, which at ~152 kb is much larger than that of the other viral vectors discussed in this chapter. The large transgene capacity allows for the inclusion of complete therapeutic genes, or even multiple genes, in addition to the necessary genomic elements required for maintenance of the transgene expression. However, an important disadvantage of HSV is that it does cause human disease and is known to cause antibody formation,[52] which can lead to a robust immune response and prevent its cellular uptake due to antibody-mediated clearance.

The natural life cycle of HSV includes two different phases of replication that utilize different host cell types and altered gene expression.[53] Briefly, HSV first comes into contact with the host epithelial cell membrane. Next, its viral envelope glycoproteins interact with epithelial cell membrane proteoglycans. The virus will then replicate within the epithelial cells and eventually cause host cell lysis, effectively releasing an increased number of virions that will be taken up by sensory nerve terminals proximal to the lysed cell. After nerve terminal uptake, the HSV are transported along the microtubule network in a retrograde manner destined for the nucleus where its genetic material will remain episomally in a latent (inactive) state.[53] This latent state is characterized by the silencing of early infection-associated genes, allowing HSV genomic material to be concealed from the host cell immune system. This provides a beneficial therapeutic function allowing long-term transgene expression. HSV vectors will likely improve with a better understanding of their biology, and their tropism for sensory neurons may make it a preferred viral vector system for neuromodulatory gene therapies.

LENTIVIRUS (RETROVIRUS)

LVs are in the family *Retroviridae*, or retroviruses, and their genome is comprised of ssRNA. The first viral vector used in clinical applications was derived from the Moloney murine leukemia virus.[54] Use of this retrovirus allowed for the subsequent development of other more widely used vectors, including LV. LV vector systems derived from human immunodeficiency virus (HIV) have been developed to transduce neurons resulting in high levels of transgene expression over prolonged periods of time, making it an excellent option for viral-mediated delivery to the nervous system.[55] LV is the second most used viral vector for gene delivery to the CNS and has shown benefit in many animal models of neurological disease. These vectors have demonstrated the ability to transduce most cell types within the CNS including neurons,[56] astrocytes,[57] adult neuronal stem cells,[58] and oligodendrocytes, as well as glioma cells.[59]

Although it has not yet been documented, since LV is derived from HIV-1, there is some concern that rearrangements during vector production could produce an infectious virus. In efforts to reduce potential risks, or appearance of risk, there have been efforts to develop LVs from feline and equine species in addition to safety modifications in human-specific types.[60,61]

As with other vector types, the two main methods for targeting the transgene expression to specific cell types are envelope protein receptor binding specificity and cell type-specific promoter activity. Alternate envelope glycoproteins from rabies virus, Mokola virus, and lymphocytic choriomeningitis virus can be used to pseudotype LVs and regulate their uptake.[62] For example, to maximize broad tissue expression LV has been pseudotyped with a glycoprotein of the vesicular stomatitis virus (VSV-G), a rabies type virus which causes flu-like illness in humans.[63] Following striatum injection and retrograde transport, rabies-G pseudotyped equine infectious anemia virus-based vector expression can be found within several brain regions such as the striatum, hippocampus, and substantia nigra. However if the same vector was pseudotyped with VSV-G instead of rabies-G it did not exhibit the same expression. After peripheral injection of VSV-G pseudotyped LV brain transduction was found, indicating retrograde transport capabilities.[64] Furthermore, this vector showed elevated expression within neurons. This neuronal preference is due to the presence of promoters that are widely found within neurons but to a much lesser degree in other CNS cell types, such as glial cells.[65] These promoter specificities have been further explored in nonhuman primates.[66,64]

Like other retroviruses, LVs can integrate into the host genome. Interestingly, host genome integration sites appear to be within genes the vast majority of the time, suggesting that altered regulation of a host gene is less likely than with other retroviruses.[67,68] Thus, there are concerns about this risk of insertional mutagenesis, particularly in light of the occurrence of leukemia in a previous use of retroviral vectors.[69,70]

NONVIRAL VECTOR-MEDIATED GENE THERAPY

DNA and RNA can be introduced in a "naked" state for delivery in various forms, including plasmid DNA (primarily gene expression), and antisense oligonucleotides, siRNA, shRNA, or miRNA (primarily gene inhibition). Physical introduction of exogenous DNA or RNA into target cells using nonviral administration can be made through a mechanical, electrical, ultrasonic, hydrodynamic, or laser-based energy.[71] Some of these methods are not amenable for use in animal models without significant toxic side effects. As these physical methods of introduction are unlikely to progress into clinical gene therapies, other types of nonviral vector systems have been developed to engineer vectors combining transgenes with lipids, polymeric structures, cell-penetrating peptides, and inorganic nanoparticles.[72]

For general application within the nervous system these vectors must be directly injected and/or have the ability to efficiently cross the blood–brain barrier after peripheral administration. Nonviral vectors designed for gene-based neuromodulation must be produced with targeting and gene expression considerations in mind. Nonviral constructs often mimic the qualities of neurotropic viruses in that they have: (1) the ability to selectively bind the neuronal cell surface and be taken up; (2) the ability to be transported by way of intracellular vesicular pathways to the soma; (3) the ability to escape the vesicular pathway upon arrival to the nucleus or perinuclear region; and (4) inherent qualities allowing entry into the nucleus and transgene expression activity.

Cationic lipids can form complexes with nucleic acids, called lipoplexes. These lipids protect the nucleic acids from degradation and aid the passage of genetic material through cellular membranes.[73] Cationic lipid systems usually have long descriptive chemical names, such as 1,2-dioleoyl-3-trimethylammonium-propane, so they are generally referred to by their acronym. Other common examples are, DOTMA, DOSPA, and DOGS.[74] This type of nonviral vector is less likely to be beneficial in diseases of the nervous system since it mainly transfects dividing cells. However, the application of these vectors has recently been explored in clinical trials for treatment of metastatic melanoma using a cationic lipid system and plasmid DNA complex (Allovectin-7).[75]

Cationic polymers are commonly used as nonviral vector systems because their wide range of molecular composition can be adapted for many types of targeting modifications. While an extremely diverse number of cationic polymers have been used, the most widely used have been poly-L-lysine (PLL) and polyethylenimine (PEI). In animal studies PEI has shown a greater ability to transfect neuronal cells better than PLL.[76] PEI polyplexes can be retrogradedly transported, making these polyplexes appealing for peripheral introduction for targeting of genetic material and other molecules to the CNS.[77] Brain and nerve injury studies have reported significant therapeutic benefit when therapeutic genes are delivered by complexes comprised of neurotropic ligands in combination with PLL, PEI, and lipid-based vector systems.[78,79] Furthermore, one study improved

Parkinson disease (PD)-related motor deficits through a neuromodulatory approach by the delivery of the gene for tyrosine hydroxylase (TH), a rate-limiting enzyme in dopamine production, within liposomes coated with polyethylene glycol (PEG) and antibodies that conferred CNS targeting.[80]

Polypeptides and proteins are also being evaluated in the development of neurotropic targeting molecules. Neurons express a number of different classes of receptors, including neuropeptide, neurotrophin, and neurotoxin receptors. Proteins and specific motifs known to have strong affinity for neuronal cell interactions and binding have been investigated. These peptides can be combined with lipoplexes, polyplexes, and other potential vector structures to greatly increase the transfection efficiency of these vectors in neuronal cell populations. Tetanus toxin was one of the first peptides studied and used as a potential targeting vehicle. Short tetanus toxin-like moieties exhibit receptor binding, cellular uptake, and transport properties similar to the toxin itself.[81–83] Fusion of these peptides with RNA or DNA to target genetic material to specific cell populations may provide solutions for improved targeting accuracy.[82]

Synthetic nanoparticles have been promising candidates for neurotherapeutic development since gold nanoparticles coated with plasmid DNA were reported to be taken up by cultured neurons. Nanoparticles can be made of a variety of materials, from lipids to polymers, and by way of their "nano," or relatively small size, are designed to efficiently cross the blood–brain barrier.[84] Combinations of materials can be used to provide increasingly specialized delivery to targeted treatment sites. For example, iron oxide particles have been coated with PLL for gene delivery to the CNS which can be monitored by MRI to validate targeting.[85] Silica nanoparticles have also been shown to provide targeted expression within neuronal cells rivaling the expression of HSV, but without the associated toxicity.[86] Poly(butylcyanoacrylate) nanoparticles have also been shown to efficiently cross the blood–brain barrier and have been used in nervous system in vivo applications.[87] Finally, nanogels are hydrophilic or amphiphilic polymer chain networks that can bind drugs, proteins, DNA, RNA, and other small molecules and are being evaluated for therapeutic utility as they have shown brain targeting specificity.[88,89]

While there is plenty of published evidence supporting the potential translational utility of nonviral delivery of gene-based therapy, it is important to note that most data in neuronal applications were generated through in vitro experimentation and have yet to be robustly tested in vivo. These nonviral methods are generally less toxic than viral-derived constructs but are less effective at expressing therapeutic transgenes within targeted tissues. A primary reason these synthetic nonviral vectors remain inferior is that they do not exhibit an equivalent to the harnessed natural neurotropism found in modern viral vector delivery systems.[90] However, if these issues are resolved, the nonviral vector system's superior safety profile (i.e., replication incompetency: lack of integration into host genome; relatively mild immune response) could influence the aims of future therapeutic development.

VIRAL-MEDIATED NEUROMODULATION AND GENE THERAPY FOR NEUROLOGICAL DISEASE

Therapeutic neuromodulation provides an effective way to manipulate and control synaptic function via intact neural pathways that maintains, improves, or restores normal neural output. While there are a multitude of studies that utilize viral vector-mediated gene expression of growth factors to treat neurodegenerative diseases, such as Alzheimer disease or amyotrophic lateral sclerosis, most do not constitute gene-based "neuromodulation." In this chapter we will limit our discussion primarily to viral-mediated therapies that focus on altering synaptic activity to control signal transduction within disease-associated neural pathways.

The vast majority of the studies incorporating gene-based neuromodulatory approaches remain in the early stages of development. However, many preclinical studies using viral vector-mediated gene expression have been advanced to clinical trials and scrutinized for safety and efficacy in human patients. Table 9.1 contains information about the clinical trials that represent the clinically tested neuromodulatory strategies in PD and chronic pain. The subsequent sections of this chapter will present examples of viral vector-mediated neuromodulation in clinical trials and the exciting preclinical research conducted in PD, chronic pain, epilepsy, and psychiatric disorders.

PARKINSON DISEASE

PD pathology is caused by the dysfunction or death of nigrostriatal neurons leading to the subsequent loss of dopamine signaling. Loss of dopaminergic signaling is closely related to the onset of PD and other movement disorders. Currently dopamine therapies are meant to treat the symptoms of PD but do nothing to slow the degeneration of dopaminergic neurons of the substantia nigra. The majority of the clinical trials in CNS gene therapy have involved PD. To date there have been five different vector systems tested for PD gene therapy in clinical trials.[91] All of these trials have used either AAV or LV to deliver the therapeutic transgene. These therapies have focused on three main approaches: (1) reduction of PD symptoms through the elevation of dopamine synthesis; (2) inhibition of disease progression by providing additional neurotrophic

TABLE 9.1 Clinical Trials in Therapeutic Neuromodulation

Neurological Disease	Clinical Phase/ID	Years Conducted	# Patients	Viral Vector	Transgene Insert	Route of Administration	Trial Objective	Significant Outcomes
Parkinson disease	Phase I NCT0195143	2003–05	12	AAV	GAD	Single infusion into subthalamic nucleus	Safety and tolerability; clinical status	GAD expression improved motor scores
	Phase II NCT00643890	2008–10	55	AAV2	GAD	Bilateral infusion into subthalamic nucleus	Evaluate effects on UPDRS motor scores	GAD express improved scores over baseline
	Phase I NCT0229736	2004–13	10	AAV2	AADC	Single infusion into putamen	Safety and tolerability; clinical status; dosage and expression	AADC expression correlated with a 30% increase in motor score
	Phase I NCT0197543	2013–ongoing	10	AAV2	AADC	MRI-guided convective infusion into putamen	Safety and tolerability; clinical status; expression versus viral biodistribution	N/A
	Phase I/II NCT0627588	2008–12	15	LV	TH AADC GCH	Single infusion into striatum	Safety and tolerability; dose response and clinical status	Improved all patient motor scores at 6 months
	Phase I/II NCT01856439	2011–ongoing	15	LV	TH AADC GCH	Single infusion into striatum	Long-term safety and tolerability; long-term clinical status	N/A
Chronic pain	Phase I NCT00804076	2008–13	10	HSV	hPPE	Intradermal injection in the area of pain	Safety and tolerability; dosage and clinical benefit	Elevated dosages were able to provide pain relief
	Phase II NCT01291901	2011–13	33	HSV	hPPE	Intradermal injection in the area of pain	Clinical benefit	N/A

factor support; and (3) inhibition of neural activity by increasing inhibitory neurotransmitter production.

The first human trial in PD utilizing viral-mediated gene therapy was in patients with moderately advanced PD. An AAV2 vector was employed to deliver glutamic acid decarboxylase (GAD), a rate-limiting enzyme in the production of the neurotransmitter γ-aminobutyric acid (GABA), to the substantia nigra. GABA is one of the main inhibitory neurotransmitters present in the brain that is involved in many neurological processes including the regulation of motor function. Motivation for movement into clinical trials was provided by preclinical studies of subthalamic AAV-mediated GAD expression. Models reported strong evidence of neuroprotection of nigral dopamine neurons and rescue of the Parkinsonian behavioral phenotype through inhibition of the subthalamic nucleus (STN) activity and output.[92,93] Additionally, AAV-GAD was found to be effective and safe in a nonhuman primate model of PD.[94] The goals of this clinical trial were to validate AAV-mediated gene delivery as safe and to regulate the firing rates within the STN of the PD brain in order to improve motor function (NCT00643890). Patients received one of three doses of AAV2-GAD that were directly injected unilaterally to the STN. The study results showed patients exhibited no adverse reaction to the treatment and no detectable immune response. Motor scores were improved in patients after 3 months as determined by the unified Parkinson's disease rating scale (UPDRS). These improvements were believed to be associated with increased metabolism in the premotor cortex, an area of the brain that regulates movement.[95]

Progression of AAV2-GAD into phase II clinical trials (NCT00643890) were conducted to evaluate the highest dose of AAV2-GAD in 21 patients compared to 23 sham control patients who were injected with sterile saline. This phase II trial supported the phase I findings that no adverse effects were associated with the surgical delivery method or gene therapy by AAV2-GAD, which was sustained through 12 months. Furthermore, the AAV2-GAD-treated group exhibited improvement in UPDRS motor scores when compared with the sham control group, providing evidence that AAV2 could be safely administered directly to the brain and that the GAD gene expression was potentially therapeutic.[96] A long-term follow-up study was proposed and approved but the company conducting the trial (Neurologix, Inc.) fell into bankruptcy and these trials were terminated.

The second example of viral-mediated neuromodulation for PD involved increasing the activity of aromatic L-amino acid decarboxylase (AADC), an enzyme that can convert levodopa to dopamine. Levodopa can increase dopamine levels and improve PD symptoms in the short term. This treatment, however, relies on endogenous enzymatic function of AADC to convert levodopa to dopamine. Researchers were motivated to understand whether elevated AADC expression could potentially provide therapeutic benefit. AAV-mediated delivery of AADC to improve levodopa therapy was established in rat PD models and was reported to increase dopamine production concomitant with behavioral improvement.[97] Furthermore, a study using a neurotoxin model of PD in nonhuman primates reported animals that received AAV-AADC, when compared to those animals that received the control gene, exhibited long-term behavioral improvement, decreased levodopa side effects, and elevated AADC expression that persisted for 6 years.[98] Elevation of AADC in striatal neurons could enable clinicians to utilize levodopa with greater efficacy and better modulate neurotransmission in PD and other dopaminergic movement disorders. To establish the safety and efficacy of AAV2-AADC treatment in humans a phase I clinical trial (NCT00229736) was launched by Avigen (subsequently bought by Genzyme). This trial was comprised of 10 patients who received a direct putaminal infusion of either a low or high dose of AAV2-AADC while concurrently taking oral levodopa. No adverse effects were reported in association with AAV2-AADC in any of the trial patients, providing evidence that this vector system was safe and tolerable for therapeutic utility. AADC activity was increased in the striatum after 6 months which positively correlated with about a 30% increase in UPDRS motor scores.[99] Because clinical improvements were detected at time points when the patient was both on or off levodopa it suggested that gene therapy was effective in converting both endogenous and exogenous levodopa. It is important to highlight the idea that expression of AADC could provide improvement on its own through maintenance of dopaminergic signaling, which could be further regulated by levodopa administration. This was further supported by the fact that all patients who received high-dose AAV2-AADC required less levodopa. This suggested that AAV2 could safely express genes of therapeutic interest and could be again used in the future to validate other targets.[100] Bolstered by these results a phase I clinical trial (NCT01973543) has been recently initiated where PD patients that are on levodopa receive putaminal AAV2-hAADC MRI-guided injections through convective infusion. Results are not yet available.[101]

Another example of viral-mediated neuromodulation in PD utilized transduction of multiple therapeutic genes all encoded within one LV construct. These three genes, intended to increase the production of dopamine, were AADC, TH, and guanosine triphosphate cyclohydrase (GCH). TH and GCH convert dietary tyrosine into levodopa, which is then converted to dopamine by AADC. This multiple-gene LV construct was preceded by an early study reporting multiple gene expression increased dopamine production when three AAV constructs expressing TH, AADC, and GCH were used in conjunction.[102] Furthermore, a large animal preclinical study found that coexpression of these enzymes using three separate constructs in the striatum of primates led to improved motor functions.[103]

These studies led to the development of a single LV vector that expressed TH, AADC, and GCH (LV-TH-AADC-GCH, or ProSavin [Oxford BioMedica]). This construct was modeled after one used in a study that reported functional improvement in a rat PD model after administration of a single LV vector expressing three catecholaminergic enzymes, including AADC and TH.[104] No reported toxic effects due to genomic insertion were observed. The phase I/II clinical trial (NCT00627588) tested three doses of ProSavin in a cohort of 15 moderate-to-advanced PD patients. No evidence of adverse events was found associated with the therapy at either 6 months or 3 years following administration.[105] These patients were then transferred into a separate phase I/II trial (NCT01856439) that is currently ongoing to assess the long-term tolerability and efficacy (10 years) of ProSavin. The results of these studies are expected to be completed in 2022.

Currently, preclinical studies are evaluating a similar approach. A single AAV vector, AAV-TH-GCH, construct has been produced and has shown promising results in a rodent model of PD.[106] However, dose-dependent toxicity must be further evaluated before significant progress into a clinical setting can be made. Additionally, it must be shown that this vector provides superior therapeutic benefit when compared to previous treatments such as ProSavin.

There is a large body of research that utilizes viral vector systems to deliver genes to increase expression of proteins believed to be lacking or dysfunctional in PD. Both neuromodulatory and neuroprotective strategies are being evaluated for clinical translation. It is important to mention, while not neuromodulation per se, that there have been clinical trials conducted using viral vectors to express neurotrophic factors to support neuronal viability and axon integrity. For example, following validation at the preclinical level a recent clinical trial (NCT00985517) utilized AAV2 to express Neuturin, a glial-derived neurotrophic factor family member (CERE-120). While it received promising results from the phase I safety validation, the subsequent expanded trial did not show significant improvement as determined by motor function scoring. Unfortunately, CERE-120 was also reported to cause adverse events in over one-third of the patients that received the therapeutic vector. A follow-on trial attempted to administer this promising therapeutic into an additional area of the brain but did not show any motor score improvements. There are a great many studies that are attempting to utilize growth factors, neurotrophic support factors, and neuromodulators for therapeutic development in PD and many other neurodegenerative diseases.

Most of these strategies are still in the early stages and it is too early to determine whether they will eventually advance all the way to clinical testing. However, the validation of improved viral-vector safety and their ability to deliver gene-based neuromodulation in both preclinical and clinical trials can be adapted for therapeutic intervention whenever promising gene targets are identified.

CHRONIC PAIN

Chronic pain can be attributed to many causes but is likely to result from localized inflammation near the nerve tissue or damage to the nerve tissue itself. There are two main classifications of chronic nerve pain: nociceptive and neuropathic. Chronic nociceptive pain involves intact nerve function and is typically caused by inflammatory induction near the nerve sending the pain signal.[107] This type of pain can be a result of other chronic disease processes such as types of arthritis, pancreatitis, or inflammatory bowel disease. Inflammation in these diseases occurs as a result of an overactive immune response generating the presence of inflammatory cytokines secreted by either immune cells and/or glial cells.[108] The other type of chronic pain, neuropathic pain, is caused by damage to the nerve tissue that elicits an aberrant pain signal that can occur without any detected injury to the tissue it innervates.[109] Neuropathic pain is seen in cases of spinal cord injury, peripheral nerve injury, anticancer treatment, and postherpetic neuralgia.[110] As pain is divided into two main phases, therapies must be designed to address each of these if effective treatment is to be successful. The nerve fibers responsible for the relay of the initial pain stimuli, which is transmitted by the Aδ-afferents, are exclusive from the prolonged secondary pain signal, which utilizes C-afferents for signal transduction.[111,112] A schematic representation of the pain pathway and the specialized fibers involved in pain signal transduction can be found in Fig. 9.4. These signals arrive at the cortex and a response signal descends from the higher brain regions back to the spinal cord where the signal can mediate the natural release of peptides to provide an analgesic effect.[113] These peptides act effectively to block pain signaling at the spinal cord and include enkephalins (ENKs), endorphins, dynorphins, and endomorphin.[114]

The development of therapies for chronic pain remains a complex process. In nociceptive pain, therapies must first deal with the primary insult that induces pain in addition to the subsequent factors that affect the chronic pain state. The first, second, and third line of pharmaceutical intervention include cyclooxygenase inhibitors such as aspirin and ibuprofen, less potent opioids (codeine),[115] and more potent opioids (morphine, fentanyl).[115] However these methods are not always effective against more severe pain and can produce unwanted side effects within the kidneys and gastrointestinal tract. Opioid treatment is effective against chronic pain states but opioids have significant tolerance issues and are commonly abused.[116,117] Additionally, high percentages of

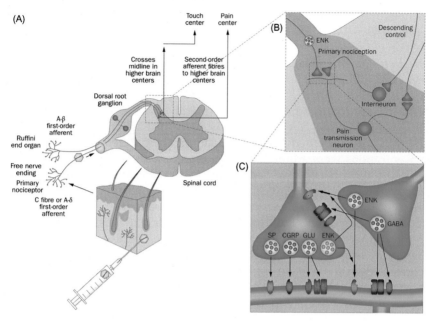

FIGURE 9.4 Gene therapy for pain using an HSV vector. (A, B) Pain signaling is mediated by primary sensory afferents that connect via synapses in the spinal cord to release neurotransmitters and peptides, including glutamate, substance P, and CGRP. After injection into the skin, the HSV vector is delivered to the cell bodies of primary afferents by retrograde axonal transport, enabling production and release of the transgene product (in this case ENK) from nerve terminals in the dorsal horn. (C) ENK released from the transduced primary afferents inhibits nociceptive neurotransmission through binding to opioid receptors at presynaptic and postsynaptic sites. CGRP, calcitonin gene-related peptide; ENK, enkephalin; GAD, glutamic acid decarboxylase; GLU, glutamate; HSV, herpes simplex virus; SP, substance P.

patients are refractive to pharmacological management of their pain and this provides the motivation for the development of gene therapy strategies to fill that need.

Chronic pain research has explored designing vector strategies that provide the ability to peripherally inject therapeutics at the site of pain to be transported in a retrograde fashion to the nerve root ganglion, the region in the peripheral nerve system that contains the cell bodies of the primary sensory neurons.[118,119] Preclinical studies of chronic pain have utilized many viral vectors including Ad, AAV, HSV, and LV.[118,120–122]

A successful pain management approach harnesses the action of endogenous opioid peptides that are increased naturally within the body after pain induction. These peptides include ENK, adrenocorticotropic hormone, melanocyte-stimulating hormone, and endorphin. HSV vectors that express ENK have been utilized to provide analgesic effects in nociceptive pain models as well as neuropathic pain models.[123–126] Clinical trials have been conducted for the treatment of chronic pain in the context of cancer pain.[127] The first clinical phase I trial (NCT00804076) was to test dose-escalation effects in patients diagnosed with primary or metastatic cancer. The vector used was a replication-defective HSV vector encoding ENK from the hPPE gene (human pre-pro-enkaphalin), named NP2. In addition to other exclusion criteria, patients who had previous HSV-related disease may have already developed antibodies against HSV and thus were excluded from participation. Three different doses of NP2 concentrations were administered through ten 100 μL intradermal injections at the corresponding dermatome in 10 patients. Additionally, pain scores were monitored in each patient for 4 weeks after injections. The safety of NP2 was verified as none of the 10 patients exhibited adverse effects associated with the treatment. Although NP2 was confirmed safe as the primary endpoint of the phase I trial, there also appeared to be therapeutic efficacy in this small patient cohort. Numeric rating scale pain scores seen in the low-dose group fell from 8 to 6 over 4 weeks while the medium-dose group saw a decrease in score from 9 to 1 in the first 2 weeks that rose back to 4 by the 4-week time point. The largest effect was seen in the high-dose group that exhibited scores that fell from 8 to 1 at 2 weeks that only reached a level of 2 by the end of the 4-week period.[127] A phase II trial (NCT01291901) has recently been completed that sought to determine the impact of intradermal delivery of NP2 on pain scores and pain medication usage in subjects with intractable pain due to malignant disease. No results from this study are currently available.

In a similar methodology HSV vectors have been employed to express endomorphin-like peptides that have been reported to effectively inhibit pain in inflammatory pain models and sciatic nerve ligation.[128,129] Additionally, there are strategies that have employed HSV and AAV constructs expressing the mu opioid receptor, to potentiate opioid effects. This approach shows promise in modulating morphine treatment.[130,131]

There are also approaches to modulate neurotransmitters to alter synaptic circuits in the CNS to inhibit neuropathic pain. GABA and glycine affect the dorsal horn of the spinal cord and it has been shown that GABA agonists can block neuropathic pain. Based on the safety and efficacy data from the first two clinical trials for NP2, a new phase I/II trial studying the effects of an HSV replication defective vector expressing GAD67 on patients experiencing diabetic neuropathy will be launched soon.[107] Viral-mediated overexpression of the enzyme GAD is reported to increase the conversion of glutamate into GABA and has been shown to reduce both neuropathic and nociceptive pain.[132,133]

Similar to alternate gene therapy strategies described in PD research, a common approach in chronic pain is to use viral constructs to express neurotrophic factors and growth factors to support neuronal health and structure. Brain-derived neurotrophic factor (BDNF) expression by grafted cells was shown to decrease pain state in rodents, thus providing the proof of principle that expression growth factors can bring about an analgesic effect.[134] Viral vectors using Ad, AAV, LV, and HSV have been employed to express growth factors and potential therapeutic targets with reported analgesic effects.[122,135–137] However, while the exact mechanisms for their analgesic benefit remain unknown, it is speculated that these factors may inhibit the cytokine response through an unknown mechanism that may be unrelated to their growth-promoting functions.

EPILEPSY

Epilepsy is characterized by the development of seizures that are caused by an imbalance in the excitatory or inhibitory neurotransmission pathways in various areas of the brain. The development of epileptic seizures can be caused by a multitude of factors, including inducible events such as head trauma, stroke, and brain infection. Unfortunately, many patients are refractive to current pharmacological intervention; or, if treatment is effective, they may develop significant side effects. Drug resistance for patients experiencing epileptic seizures poses a need for intervention that may be met by gene therapy strategies. Invasive surgical options involving the removal or ablation of the epileptic region of the brain are available but are used as a last resort in clinical settings. Gene therapies are currently being evaluated in models of epilepsy because they can provide the ability for targeted long-term gene expression within the susceptible tissue.[138] Advances in neuroimaging techniques could also be used to provide patient-specific data that can help to identify the brain regions of interest for therapeutic intervention. However, because epilepsy is multifactorial it is necessary to identify the specific genes that require expression for therapeutic benefit and as well as the specific delivery methods that are optimal for transduction of the targeted tissue.

Currently, preclinical models have been developed to address the variability within the epileptic disease sequela. One such type model involves use of electrical stimulation to areas of the brain to induce seizures that initiate focally and spread to general symptoms. This type of model is referred to as kindling and can be achieved through stimulation of many regions of the brain, including the hippocampus, amygdala, and the piriform cortex. Additional models utilize chemical or electrically induced epileptogenic insult. After insult there will be a period of time in which animals do not exhibit symptoms but will subsequently be followed by spontaneous recurrent seizures that closely mimic the human condition.

Inhibitory and excitatory signals associated with the development of seizures can be altered through viral-mediated gene expression to provide decreased seizure intensity or number of seizure events. Chemically induced epilepsy models can effectively downregulate the expression of the GABA receptor subunits alpha-1 while upregulating another subunit, alpha-4. An AAV vector, using the alpha-4 promoter sequence to express the alpha-1 subunit, showed increased alpha-1 expression concomitant with decreased frequency of seizure development in pilocarpine-treated rats.[139] This is a good example of developing a therapeutic construct with the knowledge of specific promoter activity of the target tissue. Using the promoter of the upregulated alpha-4 subunit increases expression of the alpha-1 subunit to restore nonepileptogenic GABA-dependent neural activity.

Reduction of excitatory activity has been further explored by the use of AAV vectors to manipulate N-methyl-D-aspartate receptors in excitatory and inhibitory neuronal cells. Cell-specific promoters were selected to target separate cell populations with the goal of increasing NMDA currents, which are considered critical modulators of the epileptic signaling. This study reported that vectors with a CMV promoter resulted in decreased seizures, whereas vectors with the tetracycline-off regulatable promoter caused an increased sensitivity to seizures.[140] This divergence was speculated to involve the unexpected participation of interneuron expression and signaling. Another study used LV vector to express the potassium channel Kv1.1 in excitatory neurons that reduced intrinsic excitability of transduced pyramidal neurons and provided suppression of epileptic activity over several weeks without behavioral side effects.[141] Other studies have reported that viral-mediated expression of the ion-channel Kir2.1 can induce neuronal inhibition, an effect that could be applied to many types of neurological pathways including those relating to epilepsy.[34,120]

Galanin (GAL) is a neuromodulatory peptide that is released during seizures and is known to inhibit glutamate release in the hippocampus. Deletion of GAL in mouse models has shown increased seizure occurrence while overexpression of GAL in seizure pathways displays epileptic resistance. One study used an AAV vector expressing GAL into the hippocampus of animals treated with a proepileptic chemical. This study reported viral-mediated expression of GAL led to increased cell viability and reduced both severity and frequency of seizure.[142] This study provides proof that GAL can be used to restore the balance of neural activity. Injection into other areas of the brain, such as the piriform cortex and the inferior colliculus, has also shown promising therapeutic effects. This AAV-mediated inhibition within the hippocampus has also been achieved with a fibronectin secretory signal sequence inserted in front of the GAL sequence and was shown to be effective in multiple epileptic models.[143] Similar to GAL, overexpression of the neuropeptide Y (NPY) using both AAV-2 and chimeric AAV-1/2 vectors to provide constitutive expression of NPY has been shown to provide antiseizure effects in multiple rat studies.[144,145] NPY is an endogenously expressed protein found to be at elevated levels within the hippocampus during seizure events and exhibits evidence of neuromodulatory capabilities within the epileptic phenotypes. NPY and its related receptors are engaged in a dynamic interaction within epileptic tissue and this interplay is believed to reduce epileptic events in quantity, intensity, or duration. AAV has also been used to express a receptor for NPY that was shown to potentiate the effects of NPY overexpression.[146]

In addition to the neuromodulatory strategies relevant to epilepsy, neuroprotection strategies using viral vector-mediated expression to increase protective neurotropic factors, such as fibroblast growth factor 2 (FGF-2) and BDNF, are also being tested in translational epilepsy models.[147,148] Although gene therapy in epilepsy is complicated due to the multifactorial nature of the disease, it does provide a model for developing alternatives to invasive and destructive surgical procedures. Furthermore, since electrodes are commonly placed in the areas of the brain associated with epileptic pathology, these same areas could be injected with viral vectors, without significantly more risk from the surgery.

PSYCHIATRIC DISORDERS

Although there are currently many effective therapeutic approaches to treating different psychiatric disorders, there remain significant populations of patients that remain refractive to treatment. In addition to cognitive reinforcement, current therapies employ the use an array of pharmaceutical intervention alone or in concert with surgical techniques like electrical deep brain stimulation. Psychiatric disorders have convoluted pathologies and create a complicated arena for the development of effective therapies. In order to advance the progress of viral-mediated gene therapy for the treatment of psychiatric disorders clinicians must have the ability to identify specific brain pathways and participating cell populations that underlie disease-associated symptoms. Some areas that could be potentially targeted for gene-based neuromodulation are currently being studied and explored through deep brain stimulation.[149] Advances in brain imaging techniques can provide a map for viral-mediated neuromodulation of neural pathways through the identification of specific targets. However, preclinical models are quite limited in their ability to replicate much more complex human disease processes of psychological nature. Using vector systems that have been approved safe for use in other human diseases such as PD and chronic pain can provide proof of principle that targeted gene delivery to the CNS is possible and may eventually prove their utility in the treatment of psychiatric disorders.

There are no current viral-mediated gene therapies tested in humans that are designed to induce neuromodulation to treat psychiatric disorders. Depression and addiction are disorders believed to be caused by deficits or alterations within the serotoninergic system. Imbalance in signaling controlled by the neurotransmitter serotonin and its receptors are implicated in the development of psychiatric disorders such as depression, anxiety, and fear response. Animal models of depression have shown that serotonin receptors, like p11, are essential mediators in the disease process and are considered potential gene therapy targets.[150] p11 expression is believed to be particularly important in the nucleus accumbens (NAcc), an area of the brain that is widely accepted as an affected brain region in depression and addiction. Experimental inhibition of this brain region specifically is associated with anxiety and depression-like behavior in preclinical animal models.[151] Rodents with inhibited p11 expression exhibit reduced serotonin receptor expression concomitant with associated depression-like behaviors.[152] p11 knockout mice that receive AAV-p11 within the NAcc have been reported to successfully express p11 and show an attenuation of these depression-like behaviors.[153] Moreover, a recent study has shown that p11 overexpression by AAV-p11 can also reduce addictive behaviors.[154] It is believed that these behavioral improvements are caused by neuromodulatory mechanisms that alter the synaptic activity within dysfunctional serotonergic brain pathways. Serum response factor is another molecule that is found to be reduced in the NAcc of mice that demonstrate depression and addiction-like behaviors,[155,156] and may be a future target for therapeutic neuromodulation.

Virally expressed gene-based neuromodulation has also been evaluated in the context of fear-associated behaviors. Fear is an evolutionarily conserved trait that can promote survival. However this beneficial trait can transform into a mental disorder, as seen in cases of posttraumatic stress disorder. The Boulis lab has conducted experiments to determine whether fear-associated behaviors could be altered through the introduction of an Ad construct expressing a tetanus neurotoxin peptide sequence called light chain (LC). LC degrades synaptobrevin, a protein that is necessary for synaptic neurotransmission, and thus can confer inhibition to the neuronal networks in which it is expressed. Our group was able to decrease the amplitude of acoustic startle as a measure of fear response in the animals that expressed LC compared with the control.[157] This study provides evidence that neural inhibition through gene-based neuromodulation can be used to effectively alter fear-related behaviors.

Demonstrating its widespread applicability in many different types of neurological disorders, viral-mediated gene-based neuromodulation can also be potentially applied to obsessive-compulsive disorders, eating disorders, and sleep-related disorders. Our lab conducted a study to determine whether an AAV2 construct expressing *GAD65*, a gene that can induce neuronal inhibition by increasing the production of the inhibitory neurotransmitter GABA, could alter the feeding behavior in rats. Animals that received AAV2-GAD65 hippocampal injection within the lateral nucleus, the brain region regulating feeding behavior, were observed to feed less and did not gain weight as rapidly as the control animals.[158] This study demonstrates the ability to target the specific neural tissue associated with a known behavioral function (in this case feeding behavior), which can then be altered through the introduction of a viral construct that induces synaptic inhibition. It would not be far-fetched to hypothesize similar results could be obtained if these inhibitory strategies were applied to other brain regions with respect to their behavioral associations.

The identification of additional targets in association with various psychiatric disorders must be expanded in order to adequately test gene therapy as a viable method of treatment in these disease processes. Restoration of functional serotoninergic neurotransmission by viral-mediated gene expression could potentially set the stage for controlling dysfunctional neural circuitry associated with various psychiatric disorders in order to be advanced into clinical applications.

CONCLUSIONS

The use of viral and nonviral vector systems that introduce exogenous genetic material into living cells, tissues, and organisms for prolonged therapeutic expression has expanded the possibilities for effective treatment of diseases affecting the nervous system. Gene-based neuromodulation is a fast-growing area in basic and clinical gene therapy research that could soon provide medically relevant solutions for diseases. Technological advances made in viral vector safety (i.e., removal of unnecessary viral genes or viral antigens) that limit aberrant side effects while enhancing targeting (i.e., including neurotropic peptides into viral capsid, and promoter selection) to improve tissue-specific accuracy have elevated the use of viral-mediated delivery systems as an increasingly imminent therapeutic option for many neurological diseases.

Many viral vector systems have been tested in human clinical trials for neurological diseases and are generally safe with no adverse effects attributed to the viral vectors. However, safety considerations aside, it remains unclear when these viral vector systems will provide widespread therapeutic benefit in a clinical setting. The future advancement of gene-based neuromodulation will rely on our knowledge of natural viral biology and the molecules that these viruses rely on for extracellular transport, cellular entry through plasma membrane, intracellular transport, and transgene expression following nuclear entry. Likewise it is of equal importance to understand the host response after therapeutic viral vector introduction, particularly in a diseased host, which could alter the efficacy of the viral-mediated therapy. There is a great wealth of knowledge that has been gained in clinical trials that have tested experimental gene therapies in PD and chronic pain. While robust therapeutic utility has yet to be achieved through viral vector-mediated neuromodulation, the data generated throughout the field of gene therapy have provided solid groundwork for future translation preclinical and clinical research into state-of-the-art medical interventions.

References

1. Wolff JA, Yee JK, Skelly H, et al. Adult mammalian hepatocyte as target cell for retroviral gene transfer: a model for gene therapy. *Somat Cell Mol Genet.* 1987;13(4):423–428.
2. Simonato M, Bennett J, Boulis NM, et al. Progress in gene therapy for neurological disorders. *Nat Rev Neurol.* 2013;9(5):277–291.
3. Carlton E, Teng Q, Federici T, Yang J, Riley J, Boulis NM. Fusion of the tetanus toxin C fragment binding domain and Bcl-xL for protection of peripheral nerve neurons. *Neurosurgery.* 2008;63(6):1175–1182. discussion 1182–1184.
4. Teng Q, Garrity-Moses M, Federici T, et al. Trophic activity of rabies G protein-pseudotyped equine infectious anemia viral vector mediated IGF-I motor neuron gene transfer in vitro. *Neurobiol Dis.* 2005;20(3):694–700.
5. Burger C, Gorbatyuk OS, Velardo MJ, et al. Recombinant AAV viral vectors pseudo-typed with viral capsids from serotypes 1, 2, and 5 display differential efficiency and cell tropism after delivery to different regions of the central nervous system. *Mol Ther.* 2004;10(2):302–317.
6. Duque S, Joussemet B, Riviere C, et al. Intravenous administration of self-complementary AAV9 enables transgene delivery to adult motor neurons. *Mol Ther.* 2009;17(7):1187–1196.
7. Schuster DJ, Dykstra JA, Riedl MS, et al. Biodistribution of adeno-associated virus serotype 9 (AAV9) vector after intrathecal and intravenous delivery in mouse. *Front Neuroanat.* 2014;8:42.
8. Alba R, Bosch A, Chillon M. Gutless adenovirus: last-generation adenovirus for gene therapy. *Gene Ther.* 2005;12(suppl 1):S18–S27.
9. Tomko RP, Xu R, Philipson L. HCAR and MCAR: the human and mouse cellular receptors for subgroup C adenoviruses and group B coxsackieviruses. *Proc Natl Acad Sci USA.* 1997;94(7):3352–3356.
10. Jonsson MI, Lenman AE, Frangsmyr L, Nyberg C, Abdullahi M, Arnberg N. Coagulation factors IX and X enhance binding and infection of adenovirus types 5 and 31 in human epithelial cells. *J Virol.* 2009;83(8):3816–3825.
11. Alba R, Bradshaw AC, Coughlan L, et al. Biodistribution and retargeting of FX-binding ablated adenovirus serotype 5 vectors. *Blood.* 2010;116(15):2656–2664.
12. Hacein-Bey-Abina S, Le Deist F, Carlier F, et al. Sustained correction of X-linked severe combined immunodeficiency by ex vivo gene therapy. *N Engl J Med.* 2002;346(16):1185–1193.
13. Nair V. Retrovirus-induced oncogenesis and safety of retroviral vectors. *Curr Opin Mol Ther.* 2008;10(5):431–438.
14. Shayakhmetov DM, Di Paolo NC, Mossman KL. Recognition of virus infection and innate host responses to viral gene therapy vectors. *Mol Ther.* 2010;18(8):1422–1429.

15. Huang S, Kamihira M. Development of hybrid viral vectors for gene therapy. *Biotechnol Adv*. 2013;31(2):208–223.
16. Wang J, Faust SM, Rabinowitz JE. The next step in gene delivery: molecular engineering of adeno-associated virus serotypes. *J Mol Cell Cardiol*. 2011;50(5):793–802.
17. Kwon I, Schaffer DV. Designer gene delivery vectors: molecular engineering and evolution of adeno-associated viral vectors for enhanced gene transfer. *Pharm Res*. 2008;25(3):489–499.
18. Sternson SM, Roth BL. Chemogenetic tools to interrogate brain functions. *Annu Rev Neurosci*. 2014;37:387–407.
19. Lee HM, Giguere PM, Roth BL. DREADDs: novel tools for drug discovery and development. *Drug Discov Today*. 2014;19(4):469–473.
20. Hutson TH, Foster E, Moon LD, Yanez-Munoz RJ. Lentiviral vector-mediated RNA silencing in the central nervous system. *Hum Gene Ther Methods*. 2014;25(1):14–32.
21. Wiederschain D, Wee S, Chen L, et al. Single-vector inducible lentiviral RNAi system for oncology target validation. *Cell Cycle*. 2009;8(3):498–504.
22. Raoul C, Abbas-Terki T, Bensadoun JC, et al. Lentiviral-mediated silencing of SOD1 through RNA interference retards disease onset and progression in a mouse model of ALS. *Nat Med*. 2005;11(4):423–428.
23. Chen S, Ge X, Chen Y, Lv N, Liu Z, Yuan W. Advances with RNA interference in Alzheimer's disease research. *Drug Des, Dev Ther*. 2013;7:117–125.
24. Hogg JC, Hegele RG. Adenovirus and Epstein-Barr virus in lung disease. *Semin Respir Infect*. 1995;10(4):244–253.
25. Kaufman HE. Adenovirus advances: new diagnostic and therapeutic options. *Curr Opin Ophthalmol*. 2011;22(4):290–293.
26. Benihoud K, Yeh P, Perricaudet M. Adenovirus vectors for gene delivery. *Curr Opin Biotechnol*. 1999;10(5):440–447.
27. Liu Q, Muruve DA. Molecular basis of the inflammatory response to adenovirus vectors. *Gene Ther*. 2003;10(11):935–940.
28. Raper SE, Chirmule N, Lee FS, et al. Fatal systemic inflammatory response syndrome in a ornithine transcarbamylase deficient patient following adenoviral gene transfer. *Mol Genet Metab*. 2003;80(1–2):148–158.
29. Brunetti-Pierri N, Palmer DJ, Beaudet AL, Carey KD, Finegold M, Ng P. Acute toxicity after high-dose systemic injection of helper-dependent adenoviral vectors into nonhuman primates. *Hum Gene Ther*. 2004;15(1):35–46.
30. Yang Y, Ertl HC, Wilson JM. MHC class I-restricted cytotoxic T lymphocytes to viral antigens destroy hepatocytes in mice infected with E1-deleted recombinant adenoviruses. *Immunity*. 1994;1(5):433–442.
31. Schaack J. Adenovirus vectors deleted for genes essential for viral DNA replication. *Front Biosci*. 2005;10:1146–1155.
32. Capasso C, Garofalo M, Hirvinen M, Cerullo V. The evolution of adenoviral vectors through genetic and chemical surface modifications. *Viruses*. 2014;6(2):832–855.
33. Sakhuja K, Reddy PS, Ganesh S, et al. Optimization of the generation and propagation of gutless adenoviral vectors. *Hum Gene Ther*. 2003;14(3):243–254.
34. Boulis NM, Handy CR, Krudy CA, et al. Regulated neuronal neuromodulation via spinal cord expression of the gene for the inwardly rectifying potassium channel 2.1 (Kir2.1). *Neurosurgery*. 2012;72(4).
35. Weinberg MS, Samulski RJ, McCown TJ. Adeno-associated virus (AAV) gene therapy for neurological disease. *Neuropharmacology*. 2013;69:82–88.
36. Tratschin JD, Miller IL, Smith MG, Carter BJ. Adeno-associated virus vector for high-frequency integration, expression, and rescue of genes in mammalian cells. *Mol Cell Biol*. 1985;5(11):3251–3260.

37. Louis Jeune V, Joergensen JA, Hajjar RJ, Weber T. Pre-existing anti-adeno-associated virus antibodies as a challenge in AAV gene therapy. *Hum Gene Ther Methods.* 2013;24(2):59–67.
38. McPhee S, Janson C, Li C, et al. Immune responses to AAV in phase I study for Canavan disease. *J Gene Med.* 2006;8(5):577–588.
39. McCarty DM, Monahan PE, Samulski RJ. Self-complementary recombinant adeno-associated virus (scAAV) vectors promote efficient transduction independently of DNA synthesis. *Gene Ther.* 2001;8(16):1248–1254.
40. McCarty DM. Self-complementary AAV vectors; advances and applications. *Mol Ther.* 2008;16(10):1648–1656.
41. Summerford C, Samulski RJ. Membrane-associated heparan sulfate proteoglycan is a receptor for adeno-associated virus type 2 virions. *J Virol.* 1998;72(2):1438–1445.
42. Kaludov N, Brown KE, Walters RW, Zabner J, Chiorini JA. Adeno-associated virus serotype 4 (AAV4) and AAV5 both require sialic acid binding for hemagglutination and efficient transduction but differ in sialic acid linkage specificity. *J Virol.* 2001;75(15):6884–6893.
43. Bell CL, Gurda BL, Van Vliet K, Agbandje-McKenna M, Wilson JM. Identification of the galactose binding domain of the adeno-associated virus serotype 9 capsid. *J Virol.* 2012;86(13):7326–7333.
44. Choi VW, McCarty DM, Samulski RJ. AAV hybrid serotypes: improved vectors for gene delivery. *Curr Gene Ther.* 2005;5(3):299–310.
45. Leung CH, Kliem MA, Heeke BL, et al. Assessment of hippocampal adeno-associated viral vector gene delivery via frameless stereotaxis in a nonhuman primate. *Stereotact Funct Neurosurg.* 2011;89(5):275–285.
46. Markakis EA, Vives KP, Bober J, et al. Comparative transduction efficiency of AAV vector serotypes 1-6 in the substantia nigra and striatum of the primate brain. *Mol Ther.* 2010;18(3):588–593.
47. Manfredsson FP, Rising AC, Mandel RJ. AAV9: a potential blood-brain barrier buster. *Mol Ther.* 2009;17(3):403–405.
48. Federici T, Taub JS, Baum GR, et al. Robust spinal motor neuron transduction following intrathecal delivery of AAV9 in pigs. *Gene Ther.* 2012;19(8):852–859.
49. Snyder BR, Gray SJ, Quach ET, et al. Comparison of adeno-associated viral vector serotypes for spinal cord and motor neuron gene delivery. *Hum Gene Ther.* 2011;28.
50. Asokan A, Schaffer DV, Samulski RJ. The AAV vector toolkit: poised at the clinical crossroads. *Mol Ther.* 2012;20(4):699–708.
51. Frampton Jr. AR, Goins WF, Nakano K, Burton EA, Glorioso JC. HSV trafficking and development of gene therapy vectors with applications in the nervous system. *Gene Ther.* 2005;12(11):891–901.
52. Argnani R, Lufino M, Manservigi M, Manservigi R. Replication-competent herpes simplex vectors: design and applications. *Gene Ther.* 2005;12(suppl 1):S170–S177.
53. Goins WF, Huang S, Cohen JB, Glorioso JC. Engineering HSV-1 vectors for gene therapy. *Methods Mol Biol.* 2014;1144:63–79.
54. Rosenberg SA, Aebersold P, Cornetta K, et al. Gene transfer into humans—immunotherapy of patients with advanced melanoma, using tumor-infiltrating lymphocytes modified by retroviral gene transduction. *N Engl J Med.* 1990;323(9):570–578.
55. Azzouz M, Kingsman SM, Mazarakis ND. Lentiviral vectors for treating and modeling human CNS disorders. *J Gene Med.* 2004;6(9):951–962.
56. Delzor A, Escartin C, Deglon N. Lentiviral vectors: a powerful tool to target astrocytes in vivo. *Curr Drug Targets.* 2013;14(11):1336–1346.
57. Croci C, Fasano S, Superchi D, et al. Cerebellar neurons and glial cells are transducible by lentiviral vectors without decrease of cerebellar functions. *Dev Neurosci.* 2006;28(3):216–221.

58. Geraerts M, Eggermont K, Hernandez-Acosta P, Garcia-Verdugo JM, Baekelandt V, Debyser Z. Lentiviral vectors mediate efficient and stable gene transfer in adult neural stem cells in vivo. *Hum Gene Ther*. 2006;17(6):635–650.

59. Dreyer JL. Lentiviral vector-mediated gene transfer and RNA silencing technology in neuronal dysfunctions. *Mol Biotechnol*. 2011;47(2):169–187.

60. Trabalza A, Georgiadis C, Eleftheriadou I, et al. Venezuelan equine encephalitis virus glycoprotein pseudotyping confers neurotropism to lentiviral vectors. *Gene Ther*. 2013;20(7):723–732.

61. Barraza RA, Poeschla EM. Human gene therapy vectors derived from feline lentiviruses. *Vet Immunol Immunopathol*. 2008;123(1–2):23–31.

62. Manfredsson FP, Mandel RJ. The development of flexible lentiviral vectors for gene transfer in the CNS. *Exp Neurol*. 2011;229(2):201–206.

63. Cronin J, Zhang XY, Reiser J. Altering the tropism of lentiviral vectors through pseudotyping. *Curr Gene Ther*. 2005;5(4):387–398.

64. Mazarakis ND, Azzouz M, Rohll JB, et al. Rabies virus glycoprotein pseudotyping of lentiviral vectors enables retrograde axonal transport and access to the nervous system after peripheral delivery. *Hum Mol Genet*. 2001;10(19):2109–2121.

65. Jakobsson J, Ericson C, Jansson M, Bjork E, Lundberg C. Targeted transgene expression in rat brain using lentiviral vectors. *J Neurosci Res*. 2003;73(6):876–885.

66. Yaguchi M, Ohashi Y, Tsubota T, et al. Characterization of the properties of seven promoters in the motor cortex of rats and monkeys after lentiviral vector-mediated gene transfer. *Hum Gene Ther Methods*. 2013;24(6):333–344.

67. Schroder AR, Shinn P, Chen H, Berry C, Ecker JR, Bushman F. HIV-1 integration in the human genome favors active genes and local hotspots. *Cell*. 2002;110(4):521–529.

68. Bushman F, Lewinski M, Ciuffi A, et al. Genome-wide analysis of retroviral DNA integration. *Nat Rev Microbiol*. 2005;3(11):848–858.

69. Modlich U, Baum C. Preventing and exploiting the oncogenic potential of integrating gene vectors. *J Clin Invest*. 2009;119(4):755–758.

70. Heckl D, Schwarzer A, Haemmerle R, et al. Lentiviral vector induced insertional haploinsufficiency of Ebf1 causes murine leukemia. *Mol Ther*. 2012;20(6):1187–1195.

71. Nayerossadat N, Maedeh T, Ali PA. Viral and nonviral delivery systems for gene delivery. *Adv Biomed Res*. 2012;1:27.

72. Yin H, Kanasty RL, Eltoukhy AA, Vegas AJ, Dorkin JR, Anderson DG. Non-viral vectors for gene-based therapy. *Nat Rev Genet*. 2014;15(8):541–555.

73. Koynova R, Tenchov B. Cationic lipids: molecular structure/transfection activity relationships and interactions with biomembranes. *Top Curr Chem*. 2010;296:51–93.

74. Duan Y, Zhang S, Wang B, Yang B, Zhi D. The biological routes of gene delivery mediated by lipid-based non-viral vectors. *Expert Opin Drug Deliv*. 2009;6(12):1351–1361.

75. Bedikian AY, Richards J, Kharkevitch D, Atkins MB, Whitman E, Gonzalez R. A phase 2 study of high-dose Allovectin-7 in patients with advanced metastatic melanoma. *Melanoma Res*. 2010;20(3):218–226.

76. Boussif O, Lezoualc'h F, Zanta MA, et al. A versatile vector for gene and oligonucleotide transfer into cells in culture and in vivo: polyethylenimine. *Proc Natl Acad Sci USA*. 1995;92(16):7297–7301.

77. Wang S, Ma N, Gao SJ, Yu H, Leong KW. Transgene expression in the brain stem effected by intramuscular injection of polyethylenimine/DNA complexes. *Mol Ther*. 2001;3(5 Pt 1):658–664.

78. Wang X, Wang C, Zeng J, et al. Gene transfer to dorsal root ganglia by intrathecal injection: effects on regeneration of peripheral nerves. *Mol Ther*. 2005;12(2):314–320.

79. da Cruz MT, Cardoso AL, de Almeida LP, Simoes S, de Lima MC. Tf-lipoplex-mediated NGF gene transfer to the CNS: neuronal protection and recovery in an excitotoxic model of brain injury. *Gene Ther*. 2005;12(16):1242–1252.

80. Zhang Y, Schlachetzki F, Zhang YF, Boado RJ, Pardridge WM. Normalization of striatal tyrosine hydroxylase and reversal of motor impairment in experimental parkinsonism with intravenous nonviral gene therapy and a brain-specific promoter. *Hum Gene Ther*. 2004;15(4):339–350.

81. Liu JK, Teng Q, Garrity-Moses M, et al. A novel peptide defined through phage display for therapeutic protein and vector neuronal targeting. *Neurobiol Dis*. 2005;19(3):407–418.

82. Federici T, Liu JK, Teng Q, Yang J, Boulis NM. A means for targeting therapeutics to peripheral nervous system neurons with axonal damage. *Neurosurgery*. 2007;60(5): 911–918. discussion 911–918.

83. Federici T, Liu JK, Teng Q, Garrity-Moses M, Yang J, Boulis NM. Neuronal affinity of a C7C loop peptide identified through phage display. *J Drug Target*. 2006;14(5):263–271.

84. Silva GA. Nanotechnology approaches to crossing the blood-brain barrier and drug delivery to the CNS. *BMC Neurosci*. 2008;9(suppl 3):S4.

85. Xiang JJ, Tang JQ, Zhu SG, et al. IONP-PLL: a novel non-viral vector for efficient gene delivery. *J Gene Med*. 2003;5(9):803–817.

86. Bharali DJ, Klejbor I, Stachowiak EK, et al. Organically modified silica nanoparticles: a nonviral vector for in vivo gene delivery and expression in the brain. *Proc Natl Acad Sci USA*. 2005;102(32):11539–11544.

87. Alyaudtin RN, Reichel A, Lobenberg R, Ramge P, Kreuter J, Begley DJ. Interaction of poly(butylcyanoacrylate) nanoparticles with the blood-brain barrier in vivo and in vitro. *J Drug Target*. 2001;9(3):209–221.

88. Vinogradov SV, Batrakova EV, Kabanov AV. Nanogels for oligonucleotide delivery to the brain. *Bioconjug Chem*. 2004;15(1):50–60.

89. Kabanov AV, Vinogradov SV. Nanogels as pharmaceutical carriers: finite networks of infinite capabilities. *Angew Chem Int Ed Engl*. 2009;48(30):5418–5429.

90. Bergen JM, Park IK, Horner PJ, Pun SH. Nonviral approaches for neuronal delivery of nucleic acids. *Pharm Res*. 2008;25(5):983–998.

91. Coune PG, Schneider BL, Aebischer P. Parkinson's disease: gene therapies. *Cold Spring Harbor Perspect Med*. 2012;2(4):a009431.

92. Luo J, Kaplitt MG, Fitzsimons HL, et al. Subthalamic GAD gene therapy in a Parkinson's disease rat model. *Science*. 2002;298(5592):425–429.

93. Lee B, Lee H, Nam YR, Oh JH, Cho YH, Chang JW. Enhanced expression of glutamate decarboxylase 65 improves symptoms of rat parkinsonian models. *Gene Ther*. 2005;12(15):1215–1222.

94. Emborg ME, Carbon M, Holden JE, et al. Subthalamic glutamic acid decarboxylase gene therapy: changes in motor function and cortical metabolism. *J Cereb Blood Flow Metab*. 2007;27(3):501–509.

95. Kaplitt MG, Feigin A, Tang C, et al. Safety and tolerability of gene therapy with an adeno-associated virus (AAV) borne GAD gene for Parkinson's disease: an open label, phase I trial. *Lancet*. 2007;369(9579):2097–2105.

96. LeWitt PA, Rezai AR, Leehey MA, et al. AAV2-GAD gene therapy for advanced Parkinson's disease: a double-blind, sham-surgery controlled, randomised trial. *Lancet Neurol*. 2011;10(4):309–319.

97. Sanchez-Pernaute R, Harvey-White J, Cunningham J, Bankiewicz KS. Functional effect of adeno-associated virus mediated gene transfer of aromatic L-amino acid decarboxylase into the striatum of 6-OHDA-lesioned rats. *Mol Ther*. 2001;4(4):324–330.

98. Bankiewicz KS, Forsayeth J, Eberling JL, et al. Long-term clinical improvement in MPTP-lesioned primates after gene therapy with AAV-hAADC. *Mol Ther*. 2006; 14(4).

99. Muramatsu S, Fujimoto K, Kato S, et al. A phase I study of aromatic L-amino acid decarboxylase gene therapy for Parkinson's disease. *Mol Ther*. 2010;18(9):1731–1735.

100. Christine CW, Starr PA, Larson PS, et al. Safety and tolerability of putaminal AADC gene therapy for Parkinson disease. *Neurology*. 2009;73(18):1662–1669.

101. Nduom EK, Walbridge S, Lonser RR. Comparison of pulsed versus continuous convective flow for central nervous system tissue perfusion: laboratory investigation. *J Neurosurg.* 2012;117(6):1150–1154.

102. Fan D, Shen Y, Kang D, Nakano I, Ozawa K. Adeno-associated virus vector-mediated triple gene transfer of dopamine synthetic enzymes. *Chin Med J (Engl).* 2001;114(12):1276–1279.

103. Muramatsu S, Fujimoto K, Ikeguchi K, et al. Behavioral recovery in a primate model of Parkinson's disease by triple transduction of striatal cells with adeno-associated viral vectors expressing dopamine-synthesizing enzymes. *Hum Gene Ther.* 2002;13(3):345–354.

104. Azzouz M, Martin-Rendon E, Barber RD, et al. Multicistronic lentiviral vector-mediated striatal gene transfer of aromatic L-amino acid decarboxylase, tyrosine hydroxylase, and GTP cyclohydrolase I induces sustained transgene expression, dopamine production, and functional improvement in a rat model of Parkinson's disease. *J Neurosci.* 2002;22(23):10302–10312.

105. Palfi S, Gurruchaga JM, Ralph GS, et al. Long-term safety and tolerability of ProSavin, a lentiviral vector-based gene therapy for Parkinson's disease: a dose escalation, open-label, phase 1/2 trial. *Lancet.* 2014;383(9923):1138–1146.

106. Cederfjall E, Sahin G, Kirik D, Bjorklund T. Design of a single AAV vector for coexpression of TH and GCH1 to establish continuous DOPA synthesis in a rat model of Parkinson's disease. *Mol Ther.* 2012;20(7):1315–1326.

107. Goins WF, Cohen JB, Glorioso JC. Gene therapy for the treatment of chronic peripheral nervous system pain. *Neurobiol Dis.* 2012;48(2):255–270.

108. Moalem G, Tracey DJ. Immune and inflammatory mechanisms in neuropathic pain. *Brain Res Rev.* 2006;51(2):240–264.

109. Baron R. Neuropathic pain: a clinical perspective. *Handb Exp Pharmacol.* 2009;194:3–30.

110. Gutierrez J, Raju S, Riley JP, Boulis NM. Introduction to neuropathic pain syndromes. *Neurosurg Clin N Am.* 2014;25(4):639–662.

111. Matre DA, Hernandez-Garcia L, Tran TD, Casey KL. "First pain" in humans: convergent and specific forebrain responses. *Mol Pain.* 2010;6:81.

112. Staud R, Craggs JG, Robinson ME, Perlstein WM, Price DD. Brain activity related to temporal summation of C-fiber evoked pain. *Pain.* 2007;129(1–2):130–142.

113. Ossipov MH, Dussor GO, Porreca F. Central modulation of pain. *J Clin Invest.* 2010;120(11):3779–3787.

114. Akil H, Watson SJ, Young E, Lewis ME, Khachaturian H, Walker JM. Endogenous opioids: biology and function. *Annu Rev Neurosci.* 1984;7:223–255.

115. Nicholson B. Responsible prescribing of opioids for the management of chronic pain. *Drugs.* 2003;63(1):17–32.

116. Argoff CE, Viscusi ER. The use of opioid analgesics for chronic pain: minimizing the risk for harm. *Am J Gastroenterol.* 2014;2(1):3–8.

117. Manchikanti L, Helm S. 2nd, Fellows B, et al. Opioid epidemic in the United States. *Pain Physician.* 2012;15(suppl 3):ES9–38.

118. Glorioso JC, Fink DJ. Herpes vector-mediated gene transfer in the treatment of chronic pain. *Mol Ther.* 2009;17(1):13–18.

119. Garrity-Moses ME, Liu JK, Boulis NM. Molecular biology and gene therapy in the treatment of chronic pain. *Neurosurg Clin N Am.* 2003;14(3):419–435.

120. Ma C, Rosenzweig J, Zhang P, Johns DC, LaMotte RH. Expression of inwardly rectifying potassium channels by an inducible adenoviral vector reduced the neuronal hyperexcitability and hyperalgesia produced by chronic compression of the spinal ganglion. *Mol Pain.* 2010;6:65.

121. Towne C, Pertin M, Beggah AT, Aebischer P, Decosterd I. Recombinant adeno-associated virus serotype 6 (rAAV2/6)-mediated gene transfer to nociceptive neurons through different routes of delivery. *Mol Pain.* 2009;5:52.

122. Pezet S, Krzyzanowska A, Wong LF, et al. Reversal of neurochemical changes and pain-related behavior in a model of neuropathic pain using modified lentiviral vectors expressing GDNF. *Mol Ther.* 2006;13(6):1101–1109.

123. Antunes Bras JM, Epstein AL, Bourgoin S, Hamon M, Cesselin F, Pohl M. Herpes simplex virus 1-mediated transfer of preproenkephalin A in rat dorsal root ganglia. *J Neurochem.* 1998;70(3):1299–1303.

124. Wilson SP, Yeomans DC, Bender MA, Lu Y, Goins WF, Glorioso JC. Antihyperalgesic effects of infection with a preproenkephalin-encoding herpes virus. *Proc Natl Acad Sci USA.* 1999;96(6):3211–3216.

125. Tzabazis AZ, Klukinov M, Feliciano DP, Wilson SP, Yeomans DC. Gene therapy for trigeminal pain in mice. *Gene Ther.* 2014;21(4):422–426.

126. Yang H, McNearney TA, Chu R, et al. Enkephalin-encoding herpes simplex virus-1 decreases inflammation and hotplate sensitivity in a chronic pancreatitis model. *Mol Pain.* 2008;4:8.

127. Fink DJ, Wechuck J, Mata M, et al. Gene therapy for pain: results of a phase I clinical trial. *Ann Neurol.* 2011;70(2):207–212.

128. Wolfe D, Hao S, Hu J, et al. Engineering an endomorphin-2 gene for use in neuropathic pain therapy. *Pain.* 2007;133(1–3):29–38.

129. Hao S, Wolfe D, Glorioso JC, Mata M, Fink DJ. Effects of transgene-mediated endomorphin-2 in inflammatory pain. *Eur J Pain.* 2009;13(4):380–386.

130. Gu Y, Xu Y, Li GW, Huang LY. Remote nerve injection of mu opioid receptor adeno-associated viral vector increases antinociception of intrathecal morphine. *J Pain.* 2005;6(7):447–454.

131. Xu Y, Gu Y, Xu GY, Wu P, Li GW, Huang LY. Adeno-associated viral transfer of opioid receptor gene to primary sensory neurons: a strategy to increase opioid antinociception. *Proc Natl Acad Sci USA.* 2003;100(10):6204–6209.

132. Wolfe D, Mata M, Fink DJ. A human trial of HSV-mediated gene transfer for the treatment of chronic pain. *Gene Ther.* 2009;16(4):455–460.

133. Liu J, Wolfe D, Hao S, et al. Peripherally delivered glutamic acid decarboxylase gene therapy for spinal cord injury pain. *Mol Ther.* 2004;10(1):57–66.

134. Cejas PJ, Martinez M, Karmally S, et al. Lumbar transplant of neurons genetically modified to secrete brain-derived neurotrophic factor attenuates allodynia and hyperalgesia after sciatic nerve constriction. *Pain.* 2000;86(1–2):195–210.

135. Chou AK, Yang MC, Tsai HP, et al. Adenoviral-mediated glial cell line-derived neurotrophic factor gene transfer has a protective effect on sciatic nerve following constriction-induced spinal cord injury. *PLoS ONE.* 2014;9(3):e92264.

136. Eaton MJ, Blits B, Ruitenberg MJ, Verhaagen J, Oudega M. Amelioration of chronic neuropathic pain after partial nerve injury by adeno-associated viral (AAV) vector-mediated over-expression of BDNF in the rat spinal cord. *Gene Ther.* 2002;9(20):1387–1395.

137. Hao S, Mata M, Wolfe D, Huang S, Glorioso JC, Fink DJ. HSV-mediated gene transfer of the glial cell-derived neurotrophic factor provides an antiallodynic effect on neuropathic pain. *Mol Ther.* 2003;8(3):367–375.

138. Walker MC, Schorge S, Kullmann DM, Wykes RC, Heeroma JH, Mantoan L. Gene therapy in status epilepticus. *Epilepsia.* 2013;54(suppl 6):43–45.

139. Raol YH, Lund IV Bandyopadhyay S, et al. Enhancing GABA(A) receptor alpha 1 subunit levels in hippocampal dentate gyrus inhibits epilepsy development in an animal model of temporal lobe epilepsy. *J Neurosci.* 2006;26(44):11342–11346.

140. Haberman R, Criswell H, Snowdy S, et al. Therapeutic liabilities of in vivo viral vector tropism: adeno-associated virus vectors, NMDAR1 antisense, and focal seizure sensitivity. *Mol Ther.* 2002;6(4):495–500.

141. Wykes RC, Heeroma JH, Mantoan L, et al. Optogenetic and potassium channel gene therapy in a rodent model of focal neocortical epilepsy. *Sci Transl Med.* 2012;4(161):161ra152.

142. Haberman RP, Samulski RJ, McCown TJ. Attenuation of seizures and neuronal death by adeno-associated virus vector galanin expression and secretion. *Nat Med.* 2003;9(8):1076–1080.

143. McCown TJ. Adeno-associated virus-mediated expression and constitutive secretion of galanin suppresses limbic seizure activity in vivo. *Mol Ther.* 2006;14(1):63–68.

144. Richichi C, Lin EJ, Stefanin D, et al. Anticonvulsant and antiepileptogenic effects mediated by adeno-associated virus vector neuropeptide Y expression in the rat hippocampus. *J Neurosci.* 2004;24(12):3051–3059.

145. Noe F, Frasca A, Balducci C, et al. Neuropeptide Y overexpression using recombinant adeno-associated viral vectors. *Neurotherapeutics.* 2009;6(2):300–306.

146. Woldbye DP, Angehagen M, Gotzsche CR, et al. Adeno-associated viral vector-induced overexpression of neuropeptide Y Y2 receptors in the hippocampus suppresses seizures. *Brain.* 2010;133(9):2778–2788.

147. Binder DK. The role of BDNF in epilepsy and other diseases of the mature nervous system. *Adv Exp Med Biol.* 2004;548:34–56.

148. Paradiso B, Marconi P, Zucchini S, et al. Localized delivery of fibroblast growth factor-2 and brain-derived neurotrophic factor reduces spontaneous seizures in an epilepsy model. *Proc Natl Acad Sci USA.* 2009;106(17):7191–7196.

149. Morishita T, Fayad SM, Higuchi MA, Nestor KA, Foote KD. Deep brain stimulation for treatment-resistant depression: systematic review of clinical outcomes. *Neurotherapeutics.* 2014;11(3):475–484.

150. Warner-Schmidt JL, Flajolet M, Maller A, et al. Role of p11 in cellular and behavioral effects of 5-HT4 receptor stimulation. *J Neurosci.* 2009;29(6):1937–1946.

151. Warner-Schmidt JL, Schmidt EF, Marshall JJ, et al. Cholinergic interneurons in the nucleus accumbens regulate depression-like behavior. *Proc Natl Acad Sci USA.* 2012;109(28):11360–11365.

152. Li X, Frye MA, Shelton RC. Review of pharmacological treatment in mood disorders and future directions for drug development. *Neuropsychopharmacology.* 2012;37(1):77–101.

153. Alexander B, Warner-Schmidt J, Eriksson T, et al. Reversal of depressed behaviors in mice by p11 gene therapy in the nucleus accumbens. *Sci Transl Med.* 2010;2(54):54ra76.

154. Arango-Lievano M, Schwarz JT, Vernov M, et al. Cell-type specific expression of p11 controls cocaine reward. *Biol Psychiatry.* 2014;76(10)

155. Ramanan N, Shen Y, Sarsfield S, et al. SRF mediates activity-induced gene expression and synaptic plasticity but not neuronal viability. *Nat Neurosci.* 2005;8(6):759–767.

156. Vialou V, Maze I, Renthal W, et al. Serum response factor promotes resilience to chronic social stress through the induction of DeltaFosB. *J Neurosci.* 2010;30(43):14585–14592.

157. Zhao Z, Davis M. Fear-potentiated startle in rats is mediated by neurons in the deep layers of the superior colliculus/deep mesencephalic nucleus of the rostral midbrain through the glutamate non-NMDA receptors. *J Neurosci.* 2004;24(46):10326–10334.

158. Noordmans A, Song D, Noordmans C, et al. Adeno-associated viral glutamate decarboxylase expression in the lateral nucleus of the rat hypothalamus reduces feeding behavior. *Gene Ther.* 2004;11:797–804.

INNOVATIVE THINKING

CHAPTER

10

Neuroprosthetic Advances

W. Mayr[1], M. Krenn[1] and M.R. Dimitrijevic[2,3]

[1]Medical University of Vienna, Vienna, Austria; [2]Foundation for
Movement Recovery, Oslo, Norway; [3]Baylor College of Medicine,
Houston, TX, United States

INTRODUCTION

Numerous applications of neuroprosthetic devices improve neural
impairments in humans. Popular neuroprostheses include but are not
limited to cardiac pacemakers, hearing aids, deep brain stimulation, and
spinal cord stimulation (SCS) for the neuromodification of pain. Here, we

Innovative Neuromodulation.
DOI: http://dx.doi.org/10.1016/B978-0-12-800454-8.00010-0

focus on neuroprostheses for improvement of motor control of muscle tone, volitional and externally controlled movement by external electrical neuromodification of peripheral nerves and/or neuromodification of spinal cord inputs by epidural or transcutaneous stimulation of posterior roots/posterior columns.

Electrical stimulation of peripheral nerves became widely possible when the first bipolar transistors became commercially available in the 1950s. The new generation of stimulators could generate pulse forms having sufficient accuracy, and the design was more compact and lighter. The new technology allowed portable devices which could be mounted on the body or implanted to provide neuromodulation by external control of peripheral nerves, as demonstrated by Liberson et al. in 1961[1] and in a patent in 1967.[2] Later in the 1960s implantable systems for epidural stimulation of the posterior structures of the spinal cord became available.[3]

In this chapter, we outline the neuroprosthetic advances for restoration of nerve functions in patients by electrical peripheral nerve, and SCS observed in the last 55 years. Clinical applications of functional electrical stimulation (FES) and SCS are starting to be used for neuromodulation and augmentation of altered motor control based on upper motor neuron dysfunctions. Finally, we discuss how we shall facilitate the development of clinical practice of functional neurosurgery of peripheral nerves and sensory–motor integration mechanisms of the spinal cord. There is a need for biomedical engineering laboratories within functional neurosurgery programs in order to advance innovation on how to interface with the noninjured central nervous system in restoration of impaired neurological function, a practice of contemporary restorative neurology.

FROM AN ELECTROPHYSIOLOGICAL "BRACE" TOWARD A NEUROPROSTHETIC DEVICE

Vladimir Theodore Liberson, MD, PhD (1904–94) was probably not the only one who thought to use electricity in improving impaired muscle functions and controlling movement. With his contribution, what he called at the time "functional electrotherapy" in his presentation at the International Congress of Physical Medicine and Rehabilitation, Washington DC, United States, in 1960,[4] Liberson opened a new approach to electrophysiological "bracing" in clinical practice. With this initiative he provided the foundation for people with motor deficits due to stroke, head and spinal cord injury, multiple sclerosis (MS), cerebral palsy, and other neurological disorders with upper motor neuron dysfunctions, to consider a neuroprosthetic approach. Instead of restriction of joint movement by a mechanical brace, Liberson used electrical stimulation of the peroneal nerve to activate paralyzed dorsal flexors of the ankle. With proper synchronization with the gait cycle, the electrically evoked contraction corrected drop foot in real-time. In his biography[4] Liberson describes many of his demonstrations of peroneal FES in conferences and at hospitals thus:

> Now when I turned the switch on, and the patient walks with the gait of a soldier. Now, I am going to turn switch off, and the patient will return instantaneously to the same clumsy gait.[1]

In later years his words coining "functional electrical therapy" were adapted to "functional electrical stimulation" by the scientific community.

The FES application of Liberson has been applied instead of classical braces and splints for the purpose of training patients with ambulatory hemiparesis. His findings have been repeated in several other research groups (coming and going industry products of noninvasive devices and implants: Ljubljana/Gorenje microFES, KHD Foot-Lifter Aarhus, NESS L300, Odstock Medical/Finetech Medical Salisbury, Otto Bock MyGait, ActiGait), demonstrating effective dorsal flexion of drop foot, as occurring due to an upper motor neuron lesion, achieving a satisfactory correction of the walk, as described by Vodovnik et al. in 1966.[5] In addition to acute correction of foot drop during locomotion, it was noticed by Liberson and also reported by others, that some of the patients, after an application session of such electrophysiological braces, did not resume a clumsy gait, but instead the foot drop impairment vanished for about 10–20 minutes. Obviously FES can either control functional movement patterns directly or provide a positive influence in abnormal neuromuscular coordination by eliciting action potentials simultaneously in the efferent and afferent peripheral nerves fibers. Furthermore, as Vodovnik states in 1985, FES may also improve volitional motor control of the paretic extremity and reduced spasticity even when electrical stimulation increases the contractile force of a hypotrophic muscle.[6]

Long-term use of a foot-drop stimulator applying FES to the common peroneal nerve improves walking performance even when the stimulator is off. Everaert et al. concluded in 2010 that this therapeutic effect might result from neuroplastic changes.[7] Fig. 10.1 shows the surface electromyography (EMG) recordings from ankle dorsal flexors that the voluntary muscle control changed from before and after 6 weeks of stimulation of the peroneal nerve in an individual with hemiparesis and pronounced foot-drop impairment.

According to Dimitrijevic and Dimitrijevic,[8] in general, FES of peripheral nerves can be applied in neurological rehabilitation of upper motor neuron dysfunctions for the following therapeutic goals:

- To facilitate recovery processes;
- To maintain or to enhance the trophic state of the muscle;
- To modify altered patterns of automatic and volitional functional movement;

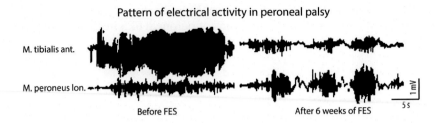

Pattern of electrical activity in peroneal palsy

FIGURE 10.1   Electromyography of a patient with hemiparesis, before and after 6 weeks of training with functional electrical stimulation of peroneal nerve. *Source: Adapted from Gracanin F, Prevec T, Trontelj J. Evaluation of use of functional electronic peroneal brace in hemiparetic patients. In: Popovic DB, ed. Proceedings of Advances in External Control of Human Extremities II. Dubrovnik: CRO, 1967: 198–205; Volumes I–X republished by Aalborg University, Denmark, May 2002.*[9]

- To enhance functional movement of a single joint;
- To modify altered neurocontrol of posture, locomotion, and skillful movements.

More sophisticated stimulators have multiple channels to activate various muscle groups in preprogrammed sequences. It has been found that the stimulation of agonist muscle groups inhibits the activation of the antagonists. This effect can be used to control the excitability of antagonists in several lower limbs muscle groups. The stimulation systems generate specific activation patterns for each channel in order to perform certain tasks, like standing, sitting down, or walking.[10–12] It has been found that by multisite stimulus systems for walking, as published by Thoma et al.[13,14] it is possible to trigger reflex patterns at various segments of the spinal cord and then produce complex movement. Such systems have been used in specialized rehabilitation centers and can be used as a simple solution for mobility in approximately 10% of paraplegic patients (Fig. 10.2).

FES can be performed in two fundamentally different ways, as efferent or afferent stimulation. The former is stimulation of the peripheral motor nerves of the paralyzed muscles to evoke their contraction. The latter is stimulation of the afferent sensory nerves of a limb as inputs for monosynaptic and polysynaptic spinal reflex arcs. This has been developed with the aim of making use of the preserved spinal reflex integration and in turn plasticity of movements.[15]

Clinical practice of using FES in patients with chronic upper motor neuron disorders can be very successful if we respect the following basic rules:

- Treat individual patients with specific motor disorders;
- Establish support from biomedical engineers;
- Apply FES only after conducting a clinical assessment of motor function.

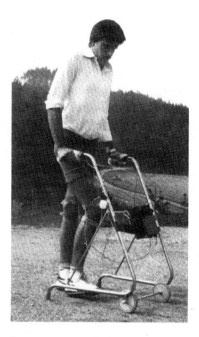

FIGURE 10.2 External restoration of movement. A paraplegic subject uses preprogrammed multichannel stimulators in order to activate the paralyzed muscles.[16]

NEUROPROSTHETIC DEVICES FOR CONTROL OF MOVEMENT VIA PERIPHERAL SENSORY NERVE STIMULATION

Electrical stimulation of sensory fibers of peripheral nerves is another neuroprosthetic approach for external support of recovery of upper motor neuron function in impaired movement. In this case, externally controlled afferent volleys in the sensory segment of the paralyzed muscles generate an additional input for the missing facilitation due to insufficiency of the corticospinal excitatory pathways.

Probably the easiest way to explain the functionality of afferent FES is by using the following example: A hemiplegic patient with "wrist drop" is unable to extend the wrist voluntarily, as shown in Fig. 10.3A. However, when an afferent electrical stimulation was added along the sensory pathway of the paralyzed muscles, extension of the wrist is feasible (Fig. 10.3C, D).

Furthermore, it was reported by McDonnell et al. that targeted afferent stimulation may facilitate the response to conventional rehabilitation

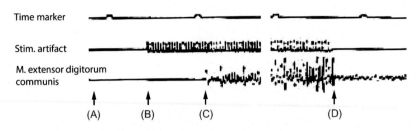

Time marker

Stim. artifact

M. extensor digitorum
communis

(A)   (B)   (C)   (D)

FIGURE 10.3   Electromyographic recordings from the extensor digitorum communis in a patient with wrist drop due to cerebral stroke. In (A), the patient was asked to extend his wrist. EMG silence means that the patient is incapable of volitional control of this muscle. In (B), a continuing train of electrical stimuli is applied to the radial nerve above the elbow while the patient is asked to relax. The further absence of EMG activity proves that the applied stimulation was purely afferent. In (C), the patient was again requested to perform voluntary extension of the wrist while stimulation was continued. He succeeds, this produces an EMG response in the muscle. In (D), voluntary effort of the patient is continued but stimulation is discontinued. There is an immediate break of EMG activity, with persistence of some small-amplitude action potentials insufficient to produce a movement. *Source: Adapted from Gracanin F, Marincek I. Development of new systems for functional electrical stimulation. In: Popovic DB, ed. Proceedings of Advances in External Control of Human Extremities III. Dubrovnik: CRO, 1970: 495–501; Volumes I–X republished by Aalborg University, Denmark, May 2002.*[17]

in patients with hemiparesis due to stroke.[18] It should be mentioned that other kinds of external input might also be successfully used along with afferent FES. Adjunctive vibration seemed to be the most promising, according to Hagbarth and Eklund.[19]

Electrical stimulation using a mesh glove is an example of a neuroprosthetic device for afferent FES. It has been shown that impaired movement of the arm and hand caused by upper motor neuron dysfunction can be ameliorated by using a wire mesh glove (Fig. 10.4) as a whole-hand surface electrode in order to stimulate afferents from the hand.

The effectiveness of this approach has been demonstrated by Dimitrijevic et al. in a study on modification of motor control by electrical afferent stimulation in 14 stroke patients over a period of more than 6 months.[20]

The effect on motor control was studied by recording surface EMG from the forearm muscles and kinematics of voluntary wrist movements at three time points: before and immediately after the initial session and at the end of the mesh-glove stimulation program conducted over several months. After applying mesh-glove stimulation daily, the range of wrist extension movement and amplitude of wrist extensors integrated EMG were significantly increased, while coactivation of biceps brachii was decreased. However, a single initial mesh-glove application had no effect on outcome measures. These findings were most prominent in subjects

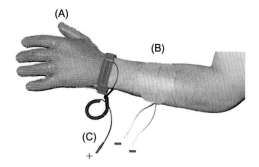

FIGURE 10.4   Mesh glove (A). Surface electrodes (B) placed over arm extensors and flexors. Wire connections to a two-channel stimulator (C). *Source: Adapted from Dimitrijevic MM, Sorokar N, Polo FE. Mesh glove eletrical stimulation. Sci Am Sci Med 1996; May/June:32–41.*[21]

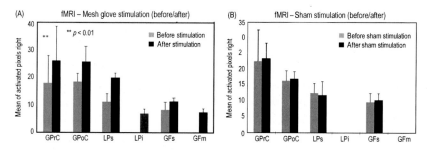

FIGURE 10.5   (A) Mean of activated pixels of the right hemisphere in all six subjects studied during test motor task (TMT) of the left hand before mesh-glove stimulation. A statistically significant increase of activation ($p < 0.01$) after mesh-glove stimulation is found for the gyrus pre- and postcentralis (GPrC and GPoC), superior and inferior parietal lobules (LPs and LPi), and superior and medial frontal gyrus (GFs and GFm). (B) Mean of activated pixels of the right hemisphere in all six subjects during TMT of the left hand before mesh-glove stimulation, and during conditioned motor task (CMT) after sham mesh-glove stimulation. There is no statistically significant increase ($p > 0.02$) of activation for the gyrus pre- and postcentralis (GPrC and GPoC), superior parietal lobule (LPs), and superior frontal gyrus (GFs). *Source: Adapted from Golaszewski S, Kremser C, Wagner M et al. Functional magnetic resonance imaging of the human motor cortex before and after whole-hand afferent electrical stimulation. Scand J Rehabil Med 1999;31:165–173.*

with chronic neurological deficits. Fig. 10.5 summarizes the results of a functional magnetic resonance study by Golaszewski et al. on human motor cortex modification by whole-hand afferent electrical stimulation.[22]

The whole hand, mesh-glove stimulation with below sensory perception intensity has a buildup and carryover effect on the level of excitability in the related motor cortex area. This has been confirmed in tests in three

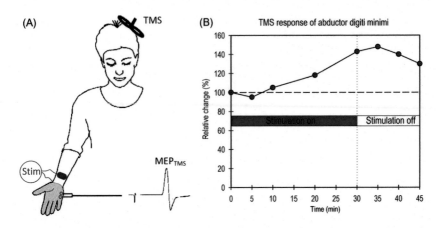

FIGURE 10.6   (A) Sketch of the research design. (B) Time course of motor cortex excitability modification by the whole-hand, mesh-glove electrical stimulation of hand afferents. *Source: (A) Adapted from Sarabon N. Transcranial magnetic stimulation offers new possibilities for the study of motor control. Kinesiol Slov 2004;10:78–104.*[23]

healthy adults with transcranial magnetic stimulation of the motor cortex. In an acute session with the whole hand by mesh-glove stimulation, it takes 30 minutes for motor cortex to reach a plateau of cortical excitability. After the cessation of hand stimulation, the increased excitability in the motor cortex was found to persist for 10–15 minutes (Fig. 10.6).

Fig. 10.6A shows the test setup for the monitoring modulation of motor cortex excitability by the whole-hand mesh-glove stimulation in a study on three adult healthy subjects. Test stimuli were applied via transcranial magnetic stimulation, monitored by continuous EMG recording, at minutes 5, 10, 20, and 30 of whole-hand afferent stimulation and minutes 5, 10, and 15 after cessation of stimulation. Fig. 10.6B shows the time course of conditioning motor cortex excitability by mesh-glove whole-hand stimulation monitored via recording of magnetic cortical stimulation induced hand EMG responses.

When a neuroprosthetic device is applied for stimulation of the peripheral nerve of an agonist muscle group, it is possible to elicit inhibition of antagonistic spinal motor cells in the spinal cord and their corresponding muscle group. An illustrative example is shown below in Fig. 10.7. Remarkably, it is possible to see a full suppressive effect of sustained ankle clonus oscillatory contractions of 7 Hz when a train of stimuli with 50 Hz and a duration of 0.4 seconds is applied to the common peroneal nerve. However, a 30- and 40-Hz train of stimuli has some relative suppressive effect, with noticeable differences between those two frequencies. It is of general interest that similar suppressive effects can also be seen in

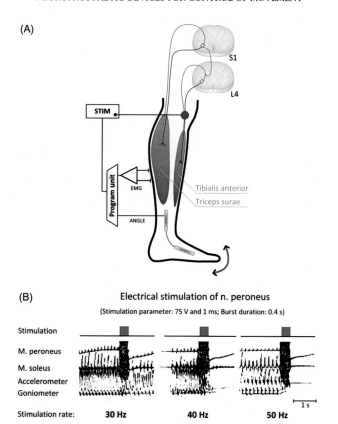

FIGURE 10.7 (A) Anticlonus model. A clonus in triceps surae (detected by an electrome-chanical or a bioelectrical clonus detector) triggers a stimulator, which delivers stimuli to the afferent fibers of the peroneal nerve. These evoke slight contraction in the tibialis anterior muscle and at the same time inhibit clonic activity in antagonistic triceps surae muscle. (B) Dependency of the anticlonus effect upon the frequency of the stimuli within the train. This proves that the effect of stimulation depends on specific electrical afferent stimulation parameters. *Source: Adapted from Gracanin F, Marincek I. Development of new systems for functional electrical stimulation. In: Popovic DB, ed. Proceedings of Advances in External Control of Human Extremities III. Dubrovnik: CRO, 1970: 495–501; Volumes I–X republished by Aalborg University, Denmark, May 2002.*

epidural stimulation in evoked tonic activity outputs with trains of stimuli with 50, 80, 100, and 120 Hz.

Any by the volitional neuro control organized movement results from an interplay of two types of nervous activity—excitation and inhibition. This caused us to begin thinking about externally controlled inhibition in addition to already-obtained successes with afferent and efferent controlled excitation and facilitation. The first step in the external electrical control of inhibition was the demonstration of an "anticlonus" model, designed by Dimitrijevic et al.[24] External electrical-controlled inhibition with functional intent was realized by afferent electrical stimulation of the peroneal nerve with a train of stimuli above the threshold for indirect motor responses. This kind of electrical stimulation evokes sustained activity in the monosynaptic reflex arc, which results in slight tonic contraction of the tibialis anterior innervated by the peroneal nerve.

At the same time, reciprocal inhibition occurs in the antagonistic triceps surae and stops the clonus in this muscle. The consistency of this effect in all patients in whom this procedure was examined suggests that the inhibition occurred through an oligo synaptic connection. This model could describe a design principle for an anticlonus device consisting of a stimulator delivering H-reflex stimuli, triggered by an electromechanical or myoelectrical clonus detector.

The above illustrated "anticlonus effect" with a specific train frequency was effective on this particular subject with an individually optimal frequency. For other subjects, though, with clinically identical neurological deficits, it will be necessary to apply different specific parameters of electrical stimulation. Thus, if clinically similar neurological deficits, like foot drop or wrist drop, are observed, the functional profiles of residual motor control can be vastly different. However, an effective frequency of the stimulation train was always found for clonus suppression in a particular subject, even when the procedure was applied within the same and other days, weeks, and months later. Moreover, through longer periods of applying an "anticlonus device," sustained clonus can be converted to becoming unsustained or even completely suppressed, even no longer requiring the "anticlonus procedure," as observed by Beres-Jones et al.[25] and even earlier by Dimitrijevic et al.[26]

NEUROPROSTHETIC DEVICES BASED ON SPINAL CORD STIMULATION OF POSTERIOR STRUCTURES OF THE SPINAL CORD

Another class of neuroprosthetic devices for neuromodification of motor control are those providing sustained electrical stimulation of posterior spinal cord structures by an implanted single or multisite electrode placed within the epidural space, as suggested by Cook and Weinstein in 1973[27] or transcutaneous stimulation of posterior structures of the lumbar cord as described by Minassian et al. in 2007[28] (Fig. 10.8).

The epidural SCS system consists of a single- or multipolar electrode connected to an implanted pulse generator, battery powered with autonomous control or powered and controlled via inductive coupling and an external control unit. Electrode configurations ranging from monopolar

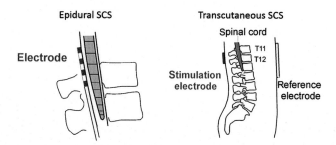

FIGURE 10.8 Schematic drawing of epidural electrodes placed close to posterior structures of the lumbar cord (left). Transcutaneous stimulation of the posterior roots of the
lumbar spinal cord applied via a large reference electrode at the lower abdominal wall and a
small active electrode dorsally close to thoracic vertebrae T11 and T12 (right). *Source: Adapted
from Minassian K, Hofstoetter US, Rattay F. Transcutaneous lumbar posterior root stimulation for
motor control studies and modification of motor activity after spinal cord injury. In: Dimitrijevic
MR, Kakulas BA, Mckay WB, et al. eds. Restorative Neurology of Spinal Cord Injury. New York,
NY: Oxford University Press, Inc.; 2012, 336.*[29]

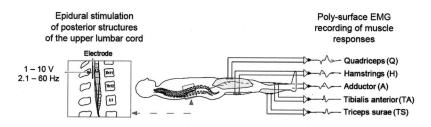

FIGURE 10.9 Epidural stimulation of lumbar posterior roots in humans with upper
motor neuron disorder. This procedure was introduced to clinical practice in 1973 for modification of spasticity and ambulation.

to up to 16 or even 32 contact points for delivery of SCS to the posterior
column and posterior roots open various possibilities to reach posterior
lumbar cord structures. Administered stimuli, usually in sustaining form,
can elicit motor unit potentials with constant and short latency from spinal cord segmental outputs (Fig. 10.9).

Epidural electrodes can be placed at any level; however, placement
closest to the somatotopographical structures of the lumbar spinal cord
is most effective for the control of spasticity in the lower limbs, particularly in posttraumatic spastic paraplegia. SCS at the spinal T1 level is
also satisfactory because an electrode inserted there is less susceptible to
displacement by movements of the spine. This location is also indicated
when it is necessary to control spasticity of the trunk and lower limbs.
Application of SCS at the cervical spine level C5–C7 is used to control

spasticity in the upper extremities, and SCS at cervical spinal level C3–C4 is used in patients with decerebrate rigidity. Sometimes spasticity and posttraumatic rigidity can be controlled more effectively by applying two electrodes at two different levels, since the stimulatory effect is restricted to position-related portions of the spinal cord, whether cervical, thoracic, or lumbar. However, we do not usually apply long-term SCS at two levels, though occasionally we have tested two levels with temporary lead placement with percutaneous test stimulation and have chosen the one with the best effect for the definite implantation while removing the other, which is a simple standard procedure in the established two-stage implantation approach.

The placement of electrodes for trial SCS is usually done by a neurosurgeon while the patient lies in the prone position. After the administration of a local anesthetic at the insertion site, catheter-type electrodes are introduced into the epidural space through Tuohy needles inserted between adjacent vertebral bodies in a manner similar to that used for lumbar puncture.

The techniques for inserting electrodes and implanting stimulation systems were described by Dimitrijevic et al.,[30] Sharkey et al.,[31] and Sherwood in 1988.[32] Once the desired location for the electrode placement is found, the position is recorded visually by fluoroscopy and through physiological markers. In addition to recording the distribution of sensations induced at stimulation rates of 10–30 Hz, both at threshold and at suprathreshold levels, we have found that it is also useful to determine motor thresholds for corresponding muscles.[31,33] To record the distribution of muscle twitches, stimulation at 1 or 2 Hz is preferable, which can be seen as single test stimuli with equally repeating twitch reactions. Once the electrodes are satisfactorily positioned, an evaluation period for pretesting the effect of permanent SCS on spasticity is undertaken before definite implantation. Transcutaneous lead extensions are provided to permit the entire electrode to be implanted, maintaining its sterility during test stimulation and throughout the procedure of the later optional coimplantation of the stimulator, after the test phase had confirmed the efficacy of application and electrode position. We have found that it is more effective to use a second set of electrodes for permanent implantation several weeks after the removal of the initial trial electrode. In this way, both the patients and the team of healthcare professionals, who participate in the procedure, have time to evaluate the effect of SCS.

The definite implantation procedure is rather simple and consists of placing a pacing device in a subcutaneous pocket and then connecting the electrode lead, after removal of the test lead extension and subcutaneous tunneling toward the pacer site. Once the connections are secure, and the device has been checked electrically, the incisions are closed.

Any patient suffering from spasticity, muscle weaknesses, chronic fatigue syndrome of MS, or poor endurance of gait locomotion is a potential candidate for SCS, particularly when other means of treatment are not effective or induce severe side effects. In the process of selecting patients it is important to consider the following:

- The patient can be a candidate for SCS if spasticity is caused by a recognized neurological condition that is stable or very slowly progressive.
- The patient can comprehend the function of SCS and monitor the operational status of the equipment.
- The patient will have available in his or her place of residence full medical and biomedical engineering support, including an attending physician knowledgeable about SCS procedures.
- The patient is otherwise healthy, without any ongoing infection or neurological complications of the primary disease.

We have experienced the most satisfactory control of spasticity in patients with severe spastic paraplegia, flexor and extensor spasms, absence of volitional movement, and severely impaired posterior column function. In such conditions, an epidural electrode placed at the somatotopic lumbar portion of the spinal cord will affect satisfactory control of the spasticity. In our study on the effectiveness of SCS for control of spasticity, we found that control of spasticity by SCS was not correlated with the severity of spasticity, the type of spasticity (flexor or extensor), or the ability to ambulate. However, stimulation was more effective in patients with incomplete cervical lesions than in complete cervical lesions. Stimulation below the lesion was more effective than above. It was concluded that SCS was effective when electrodes were properly positioned below the lesion near the posterior aspect of the spinal cord in patients with some residual spinal cord function. Dimitrijevic et al. hypothesized in 1986 that SCS controls spasticity by modification of activity of spinal–brainstem–spinal loops and suppression of segmental excitation through antidromic activation of propriospinal pathways.[34]

There has been some controversy about the benefit of SCS delivered above the damaged segment of the cord in comparison to SCS delivered below the level of injury. These two sites of stimulation will result in the eliciting of two different mechanisms. Stimulation above the lesion will predominantly activate long loop excitatory mechanisms with suppression of bulbospinal excitation or increase bulbospinal influence on segmental inhibitory interneurons. Stimulation below the spinal cord lesion, particularly when posterior column functions are severely impaired, will activate multisegmental descending branches of primary sensory neurons below the lesion level that will elicit the activity of inhibitory interneurons. In all other situations where spasticity is present along with volitional movement, the selection of patients, who can expect benefit, is not as straightforward, and a careful examination is necessary before a final decision is made.

Clinical Effects of Spinal Cord Stimulation Neuroprosthetic Devices

The term SCS is used for electrical stimulation and inducing depolarization of the posterior structures of the spinal cord in the somatotopographical lumbar, thoracic, or cervical regions, with electrode placement in the dorsal midline of the epidural space. After Cook and Weinstein reported in 1973 that SCS improved motor function in MS patients,[27] numerous publications described its effectiveness not only in MS patients but also in those with other neurological conditions—such as spinal cord injuries, head injuries, stroke, cerebral palsy, dystonia, spasmodic torticollis, and degenerative diseases.[35-38]

In his extensive review on SCS,[32] Sherwood listed the various authors who, following the lead of Cook and Weinstein,[27] used SCS for the management of MS.[39-46] However, there have also been reports on failure of SCS in MS, e.g., Refs. [47–49]. Successful management of spasticity in spinal cord-injured (SCI) patients by means of SCS has also been reported by several authors, such as Campos et al.[50], Dimitrijevic et al.[51], Richardson and McLone,[52] Waltz and Pani,[53] and Meglio et al.[54] along with the treatment of familial spastic paraplegia by Dooley in 1976.[39] We have found that SCS can be effective for the control of spasticity as well as intermittent spasms. Although the beneficial effects of SCS were reported in athetosis, dystonia, and spastic torticollis, details about patient selection are lacking.[55]

In our experience, SCSs can be effective in ambulatory patients with a benign form of MS, who report improvement of endurance when stimulated,[56] in patients with cerebral palsy, in whom muscle coordination can be improved by increasing endurance, and in selected patients with segmental dystonia, who have previously benefited from neuromuscular stimulation.[57] SCS can modify and improve volitional motor control, with increased endurance of mobility.

Gybels and Van Roost reviewed 39 publications by 19 authors in 1985 concerning SCS used for the modification of dystonic and hyperkinetic conditions in 1000 patients and found it very difficult to decide whether the authors were dealing with spasticity or other motor problems.[38] They concluded that SCS can improve bladder function in 40–50% of patients and ameliorate spasticity in 20–40%. In their later critical review on SCS used for treatment of spasticity,[36] they analyzed 16 papers describing approximately 340 patients in which the scores for improving spasticity and motor performance were reported to be high. Pinter et al. found in 2000 that efficacy of SCS for control of spasticity in chronic spinal cord injuries relies on epidural upper lumbar cord (L1, L2, L3) electrode placement.[58]

A brief review of the history of the development of SCS clearly indicates that the procedure is technically simple but physiologically poorly defined. It has been used in a variety of motor disorders, and spasticity has only been successfully controlled in a small percentage of patients. Nevertheless, it remains unclear in several neurological conditions whether SCS is most beneficial for the control of spasticity. SCS intervention requires a team, including at least an informed physiatrist on clinical practice of external control of upper motor neuron functions, a functional neurosurgeon, a clinical neurophysiologist, and a biomedical engineer. Such a multifunctional professional team can assess qualitatively and quantitate in order to convert spasticity to functional motor control of residual motor function. Goals of SCS should be not only control of muscle hypertonia, but conversion of spasticity to movement control. Therefore, an SCS intervention for modification of altered upper motor neuron functions is not just placement of epidural electrodes under X-ray fluoroscopy anatomical monitoring and connection to an electrical stimulus generator, but also extensive neurophysiological monitoring of underlying spinal cord mechanisms of altered upper motor neuron function and comprehensive assessment of effects of SCS, which should be the background information for designing the intervention protocol and definition of goals. Thus, the observed decline in the use of epidural stimulation for treatment of spasticity is not directly due to lack of long-term efficacy for relieving spasticity and not being cost-effective, as claimed by Midha and Schmitt,[59] but rather due to its application in incompletely developed professional environments.

Neuromodulation of Lumbar Cord Processing by External Control of Afferents

Electrical SCS of posterior structures of the lumbar cord in human, after accidental SCI above the lumbar cord, opens the possibility to control spasticity and to enhance residual motor control, in parallel with the "therapeutic procedure" to study processing capabilities of lumbar network parts being deprived of brain control. Furthermore, as we try to visualize an illustrative sketch in Fig. 10.10, we face a strong interaction between science and technology, as well as a high integration of technology in medicine in clinical practice. These two aspects are outlined in the two subheadings: "Clinical effects of spinal cord stimulation neuroprosthetic devices," and "Neuromodulation of lumbar cord processing by external control of afferents." We are trying to stress that the approach "medicine and technology" was developed through empirical findings of effects of SCS for neuromodulation; however, clinical practice in this case did not provide sufficient long-term progress. On the other hand,

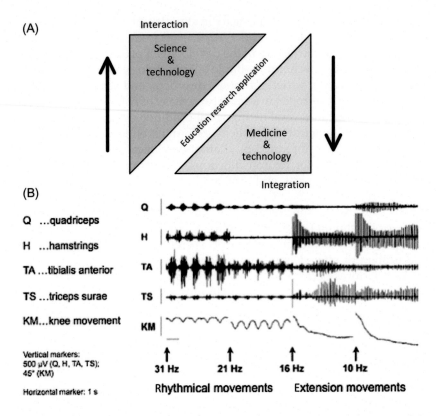

FIGURE 10.10   (A) Sketch of two alternative approaches in innovative neuromodulation: (1) medicine and technology; (2) science and technology. (B) Lumbar spinal cord can respond with different processing of posterior root inputs. Records show that depending on input frequency, lumbar cord output can be tonic or rhythmical. *Source: (B) Adapted from Jilge B, Minassian K, Rattay F, et al. Initiating extension of the lower limbs in subjects with complete spinal cord injury by epidural lumbar cord stimulation. Exp Brain Res. 2004;154:308–326.*

following the approach "science and technology" is leading to significant advancement in human neurosciences of motor control of intact and altered spinal cord.

Fig. 10.10 shows a modification of processing lumbar cord network capabilities caused by two different parameters of epidural electrical stimulation.[60] This is clearly visible in the electromyographical recordings from motor units in quadriceps, hamstrings, tibialis anterior, and triceps surae muscles, and monitoring of knee movement, during continuous lumbar epidural stimulation with frequencies of 31, 21, 16, and 10 Hz, and otherwise constant parameters. It is obvious that lower frequency or sustained higher stimulation frequency causes input responses with tonic output and contralateral rhythmical output in an unchanged stimulation setup.

Nearly 30 years after the first clinical applications of SCS for modification of spasticity and movement by Cook and Weinstein[27] various series of neurophysiological studies on lumbar motor control were initiated. An early one in 1998 examined nonpatterned electrical stimulation of the posterior structures of the caudal cord in subjects with complete, long-standing spinal cord injury. This study showed that epidural SCS can elicit step-like EMG activity and locomotor synergies in paraplegic subjects. An electrical train of stimuli applied to the second lumbar segment with a frequency of 25–60 Hz and an amplitude of 8–9 V was effective in inducing rhythmic, alternating stance and swing phases of the lower limbs. As concluded by Dimitrijevic et al. in 1998, this finding suggested that spinal circuitry in humans has the capability of generating locomotor-like activity even when isolated from brain control, and the externally controlled sustained electrical stimulation of the spinal cord can replace the tonic drive generated by the brain.[61] These findings have since been confirmed by others and further extend our understanding of sensory–motor processes of the caudal spinal cord involved in motor control.[62,63]

Summarizing all observations of epidural stimulation on input–output relations within the caudal regions of the cord, isolated by accidental injury from brain motor control, clearly shows that the circuitry there is more than a "relay system" carrying impulses between brain motor structures and spinal motor nuclei. Its role can be seen as that of helping integrate control over the reflex and volitional activity as well as over posture and gait. However, the area is functionally isolated from brain motor control, then epidural stimulation can elicit varieties of tonic and rhythmical movements. In fact, these caudal segments have a large population of interneurons, which respond to external epidural nonpatterned electrical stimulation by forming neural circuits. Those circuits represent the functional organization, which is flexible, and give it a multifunctional character that can generate modular actions, reconfiguration, and flexible operation. Under varieties of input by epidural stimulation, and isolated from brain, the region can not only be considered to act as a central pattern generator for locomotion but in a functional extension react to external responses with a variety of movement synergies. Responses to external neuromodification by developing control of motor activities in varieties of movements suggests it may be a kind of "spinal cord brain."

NEUROPROSTHESIS FOR MOTOR CONTROL AVAILABLE TODAY

Though numerous approaches for application of FES for movement restoration have been demonstrated in clinical research only a few have become established methods with associated equipment remaining continuously available as commercially successful or at least stable products. Today we can roughly see three indications where FES can provide valuable improvements for individuals with paralysis. The first is gait correction by lifting a dropped foot and triggering withdrawal reflex activity, one of these products was just recently extended to additional thigh stabilization support. The second is gait facilitation by modification of spasticity and the third is activation of hip and knee extensors for health-relevant exercising to gain tissue conditioning and cardiovascular fitness.

As described above, peroneal nerve stimulation has the longest tradition in both technical and methodological developments, still building on Liberson's early achievements. Over the years several times commercial equipment has appeared on the market and disappeared soon after, without achieving persistent relevance. Recently, we have observed a growing awareness of the need for careful individual assessment of altered physiological conditions, as occurs following an injury, along with dedicated training and supervision follow-up programs that have finally led to successful establishment of beneficial clinical programs. An impressive example is the Odstock Dropped Foot stimulation system (ODFS, Odstock Medical Limited, Salisbury, Wiltshire, United Kingdom), technically similar to the early noninvasive gait correction systems, but embedded in an intensive clinical supervision program in the National Clinical FES Centre, Salisbury District Hospital, Salisbury, United Kingdom. Meanwhile the program offers an additional implant-based system (STIMuSTEP, Finetech Medical Ltd., Hertfordshire, United Kingdom) capable of improving application comfort as soon as satisfactory functional improvement has been convincingly accomplished with the noninvasive but less comfortable external system. A main advantage is that the implanted electrodes are permanently ready for immediate use, whereas skin-attached electrodes require accurate placement and often time-consuming search for optimal position, which can result in discontent and loss of interest for permanent use.

Based on a parallel concept of a noninvasive (MyGate) and an implantable (ActiGait) is a solution offered by Otto Bock Inc. (Duderstadt, Germany). All main components of the MyGate stimulator, including preadjusted electrode configuration, are integrated in a below-knee cuff with anatomically shaped contours for reproducible placement. The control switch, placed below the ipsilateral heel, is a standalone module with wireless data link to the stimulator, a wireless remote control acts as the main user interface. The implantable version has a similar system architecture, the implanted stimulator is supplied and controlled via inductive coupling and placed in the proximal thigh with electrode placement at the peroneus nerve above knee. Bioness Inc., Valencia, CA, United States, offers the L300, which has a similar system design as Otto Bock's MyGate, but is extendable with L300+, an external cuff for the thigh with integrated surface stimulation electrodes for quadriceps and hamstring muscles. This additional module is controlled by the L300 gait sensors with coordinated neuromuscular activation of muscle groups through the gait cycle and is especially helpful in case of weaknesses in the thigh muscles. All these available systems can provide direct functional improvements in gait augmentation and correction for individuals with central paralysis from stroke, head injury, or incomplete spinal cord injury. Indirectly, reduction in spasticity can develop from prolonged use of these FES devices for modification of movement patterns in long-term applications.

A second family of devices that has gained relevance in restoration efforts for impaired movement comprises implants for epidural stimulation. The mode of operation is an indirect one: the actually declared "intended use" is still "pain relief," but more and more they find application for modification of spasticity. In principle, both pain and spasticity have adverse influence on voluntary movement and consequently their reduction can have a strong impact on better and more efficient controllability of movement functions. Simple battery-powered and radio frequency (RF)-powered single-channel stimulation implants had been available since introduction of the method in the 1980s, more or less without much innovation over decades. In recent years all the main providers (Medtronic Inc., Minneapolis, MN, United States; Saint Jude Medical Inc., Plano, TX, United States; and Boston Scientifics, Marlborough, MA, United States) have developed their products toward multipolar electrode arrays with multichannel stimulus control and toward rechargeable batteries by induction. Anchoring is provided to prevent electrode dislocation with movement, which has been a frequent complication in earlier applications. These innovations provide more flexibility in delivering stimuli to optimized locations, prevent electrode dislocations and extend lifetime of implants from what had been 2–3 years average battery life to at least 10–15 years. Current systems provide paddle arrays on an insulation sheet or axial lines of cylindrical contacts with up to 32 independent electrodes. In addition to the legally declared "intended use" for pain treatment, the systems are meanwhile successfully applied for modification of spasticity, as efficiency has been clearly demonstrated in published scientific studies, though this important application field is still not yet included in manufacturers' "intended use" statements. All systems have in common that individual effectiveness is first tested with temporary electrode placement and percutaneous lead extensions. In cases of obvious and stable symptom improvements, the definite implantation is completed with removal of the percutaneous extension lead and subcutaneous placement of the programmable IPG.

Finally, we have established methods and equipment for applications wherein the restoration of movement provides important health benefits, but more or less no daily life mobility support. This concerns mainly maintenance and metabolic nutrition of tissue in the paralyzed lower extremity as a countermeasure against decubitus ulcers, hypoperfusion, and early severe osteoporosis and, if upright posture exercises are included, can substantially improve cardiovascular fitness.

In practical applications, we need a clear differentiation between upper and lower motor neuron lesions. In the first case we can rely on motor nerve and neuromuscular stimulation, in the second we need to elicit action potentials in muscle fibers directly, as the peripheral motor nerve lesion leads to loss of nerve supply of the muscles, with direct muscle stimulation as the only option. For neuromuscular stimulations we find a large variety of general-purpose stimulators capable of inducing strong and effective muscle contraction, which can train and maintain muscle function and tissue. We are only aware of one medical product currently offered with the intended use of supporting standing and ambulatory stepping maneuvers, providing programmability of controlled multichannel stimulus patterns as required for guided movements: Motionstim-8, Kraut-Timmermann GmbH, Hamburg, Germany. The device comprises eight channels for stimulation via surface electrodes, is freely programmable, and is also useful for functional upper-extremity applications. Other similar systems have been on the market and in research, but to the best of our knowledge nothing comparable is offered at present as a certified medical product.

Direct muscular stimulation, in the absence of motor nerves, requires specific stimuli, long-duration impulses with a pulse width of at least 30 ms without significant atrophy or degeneration of the muscle or more, if muscles are pronouncedly damaged by degenerative processes. Currently there is only one device on the market that can effectively rebuild and maintain denervated muscles and induce functional movements including standing maneuvers—the Den2x, Schuhfried GmbH, Moedling, Austria. Other stimulators are offered for delaying degenerative processes but their stimuli are not strong enough to induce sufficient motor activity for functional training and usable movement patterns.

To summarize, there are established methods and associated equipment for three application lines in restoration of movement, direct augmentation and support of gait improvement with foot-drop neuroprostheses, indirect improvement of movement patterns by SCS-induced pain or spasticity reduction, and decubitus prophylaxis and training of cardiovascular fitness by noninvasive neuromuscular and muscular electrical stimulation. Beneficial and economical permanent use is strongly dependent on an established appropriate clinical environment with integrated technical expertise and support, and careful long-term supervision of regular home-based application.

Neuroprothesis for Motor Control Under Development

Developments and innovations for widely available neuroprostheses in the coming years are difficult to predict. We can foresee that the three application fields described above will develop toward easier handling of equipment and a growing number of clinical programs to provide improved assessment, planning, guidance, and support for individualized long-term application in the home environment. These structural developments are long overdue and seem to find better border conditions in the present socioeconomic background that tends to reduce central public institution services and promote professionally supervised and self-responsible home-based treatment for chronic health concerns and outpatient rehabilitation programs. Actual medical product regulations delay the availability of most recent technological innovations in healthcare as certification of novel equipment has become extremely time-consuming and costly. Therefore stepwise derivative developments of established products are more realistic than transfer of most recent technology prototypes to the medical product market. Innovations building on actual equipment will most likely include improvements in general design and physical handling, wireless control, automated control features, segmentation of electrode surfaces to arrays, improved power supply solutions with wirelessly rechargeable lighter batteries and longer operation time, and integrated compliance monitoring systems, with direct and remote graphical interfaces, for safety monitoring, guidance, and optimization of procedures and also collection of data for "evidence-based medicine," along with ethical and economic justification of the treatment.

Specifically referring to the product and application lines available today, as discussed in the respective section above, and actual observed research and development activities we can identify trends and potential innovations in all three categories currently supporting restoration of movement. In gait correction systems for foot drop conditions we can expect further simplification of equipment handling and improvements in control and reliability. In noninvasive systems, feedback sensors will extend from the classical heel switch to multiple sensors, presumably embedded in insoles or garment components with wireless data transmission, providing more detailed information on foot position and movement dynamics to be used for optimizing gait patterns. Stimulation electrodes will be electrode arrays that allow simpler and only approximate placement of the array itself or integrated in a below-knee cuff stimulator. Selection algorithms for optimal array contacts or groups of contacts to be activated for administering stimuli and automated adaptive parameter adjustments are foreseeable important innovation steps to increase comfort and user acceptance. Compliance monitoring systems with direct and remote data access will support both motivation of better-informed users and more efficient external support. Extension to additional functional modules for knee and hip extensor muscles, as recently offered by NESS could widen the indication spectrum. Provision of compatible noninvasive and implantable systems with similar functionality is sound, as it allows extensive functional testing and supports decision-making for a potential implantation, which can provide clear additional benefits in comfort and reliability of daily use. This parallel approach could become a standard offer providing more efficiency and cost-effectiveness in management of implant applications in general.

Similar technical developments will most likely occur in the field of SCS but, perhaps more importantly, the long overdue extension of the certified application spectrum will come and lead to wider integration of epidural stimulation in clinical programs for restoration of movement. As research studies have clearly shown notable evidence for therapeutic and functional benefit, spasticity treatment as well as amelioration of residual movement patterns will very likely become established clinical application fields. The combination of already-established test implantations and the versatile recently presented multichannel implantable systems for epidural stimulation will extend to noninvasive systems for advantageous use in functional assessment and trial applications. In particular, functional assessment for intervention planning and monitoring, e.g., lesion profiles after spinal cord injury, will be upgraded to acquiring electrophysiological and biomechanical reactions on artificial afferent inputs—electrical stimuli—in the central and peripheral neural system, which can be administered noninvasively or via implanted electrode configurations. Activation of intact, but postlesion inactive, spinal neural networks by afferent inputs has been successfully demonstrated in research studies and will enhance the armamentarium for restoration of impaired movement efforts.

Finally, not least, the spectrum of functional therapy, activation of paralyzed functions for maintenance of tissue quality and metabolic nutrition—soft tissue as well as bone—and of cardiovascular fitness—regular verticalization to upright posture—will gain more importance. There is clear benefit in decubitus prophylaxis and general health, especially for spinal cord-injured patients. This field has just recently been extended to peripheral lesions and direct muscle stimulation, a novel and efficient option with insufficient but growing awareness in rehabilitation medicine. Associated equipment will also develop to yield easier and more attractive handling and monitoring functions, as outlined for the above-discussed stimulation systems. Taking advantage of unquestionable proven health and economical benefits with these systems will become more and more paramount as improvements accelerate both technically and in their support and training.

References

1. Liberson WT, Holmquest HJ, Scot D, et al. Functional electrotherapy: stimulation of the peroneal nerve synchronized with the swing phase of the gait of hemiplegic patients. *Arch Phys Med Rehabil.* 1961;42:101–105.

2. Offner FF, Liberson WT. Method of muscular stimulation in human beings to aid in walking. 1967. Patent: US 3,344,792.

3. Shealy CN, Mortimer JT, Reswick JB. Electrical inhibition of pain by stimulation of the dorsal columns: preliminary clinical report. *Anesth Analg.* 1967;46(4):489–491.

4. Liberson WT.. In: Cohn R, Liberson CW, eds. *Brain, Nerves, Muscles and Electricity: My Life in Science.* New York: Smyrna Press; 1999.

5. Vodovnik L, Dimitrijevic MR, Prevec TS, et al. Electronic walking aids for patients with peroneal palsy. *Proc World Symp Med Electron.* 1966;4:58–61.

6. Vodovnik L. Modification of abnormal motor control with functional electrical stimulation of peripheral nerves. In: Eccles J, Dimitrijevic MR, eds. *Recent Achievements in Restorative Neurology: Upper Motor Neuron Functions and Dysfunctions.* Basel, Switzerland: Karger; 1985:346.

7. Everaert DG, Thompson AK, Chong SL, et al. Does functional electrical stimulation for foot drop strengthen corticospinal connections? *Neurorehabil Neural Repair.* 2010;24:168–177.

8. Dimitrijevic MM, Dimitrijevic MR. Clinical elements for the neuromuscular stimulation and functional electrical stimulation protocols in the practice of neurorehabilitation. *Artif Organs.* 2002;26:256–259.

9. Gracanin F, Prevec T, Trontelj J. Evaluation of use of functional electronic peroneal brace in hemiparetic patients. In: Popovic DB, ed. *Proceedings of Advances in External Control of Human Extremities II.* Dubrovnik, CRO, 1967, pp. 198–205; Volumes I–X republished by Aalborg University, Denmark, May 2002.

10. Bijak M, Mayr W, Rakos M, et al. The Vienna functional electrical stimulation system for restoration of walking functions in spastic paraplegia. *Artif Organs.* 2002;26: 224–227.

11. Keller T, Popovic MR, Pappas IPI, et al. Transcutaneous functional electrical stimulator "Compex Motion". *Artif Organs.* 2002;26:219–223.

12. Simcox S, Davis G, Barriskill A, et al. A portable, 8-channel transcutaneous stimulator for paraplegic muscle training and mobility—a technical note. *J Rehabil Res Dev.* 2004;41:41–52.

13. Thoma H, Frey M, Holle J, et al. State of the art of implanted multichannel devices to mobilize paraplegics. *Int J Rehabil Res.* 1987;10:86–90.

14. Thoma H, Frey M, Gruber H, et al. First implantation of a 16-channel electric stimulation device in the human body. *Trans Am Soc Artif Intern Organs.* 1983;29:301–306.

15. Dimitrijevic MR. Use of physiological mechanisms in the electrical control of paralyzed extremities. In: Popovic DB, ed. *Proceedings of Advances in External Control of Human Extremities II.* Dubrovnik, CRO, 1967, pp. 27–41; Volumes I–X republished by Aalborg University, Denmark, Popovic DB (ed.), May 2002.

16. Kralj AR, Bajd T. ISBN 0-8493-4529-4. *Functional Electrical Stimulation: Standing and Walking After Spinal Cord Injury.* Boca Raton, Florida: CRC Press Inc.; 1989:175.

17. Gracanin F, Marincek I. Development of new systems for functional electrical stimulation. In: Popovic DB, ed. *Proceedings of Advances in External Control of Human Extremities III.* Dubrovnik, CRO, 1970, pp. 495–501; Volumes I–X republished by Aalborg University, Denmark, May 2002.

18. McDonnell MN, Hillier SL, Miles TS, et al. Influence of combined afferent stimulation and task-specific training following stroke: a pilot randomized controlled trial. *Neurorehabil Neural Repair.* 2007;21:435–443.

19. Hagbarth K, Eklund G. Motor effects of vibratory muscle stimuli in man. In: Granit A, ed. *Muscular Afferents and Motor Control: Proceedings of the First Nobel Symposium.* Stockholm: John Wiley & Sons Inc.; 1966:177–186.

20. Dimitrijevic MM, Stokic DS, Wawro AW, et al. Modification of motor control of wrist extension by mesh-glove electrical afferent stimulation in stroke patients. *Arch Phys Med Rehabil.* 1996;77:252–258.

21. Dimitrijevic MM, Sorokar N, Polo FE. Mesh glove electrical stimulation. *Sci Am Sci Med.* 1996;May/June:32–41.

22. Golaszewski S, Kremser C, Wagner M, et al. Functional magnetic resonance imaging of the human motor cortex before and after whole-hand afferent electrical stimulation. *Scand J Rehabil Med.* 1999;31:165–173.

23. Sarabon N. Transcranial magnetic stimulation offers new possibilities for the study of motor control. *Kinesiol Slov.* 2004;10:78–104.

24. Dimitrijevic MR, Gracanin F, Prevec TS, et al. An anti-clonus model *Proceedings of the Seventh International Conference on Medical and Biological Engineering.* Stockholm: SWE; 1967.

25. Beres-Jones JA, Johnson TD, Harkema SJ. Clonus after human spinal cord injury cannot be attributed solely to recurrent muscle-tendon stretch. *Exp Brain Res.* 2003;149:222–236.

26. Dimitrijevic MR, Nathan PW, Sherwood AM. Clonus: the role of central mechanisms. *J Neurol Neurosurg Psychiatry.* 1980;43:321–332.

27. Cook AW, Weinstein SP. Chronic dorsal column stimulation in multiple sclerosis. Preliminary report. *N Y State J Med.* 1973;73:2868–2872.

28. Minassian K, Persy I, Rattay F, et al. Posterior root-muscle reflexes elicited by transcutaneous stimulation of the human lumbosacral cord. *Muscle Nerve.* 2007;35:327–336.

29. Minassian K, Hofstoetter US, Rattay F. Transcutaneous lumbar posterior root stimulation for motor control studies and modification of motor activity after spinal cord injury. In: Dimitrijevic MR, Kakulas BA, Mckay WB, eds. *Restorative Neurology of Spinal Cord Injury.* New York, NY: Oxford University Press, Inc.; 2012:336.

30. Dimitrijevic MR, Faganel J, Sharkey PC, et al. Study of sensation and muscle twitch responses to spinal cord stimulation. *Int Rehabil Med.* 1980;2:76–81.

31. Sharkey PC, Dimitrijevic MM, Faganel J. Neurophysiological analysis of factors influencing efficacy of spinal cord stimulation. *Appl Neurophysiol.* 1982;45:68–72.

32. Sherwood AM. Spinal cord stimulationWebster JG, editor. *Encyclopedia of Medical Devices and Instrumentation,* vol. 4. New York, NY: Wiley; 1988:3022.

33. Sherwood AM, Sharkey PC, Dimitrijevic MR. Biomedical engineering specifications for epidural spinal cord stimulation to augment motor performance. *Int Rehabil Med.* 1980;2:62–67.

34. Dimitrijevic MR, Illis LS, Nakajima K, et al. Spinal cord stimulation for the control of spasticity in patients with chronic spinal cord injury: II. Neurophysiologic observations. *Cent Nerv Syst Trauma.* 1986;3:145–152.

35. Dimitrijevic MR, Faganel J. Spinal cord stimulation for the treatment of movement disorders. In: Lazorthes Y, Upton ARM, eds. *Neurostimulation: An Overview.* Futura Publishing Co Inc.; 1985:320.

36. Gybels J, van Roost D. Spinal cord stimulation for spasticity, In: Sindou MP, Abbott RI, Keravel Y, eds. *Adv Tech Stand Neurosurg.* 1987;15:63–96.

37. Cioni B, Meglio M, Zamponi A. Effect of spinal cord stimulation on motor performances in hemiplegics. *Stereotact Funct Neurosurg.* 1989;52:42–52.

38. Gybels J, Van Roost D. Spinal cord stimulation for the modification of dystonic and hyperkinetic conditions: A critical review. In: Eccles J, Dimitrijevic MR, eds. *Recent Achievements in Restorative Neurology: Upper Motor Neuron Functions and Dysfunctions.* Basel, Switzerland: Karger; 1985:346.

39. Dooley DM, Kasprak M, Stibitz M. Electrical stimulation of the spinal cord in patients with demyelinating and degenerative diseases of the central nervous system. *J Fla Med Assoc.* 1976;63:906–909.

40. Illis LS, Oygar AE, Sedgwick EM, et al. Dorsal-column stimulation in the rehabilitation of patients with multiple sclerosis. *Lancet.* 1976;1:1383–1386.

41. Krainick JU, Thoden U, Strassburg HM, et al. The effect of electrical spinal cord stimulation on spastic movement disordersWüllenweber R.Brock M, Hamer J, editors. *Lumbar Disc Adult Hydrocephalus—Advances in Neurosurgery*, vol. 4. Berlin Heidelberg: Springer; 1977:340.

42. Thoden U, Krainick JU, Strassburg HM, et al. Modulation of monosynaptic reflexes by dorsal column stimulation (DCS) in spasticity. *Pflugers Arch J Physiol.* 1976:365.

43. Hawkes CH, Fawcett D, Cooke ED, et al. Dorsal column stimulation in multiple sclerosis: effects on bladder, leg blood flow and peptides. *Appl Neurophysiol.* 1981;44:62–70.

44. Read DJ, Matthews WB, Higson RH. The effect of spinal cord stimulation on function in patients with multiple sclerosis. *Brain.* 1980;103:803–833.

45. Siegfried J. Two different aspects of neurosurgical treatment of spasticity. Cerebral intervention and stimulation of the posterior spinal cord. *Neurochirurgie.* 1977;23:344–347.

46. Abbate AD, Cook AW, Atallah M. Effect of electrical stimulation of the thoracic spinal cord on the function of the bladder in multiple sclerosis. *J Urol.* 1977;117:285–288.

47. Rosen JA, Barsoum AH. Failure of chronic dorsal column stimulation in multiple sclerosis. *Ann Neurol.* 1979;6:66–67.

48. Young RF, Goodman SJ. Dorsal spinal cord stimulation in the treatment of multiple sclerosis. *Neurosurgery.* 1979;5:225–230.

49. Duquette P, Duquette J, Bouvier G. La stimulation electrique de la moelle epiniere dans la sclerose en plaques [Electrical stimulation of the spinal cord in multiple sclerosis]. *Union Med Can.* 1980;109:890–894.

50. Campos RJ, Dimitrijevic MM, Faganel J, et al. Clinical evaluation of the effect of spinal cord stimulation on motor performance in patients with upper motor neuron lesions. *Appl Neurophysiol.* 1981;44:141–151.

51. Dimitrijevic MM, Dimitrijevic MR, Illis LS, et al. Spinal cord stimulation for the control of spasticity in patients with chronic spinal cord injury: I. Clinical observations. *Cent Nerv Syst Trauma.* 1986;3:129–144.

52. Richardson RR, McLone DG. Percutaneous epidural neurostimulation for paraplegic spasticity 1978;9(3):153–155.

53. Waltz JM, Pani KC. Spinal cord stimulation in disorders of the motor system. In: Popovic DB, ed. *Proceedings of Advances in External Control of Human Extremities VI*. Dubrovnik, CRO, 1978, pp. 545–556; Volumes I–X republished by Aalborg University, Denmark, May 2002.

54. Meglio M, Cioni B, Amico ED, et al. Epidural spinal cord stimulation for the treatment of neurogenic bladder. *Acta Neurochir (Wien).* 1980;54:191–199.

55. Waltz JM, Davis JA. Cervical cord stimulation in the treatment of athetosis and dystonia. *Adv Neurol.* 1983;37:225–237.

56. Dimitrijevic MR, Dimitrijevic MM, Sherwood AM, et al. Neurophysiological evaluation of chronic spinal cord stimulation in patients with upper motor neuron disorders. *Int Rehabil Med.* 1980;2:82–85.

57. Katz RT, Rymer WZ. Spastic hypertonia: mechanisms and measurement. *Arch Phys Med Rehabil.* 1989;70:144–155.

58. Pinter MM, Gerstenbrand F, Dimitrijevic MR. Epidural electrical stimulation of posterior structures of the human lumbosacral cord: 3. Control of spasticity. *Spinal Cord.* 2000;38:524–531.

59. Midha M, Schmitt JK. Epidural spinal cord stimulation for the control of spasticity in spinal cord injury patients lacks long-term efficacy and is not cost-effective. *Spinal Cord Off J Int Med Soc Paraplegia.* 1998;36:190–192.

60. Jilge B, Minassian K, Rattay F, et al. Initiating extension of the lower limbs in subjects with complete spinal cord injury by epidural lumbar cord stimulation. *Exp Brain Res.* 2004;154:308–326.

III. INNOVATIVE THINKING

61. Dimitrijevic MR, Gerasimenko Y, Pinter MM. Evidence for a spinal central pattern generator in humans. *Ann NY Acad Sci.* 1998;860:360–376.
62. Angeli CA, Edgerton VR, Gerasimenko YP, et al. Altering spinal cord excitability enables voluntary movements after chronic complete paralysis in humans. *Brain.* 2014;137:1394–1409.
63. Danner SM, Hofstoetter US, Freundl B, et al. Human spinal locomotor control is based on flexibly organized burst generators. *Brain.* 2015:1–12.

Neuromodulation for Memory

D.S. Xu and F.A. Ponce

St. Joseph's Hospital and Medical Center, Phoenix, AZ, United States

INTRODUCTION

Within neural circuits, memory encompasses the encoding, storage, and retrieval of data. During the past decade, exponential progress has been made in understanding the biologic underpinnings of these three

Innovative Neuromodulation.
DOI: http://dx.doi.org/10.1016/B978-0-12-800454-8.00011-2

235

processes. Through advances in biomedical technologies, imaging, and molecular engineering, the functional unit of memory has been honed from anatomic structures into cellular networks, dendritic trees, individual synapse, and finally the sequential protein cascade that constitute the physical basis of memory. At each scale of study, multiple techniques have been developed to target neural substrates with varying specificities. This chapter reviews the resultant body of work as it pertains to neuromodulation of memory with a focus on advances that have refined our understanding of memory processing as well as those with potential clinical applications.

VALIDATION OF HEMISPHERIC ENCODING-RETRIEVAL ASYMMETRY (HERA) MODEL

Functional asymmetry of the cerebral hemispheres has been a long-established tenet with the best known example being language dominance in the left hemisphere. Beginning in the early 1990s, multiple studies utilizing positron emission tomography (PET) and functional magnetic resonance imaging (fMRI) began detecting differential cortical engagement across the frontal regions during neurocognitive memory testing. Specifically, during task learning, the left prefrontal cortex was more active than the right prefrontal cortex, whereas during recall or recognition testing, the right prefrontal cortex was more engaged.[1,2] As summarized in Fig. 11.1, this generalized pattern of the right prefrontal cortex being more involved in memory retrieval and the left prefrontal cortex being more involved in memory encoding served as the basis of the hemispheric encoding-retrieval asymmetry model (HERA).[3] Corroborating HERA are several clinical observations that frontal lobe lesions, while not known to cause significant amnesia, are still associated with significant cognitive impairment during organizational memory and recall of new tasks.[4,5]

In order to further clarify the functional anatomy of the prefrontal cortex, transcranial magnetic stimulation (TMS) and direct current stimulation (DCS) have emerged as higher-resolution tools to assess the functional participation of different structures. Unlike PET and fMRI that rely on changes in metabolic activity and regional cerebral blood flow to indirectly measure cortical activity, both TMS and DCS allow selective interference and augmentation of cortical activity.[6,7] TMS employs Faraday's law by creating electromagnetic impulses, which in turn can induce focal electrical activity in regions of the brain through elicitation of action potential volleys. Low-frequency TMS can lead to inhibition of cortical excitability whereas high-frequency stimulation can lead to significant excitation of cortical activity, with both lasting beyond the duration of

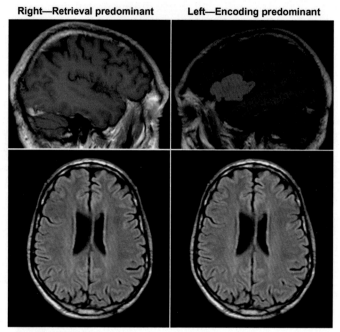

FIGURE 11.1 Prefrontal cortex asymmetry in encoding and retrieval. Sagittal T1-weighted and axial fluid attenuated inversion recovery weighted imaging are displayed with red overlay of the prefrontal cortex. The highlighted region of interest as well as the tasks associated with activation of that region from the literature are outlined below. For complete summaries, refer to Refs. [2,3]. *Source: Courtesy of the authors and Barrow Neurological Institute.*

stimulation.[8,9] On the other hand, DCS mediates its effects by producing a weak localized current, with functional effects dictated by the direction of current. Anodal stimulation leads to increased neuronal depolarization and generalized excitation, whereas the opposite is true for cathodal stimulation, which inhibits neuronal activity through hyperpolarization.[6]

Initial regional analysis by Mottaghy et al. demonstrated that low-frequency repetitive TMS across the prefrontal cortex of either hemisphere was able to produce an inhibitory response that was mirrored by decreases in regional cerebral blood flow as well as subject performance in a verbal memory task.[10] Similarly, Kincses et al. utilized DCS to target a large portion of the left prefrontal cortex during probabilistic classification testing, whereby subjects learned to predict two outcomes after being presented by a particular combination of cues, and found that performance was significantly improved during DCS stimulation.[11]

Further refinements in our understanding were made by Rossi et al. when they utilized TMS in an inhibitory fashion on 13 volunteers to target different sections of the prefrontal cortex on both hemispheres.[12] During testing of visual memory and recall, their group discovered inhibition of the right dorsolateral prefrontal cortex significantly impaired recall of pictorial data and, similarly, inhibition of the left dorsolateral prefrontal cortex significantly impaired memorization of image data. Additional work by Fregni et al. examined the effects of increasing excitability in the left dorsolateral prefrontal cortex through DCS.[13] In their study, 15 volunteers participated in memory tests involving sequential letter recognition and recall. Stimulation of the left dorsolateral prefrontal cortex during the recognition phase resulted in all subjects having dramatic performance improvements.

These results broadly validate HERA and identify the dorsolateral prefrontal cortex of both hemispheres as differentially specialized for memory processing. Selective isolation and stimulation of these relevant structures with TMS and DCS indicate neuromodulatory effects on explicit memory that have the potential for clinical translation.

MOTOR MEMORY—INTERHEMISPHERIC COMPETITION MODEL

A fundamental cognitive division of memory is the separation of explicit, or declarative memory, from implicit memory, defined as memories that aid or affect the performance of tasks without conscious awareness. Within the latter, motor memory is the most relevant example and is a prerequisite for learning new motor skills throughout life. Through anatomic and neuroimaging studies, the distributive network responsible for the functional changes involved with motor learning and adaptation have been delineated and include the primary motor cortex (M1), premotor and supplementary motor areas, striatum, thalamus, and cerebellum.[14,15] Studies evaluating neuromodulatory targets have thus far predominantly focused on the role of M1.

During motor training and learning, topographical reorganization of cortical activity occurs within the active M1.[16,17] Additional studies in humans have revealed that significant interhemispheric connectivity and activity occurs between M1s during acquisition of new motor skills. These studies utilized a double-pulse TMS paradigm whereby the amplitude of TMS induced motor-evoked potentials on one hemisphere is measured after a conditioning TMS pulse is first employed on the contralateral hemisphere. Through this model, multiple groups have demonstrated that the majority of interhemispheric coupling appears inhibitory at baseline and that excitation of the ipsilateral, active M1, coincides with inhibition of the contralateral M1.[18–20]

Based on these data, a simplified "competition" model of interhemispheric processing emerged (Fig. 11.2) where unilateral excitation of the active M1 may augment contralateral motor learning. Congruent to this model, application of excitatory regimens of TMS on the active M1 during serial finger movements was shown by Kim et al. to facilitate sequence repetition speed and accuracy.[21] Additional evidence was provided by Nitsche et al. and Boggio et al. with the use of DCS excitation of the active M1, which was found to improve subject performance on finger sequence tasks as well as the Jebsen–Taylor hand function test, a motor test used in stroke research that recapitulates activities of daily living.[22–24]

Coupled with stimulation of the ipsilateral active M1, targeted disruption or inhibition of the contralateral inactive M1 may lead to paradoxical functional gains of the active ipsilateral body, possibly through decreased interhemispheric inhibition. Initial work by Conchou et al. utilized PET imaging to demonstrate increased left-sided M1 blood flow upon inhibitory TMS applied to the right M1 during right hand movement.[62] Kobayashi et al. demonstrated both electrographical and functional consequences of TMS inhibition on M1, with resultant gains in participate performance on ipsilateral finger movement testing.[25,26]

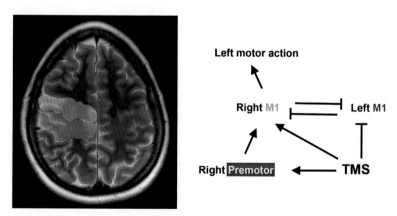

FIGURE 11.2   Interhemispheric competition for motor learning. On an axial T2-weighted MRI slice is highlighted the primary motor cortex (M1) in red and green, as well as the right premotor cortex in yellow. For left-sided motor learning and execution, a schematic flow chart depicts the interactions between these components as well as possible routes of intervention with TMS. Strategies include ipsilateral activation of the engaged M1 or premotor cortex as well as inhibition of the contralateral M1. *Source: Courtesy of the authors and Barrow Neurological Institute.*

RECOVERY OF MOTOR MEMORY AFTER STROKE

Motor recovery following stroke is a complex feat, mediated in part by learning processes that modify and enlist multiple motor networks through long-term excitation and depression.[27] Resultant adaptations include compensatory reorganization of motor areas, both local and accessory to the stroke lesion, as well as recruitment of previously silent cortical contributors in the contralateral hemisphere.[28–31] A well-documented functional barrier to stroke recovery is the disruption of previously discussed interhemispheric inhibitory balance. Work by Duque et al. and Murase et al. demonstrated that in patients with chronic stroke, inhibitory signaling from the healthy hemisphere to the lesioned side was significantly larger and that the level of inhibition correlated with the degree of motor deficit.[32,33] These data support the hypothesis that continued motor impairment poststroke may be exacerbated by a maladaptive increase in inhibition by the healthy hemisphere.

Recently, multiple efforts have been undertaken to modulate baseline interhemispheric rivalry as well as the maladaptive poststroke inhibitory response for neurorehabilitation. One of the first groups to examine this paradigm was Mansur et al. who evaluated the utility of applying inhibitory TMS to the healthy hemisphere in chronic stroke patients in order to counteract the increased inhibitory signaling originating from that side.[34] Their group ran a double-blind controlled trial on 10 stroke patients who had incurred their deficits within the past year. Patients who underwent stimulation of the contralesional hemisphere gained significant improvements in hand reaction time as well as performance on the Purdue pegboard test. Their strategy of contralateral inhibition has been validated in multiple additional studies.[35,36]

An additional approach is to strengthen excitation of the ipsilesional hemisphere in order to counterbalance excessive contralateral inhibition. The first group to test this paradigm was Khedr et al. who recruited 52 patients within the first 2 weeks after a middle cerebral artery stroke to undergo a randomized blinded clinical trial evaluating the adjunctive use of ipsilesional stimulatory TMS on motor recovery after 10 days of training. Patients who received TMS showed significantly improved disability scores posttherapy than control patients. Follow-up trials utilizing different stimulatory settings have also demonstrated similar therapeutic benefit.[36–38]

Given these strategies for targeting either hemisphere, a logical question to ask is which side of stimulation would achieve optimal benefits. Two studies by Khedr et al. and Takeuchi et al. examined stroke patients randomized to receive contralesional inhibitory TMS versus ipsilesional excitatory TMS combined with motor training.[39,40] Both study results illustrated that patients who had received contralesional inhibitory therapy exhibited greater gains in performance during hand motor training. Furthermore, Takeuchi et al. also found that patients who had received bihemispheric therapy also performed better than stimulation of the damaged hemisphere alone. These results suggest that targeted inhibition of the contralateral hemisphere in stroke patients, with or without excitatory treatment of the affected hemisphere alone, may afford greater recovery than the latter treatment alone.

The sum of current experiences with TMS and DCS demonstrate its invaluable utility in aiding our understanding of physiologic motor memory, its derangement after injury, and novel interventional strategies for improving neurorehabilitation. However, multiple avenues of unresolved questions still need further investigation including refinement of target sites, parameters for stimulation, as well as optimizing patient selection, such as the location of stroke, timing of intervention in relation to chronicity of injury, and assessment of more complex motor outcomes. This knowledge, as well as increased understanding of the physiologic and mechanistic responses underscoring TMS and DCS, will advance their role beyond experimental tools and into the clinical realm of neuromodulatory therapies for rehabilitation.

DEEP BRAIN STIMULATION FOR DECLARATIVE MEMORY AND DEMENTIA

Direct Hippocampal Stimulation

The structural foundation of episodic memory involves multiple structures along the medial temporal lobe and components of the limbic system. Compartmentalized analysis of these structures has progressed through the use of intraoperative recordings during epilepsy surgery as well as with deep brain stimulation (DBS), both of which allow selective electrical stimulation of focal targets. The nature of the cellular and circuitry response to direct electrical stimulation is still unknown, but distinct neuromodulatory effects can be elicited in a site-specific manner. A summary of the major studies evaluating DBS stimulation for memory is listed in Table 11.1.

One of the most salient targets is the mesial temporal lobe structures long known to be critically involved in memory. Interestingly, early attempts at direct electrical stimulation of these sites showed predominantly disruptive effects on memory function. Halgren et al. assessed direct electrical stimulation of the hippocampal formation and amygdala in epilepsy patients undergoing depth electrode monitoring and found that unilateral stimulation at levels high enough to cause afterdischarge activity resulted in significant performance impairment on paired

TABLE 11.1 Summary of Electrode Stimulation Trials for Memory in Humans

Year	Author	# of Patients	Pathology	Target	Results	Frequency/pulse width/stimulation
1985	Halgren	3	Epilepsy	Amygdala Hippocampus Parahippocampal gyrus	Impaired paired-association testing	NA
2004	Coleshill	6	Epilepsy	Hippocampus	Impaired word and picture recognition	50 Hz/1 μs/NA
2010	Lacruz	12	Epilepsy	Hippocampus	Impaired recognition and memory	5 s/1 ms/< 6.0 mA
2012	Suthana	7	Epilepsy	Entorhinal cortex	Improve location and spatial learning	50 Hz/300 μs/< 3.0 V
2008	Hamani	1	Obesity	Fornix-incidental	Improvement in cognitive testing and increased activity of the mesial temporal lobes	130 Hz/60 μs/< 5.0 V
2010	Laxton	6	Alzheimer	Fornix	Stability and reduction in cognitive decline	130 Hz/90 μs/3.0 V
1985	Turnbull	1	Alzheimer disease	Nucleus basalis of Meynert	Reduced decline in hemispheric PET metabolic activity	NA
2014	Kuhn	6	Alzheimer disease	Nucleus basalis of Meynert	Reduced rate of clinical decline and increased cortical PET metabolic activity in 4	20 Hz/NA/NA
2009	Freund	1	Parkinson disease	Nucleus basalis of Meynert	Dramatic improvement in neurocognitive evaluations	20 Hz/120 μs/1.0 V

NA, not available.

associate learning tasks.[41] Further studies utilizing unilateral and bilateral stimulation of the same structures revealed that even low-level stimulation below afterdischarge threshold impaired multiple aspects of episodic memory such as word recall, facial, and object recognition.[42,43]

Entorhinal Cortex Stimulation

Although stimulation of the hippocampus and amygdala has elicited deleterious effects on declarative memory, stimulation of nearby and related structures has yielded positive neuromodulatory gains. Recent work by Suthana et al. has identified the entorhinal cortex as one such target.[44] In their study, seven epilepsy patients had a combination of depth electrodes placed in the entorhinal cortex and hippocampus for seizure monitoring. Neurocognitive testing that encompassed navigation through a virtual maze was utilized to assess spatial learning and recall. All six patients that underwent entorhinal stimulation at subafterdischarge threshold during the learning phase demonstrated dramatic improvements in their ability to recite displayed paths with improved efficiency. Interestingly, four of those patients who had concurrent entorhinal and hippocampal leads demonstrated resetting of the theta rhythm (3–8 Hz) within the hippocampus, a finding known to aid memory formation in animal models.[45,46] The investigators postulate that because the entorhinal cortex is the primary cortical afferent pathway into the hippocampus, stimulation of this gateway optimizes subsequent encoding of data for storage and retrieval.

Fornix Stimulation for Alzheimer Disease

One of the most promising memory enhancement targets to garner potential clinical translation is fornix stimulation. The origins of this approach occurred incidentally during experimental treatment of a cognitively normal 50-year-old patient for obesity through DBS of his hypothalamus.[47] The patient underwent bilateral DBS electrode placement and intraoperatively, reported vivid déjà vu experiences when either electrode was stimulated. Three weeks postoperatively the patient demonstrated multiple standard deviation improvements on the California verbal learning test, as well as the spatial associative learning test. Standardized low-resolution electromagnetic tomography (sLORETA) showed that activation of the electrodes drove electrophysiologic activity in the medial temporal structures and hippocampus. Subsequent plotting of the electrode position and trajectory revealed that its ventral leads were adjacent to the columns of the fornix.

The significant, positive neurophysiologic changes seen with forniceal stimulation led the authors to hypothesize that such an approach could be leveraged in the setting of dementia to improve performance of memory circuits. They subsequently performed a phase I study enlisting six patients with early Alzheimer disease to undergo placement of bilateral DBS electrodes targeting the forniceal columns.[48] Stimulation parameters consisted of monopolar stimulation at 3–5 V, with a frequency of 130 Hz and 90 µseconds duration. Postoperative PET imaging showed increased fludeoxyglucose (FDG) uptake across the temporoparietal lobes compared to baseline at 1 month postoperatively and persisted up to 1 year after surgery. Clinically, five of six patients showed a significantly decreased decline on the mini-mental state examination during the year postsurgery compared to before surgery. Furthermore, at 6 months postsurgery, four of six patients showed improvement on the Alzheimer disease assessment scale—cognitive substrate.[49] These early pilot data demonstrate that forniceal DBS therapy is a safe means to achieve memory neuromodulation that may potentially offer clinical benefit in patients with Alzheimer disease. Additional investigation is underway through a large phase II double-blinded randomized clinical trial evaluating 42 patients with early Alzheimer disease that recently finished enrollment. Preliminary outcome data will offer further appraisal of this approach as a therapeutic strategy.

Nucleus Basalis of Meynert Stimulation

Cholinergic signaling to the hippocampus is thought to play a significant role in encoding and consolidation of nascent memories.[50] The nucleus basalis of Meynert (NBM) is a pivotal cholinergic relay, projecting widespread innervation to the cortex and medial temporal lobe structures. Degeneration of the NBM is seen both in Alzheimer disease as well as Parkinson disease, and pharmacologic therapy for both conditions consists of anticholinesterase inhibitors.[51–53] Selective DBS of the NBM in the setting of dementia has had limited and mixed results. Turnbull et al. published an early case report in 1985 of a patient with early Alzheimer disease who underwent placement of a unilateral DBS electrode in his left NBM.[54] No clinical benefit was reported 8 months after therapy, but 2-month follow-up FDG-PET imaging showed that the patient's stimulated left hemisphere had undergone metabolic decrement at half the rate of the contralateral hemisphere.

A more recent and rigorously designed study was conducted by Kuhn et al. involving six patients with clinical and biochemical evidence of Alzheimer disease.[55] All patients received NBM electrodes and first underwent a 2-week-long randomized double-blinded sham-stimulation controlled phase, followed by an open-label phase where all participants had their stimulators activated. No significant neurocognitive or clinically significant changes were seen in the double-blinded phase. However, by the end of a year of open stimulation, the mean rates of decline on patients' Alzheimer disease assessment scale as well as on the mini-mental status exam were statistically slower compared to history controls from pharmacologic studies. Furthermore, three out of four patients who were assessed by PET imaging demonstrated global increases in cortical glucose metabolism. These results suggest that NBM stimulation can be performed safely, and deserves further study as a potential intervention for stabilizing or delaying cognitive decline in Alzheimer disease.

A similar examination of NBM stimulation was undertaken by Freund et al. for Parkinson disease-related dementia.[56] The investigators treated a 71-year-old man with worsening motor and cognitive decline due to Parkinson disease, and implanted him with bilateral subthalamic nucleus (STN) and NBM electrodes to treat his motor and cognitive deficits, respectively. The patient had his STN stimulation turned on first, and 6 weeks later showed improvement in three of four neuropsychologic tests, which was interpreted as generalized mechanical gains due to improved motor function. When the NBM electrodes were subsequently activated, the patient displayed further improvement in his entire neuropsychologic battery with interval loss and recapitulation of gains when NBM stimulation was toggled. These results are encouraging regarding the role of NBM stimulation, and further studies will be needed to validate the clinical benefits and assess for neurophysiologic changes seen on imaging.

OPTOGENETIC ISOLATION OF MEMORY ENGRAMS

An engram is the biophysical embodiment of a memory. Long regarded as a conceptual entity, engrams can now be thought of as the activation of a specific neural cell population. Identification and perturbation of those cell populations is a fundamental experimental paradigm within neuroscience and previously has been limited to gross anatomic tracts and structures. However, optogenetics is an emerging molecular toolset that can be utilized within animal models to allow identification, tagging, and further manipulation of cell populations in the context of specific functional activities. An overview of optogenetic methodology and electrophysiology can be found elsewhere[57] as well as in this text. Our focus instead will be on the specific application of optogenetics on memory circuits. Within this field, one of the most robust experimental paradigms has emerged from the group led by Susumu Tonegawa who have applied optogenetics in mouse models to identify, activate, and further manipulate engrams at the cell population level.[60,61]

Early work from Tonegawa's group utilized a transgenic line of mice that had the *c-fos* promotor coupled with the tetracycline transactivator protein.[60,61] Anatomic regions of interest within the mice brain then underwent stereotactic transfection of a coding sequence of Channel Rhodopsin

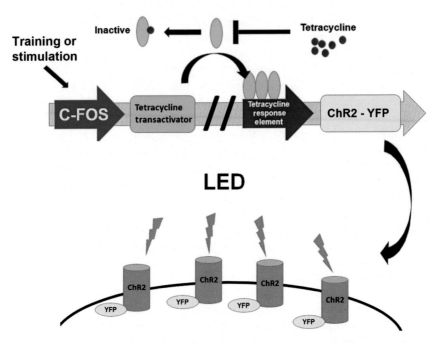

FIGURE 11.3 Optogenetic signaling system. A schematic of the molecular construct utilized to isolate and subsequently activate a subpopulation of neurons is displayed. Under experimental stimulation or training, active neurons will drive the *c-fos* promoter leading to production of the tetracycline transactivator (tTA) protein. When mice are exposed to tetracycline, tTA is inhibited, but when tetracycline is removed from the diet, the tTA will drive the tetracycline response element promoter, leading to expression of ChR2 tagged with yellow fluorescent protein (YFP), effectively labeling and isolating this active neuronal cell population. Subsequent implantation and exposure of a fiberoptic LED will light-trigger ChR2, resulting in membrane depolarization. Furthermore, YFP tagging allows histologic analysis of tissue. *Source: Courtesy of the authors and Barrow Neurological Institute.*

2 (ChR2) regulated by a tetracycline-responsive element.[58,59] A schematic of the signaling system is seen in Fig. 11.3. Briefly, *c-fos* is an immediate early gene that is expressed during neuronal activity. Upon conditioning mice without the presence of doxycycline, active neurons will express *c-fos* as well as ChR2, thereby labeling that active cell population during a function-specific context related to the conditioning. Surgical implantation of a light-emitting diode further enables specific activation of those labeled cells through light-mediated depolarization of ChR2.

This experimental model was applied to mice conditioned with foot shocks, and a subpopulation of cells in the CA1 region of the mouse hippocampus was labeled with ChR2. Subsequent light stimulation of this cell population recapitulated the phenotypic freezing response that the mice displayed when being shocked, suggesting recall of the fear memory.[60]

Following this study, the authors made additional progress by developing a variation of this methodology to create false memory associations within mice.[61] This feat was achieved by enabling ChR2 labeling when mice were exposed to red lighting. Those mice then underwent fear conditioning with foot shocks in dark lighting, but with concurrent intracranial light activation of the previously labeled cells. When these mice were put back into a red lighting context, they exhibited fear freezing despite never having received shock conditioning within a red lighting environment. Histological analysis revealed two distinct cell populations being activated within the amygdala with varying densities depending on the sequence of conditioning and stimulation, suggesting cross-recruitment of different neurons in separate circuits.

Optogenetic study of memory has only scratched the surface. Current experiences demonstrate that it is possible to isolate, label, and selectively stimulate the cells that make up the building blocks of memory engrams in animal models. These techniques allow novel insights into the functional cellular circuitry that make up memory, and permit study of their malleability and interaction with other memories. Expansion of this work will encompass evaluating other regions of the brain as well as the flow and interaction of different memory circuits. While it is still too early to foresee a direct clinical analog of this technology being applied to humans, the incoming wave of progress and discovery will likely have translational utility.

CONCLUSION

Neuromodulation has significantly advanced our understanding of the biophysical underpinnings of memory and driven its concept to evolve rapidly from theoretical constructs of thought storage and flow to an active biologic process. Continued use of evolving neuromodulatory techniques has allowed us to validate fundamental models of cognitive processing in the normal physiological state and within diseases. This in turn has led to exciting new treatment strategies for stroke rehabilitation and the treatment of dementias. As our experimental methods to selectively target neural circuitry grow, so too will the opportunities for their clinical translation and application.

KEY QUESTIONS

1. In what areas can we expand on existing progress made with transcranial and deep brain stimulation for memory neuromodulation and what are some experiments that can be designed for that aim?

2. What are the technological and ethical challenges that face further refinement of neuromodulation study within humans?

3. How can optogenetic analysis of memory engrams in animal models translate scientific or clinical discoveries for human application?

References

1. Tulving E, Kapur S, Craik FI, Moscovitch M, Houle S. Hemispheric encoding/retrieval asymmetry in episodic memory: positron emission tomography findings. *Proc Natl Acad Sci USA*. 1994;91(6):2016–2020.
2. Nyberg L, Cabeza R, Tulving E. PET studies of encoding and retrieval: the HERA model. *Psychon Bull Rev*. 1996;3(2):135–148.
3. Habib R, Nyberg L, Tulving E. Hemispheric asymmetries of memory: the HERA model revisited. *Trends Cogn Sci*. 2003;7(6):241–245.
4. Janowsky JS, Shimamura AP, Kritchevsky M, Squire LR. Cognitive impairment following frontal lobe damage and its relevance to human amnesia. *Behav Neurosci*. 1989;103(3):548–560.
5. Wheeler MA, Stuss DT, Tulving E. Frontal lobe damage produces episodic memory impairment. *J Int Neuropsychol Soc*. 1995;1(6):525–536.
6. Nitsche MA, Paulus W. Excitability changes induced in the human motor cortex by weak transcranial direct current stimulation. *J Physiol*. 2000;527(Pt 3):633–639.
7. Hallett M. Transcranial magnetic stimulation and the human brain. *Nature*. 2000; 406(6792):147–150.
8. Chen R, Classen J, Gerloff C, et al. Depression of motor cortex excitability by low-frequency transcranial magnetic stimulation. *Neurology*. 1997;48(5):1398–1403.
9. Maeda F, Keenan JP, Tormos JM, Topka H, Pascual-Leone A. Modulation of corticospinal excitability by repetitive transcranial magnetic stimulation. *Clin Neurophysiol*. 2000;111(5):800–805.
10. Mottaghy FM, Krause BJ, Kemna LJ, et al. Modulation of the neuronal circuitry subserving working memory in healthy human subjects by repetitive transcranial magnetic stimulation. *Neurosci Lett*. 2000;280(3):167–170.
11. Kincses TZ, Antal A, Nitsche MA, Bartfai O, Paulus W. Facilitation of probabilistic classification learning by transcranial direct current stimulation of the prefrontal cortex in the human. *Neuropsychologia*. 2004;42(1):113–117.
12. Rossi S, Cappa SF, Babiloni C, et al. Prefrontal cortex in long-term memory: an "interference" approach using magnetic stimulation. *Nat Neurosci*. 2001;4(9):948–952.
13. Fregni F, Boggio PS, Nitsche M, et al. Anodal transcranial direct current stimulation of prefrontal cortex enhances working memory. *Exp Brain Res*. 2005;166(1):23–30.
14. Karni A, Meyer G, Rey-Hipolito C, et al. The acquisition of skilled motor performance: fast and slow experience-driven changes in primary motor cortex. *Proc Natl Acad Sci USA*. 1998;95(3):861–868.
15. Reis J, Robertson EM, Krakauer JW, et al. Consensus: can transcranial direct current stimulation and transcranial magnetic stimulation enhance motor learning and memory formation? *Brain Stimul*. 2008;1(4):363–369.
16. Karni A, Meyer G, Jezzard P, Adams MM, Turner R, Ungerleider LG. Functional MRI evidence for adult motor cortex plasticity during motor skill learning. *Nature*. 1995;377(6545):155–158.
17. Nudo RJ, Milliken GW, Jenkins WM, Merzenich MM. Use-dependent alterations of movement representations in primary motor cortex of adult squirrel monkeys. *J Neurosci*. 1996;16(2):785–807.
18. Duque J, Murase N, Celnik P, et al. Intermanual differences in movement-related interhemispheric inhibition. *J Cogn Neurosci*. 2007;19(2):204–213.

19. Chen R. Interactions between inhibitory and excitatory circuits in the human motor cortex. *Exp Brain Res.* 2004;154(1):1–10.
20. Daskalakis ZJ, Christensen BK, Fitzgerald PB, Roshan L, Chen R. The mechanisms of interhemispheric inhibition in the human motor cortex. *J Physiol.* 2002;543(Pt 1):317–326.
21. Kim YH, Park JW, Ko MH, Jang SH, Lee PK. Facilitative effect of high frequency sub-threshold repetitive transcranial magnetic stimulation on complex sequential motor learning in humans. *Neurosci Lett.* 2004;367(2):181–185.
22. Nitsche MA, Schauenburg A, Lang N, et al. Facilitation of implicit motor learning by weak transcranial direct current stimulation of the primary motor cortex in the human. *J Cogn Neurosci.* 2003;15(4):619–626.
23. Boggio PS, Castro LO, Savagim EA, et al. Enhancement of non-dominant hand motor function by anodal transcranial direct current stimulation. *Neurosci Lett.* 2006;404(1–2):232–236.
24. Jebsen RH, Taylor N, Trieschmann RB, Trotter MJ, Howard LA. An objective and stand-ardized test of hand function. *Arch Phys Med Rehabil.* 1969;50(6):311–319.
25. Plewnia C, Lotze M, Gerloff C. Disinhibition of the contralateral motor cortex by low-frequency rTMS. *Neuroreport.* 2003;14(4):609–612.
26. Kobayashi M, Theoret H, Pascual-Leone A. Suppression of ipsilateral motor cortex facilitates motor skill learning. *Eur J Neurosci.* 2009;29(4):833–836.
27. Krakauer JW. Motor learning: its relevance to stroke recovery and neurorehabilitation. *Curr Opin Neurol.* 2006;19(1):84–90.
28. Cramer SC, Nelles G, Benson RR, et al. A functional MRI study of subjects recovered from hemiparetic stroke. *Stroke.* 1997;28(12):2518–2527.
29. Ward NS, Newton JM, Swayne OB, et al. Motor system activation after subcortical stroke depends on corticospinal system integrity. *Brain.* 2006;129(Pt 3):809–819.
30. Swayne OB, Rothwell JC, Ward NS, Greenwood RJ. Stages of motor output reorganiza-tion after hemispheric stroke suggested by longitudinal studies of cortical physiology. *Cereb Cortex.* 2008;18(8):1909–1922.
31. Chollet F, DiPiero V, Wise RJ, Brooks DJ, Dolan RJ, Frackowiak RS. The functional anatomy of motor recovery after stroke in humans: a study with positron emission tomography. *Ann Neurol.* 1991;29(1):63–71.
32. Murase N, Duque J, Mazzocchio R, Cohen LG. Influence of interhemispheric interac-tions on motor function in chronic stroke. *Ann Neurol.* 2004;55(3):400–409.
33. Duque J, Hummel F, Celnik P, Murase N, Mazzocchio R, Cohen LG. Transcallosal inhibi-tion in chronic subcortical stroke. *NeuroImage.* 2005;28(4):940–946.
34. Mansur CG, Fregni F, Boggio PS, et al. A sham stimulation-controlled trial of rTMS of the unaffected hemisphere in stroke patients. *Neurology.* 2005;64(10):1802–1804.
35. Ackerley SJ, Stinear CM, Barber PA, Byblow WD. Combining theta burst stimulation with training after subcortical stroke. *Stroke.* 2010;41(7):1568–1572.
36. Hoyer EH, Celnik PA. Understanding and enhancing motor recovery after stroke using transcranial magnetic stimulation. *Restor Neurol Neurosci.* 2011;29(6):395–409.
37. Chang WH, Kim YH, Bang OY, Kim ST, Park YH, Lee PK. Long-term effects of rTMS on motor recovery in patients after subacute stroke. *J Rehabil Med.* 2010;42(8):758–764.
38. Emara TH, Moustafa RR, Elnahas NM, et al. Repetitive transcranial magnetic stimula-tion at 1 Hz and 5 Hz produces sustained improvement in motor function and disability after ischaemic stroke. *Eur J Neurol.* 2010;17(9):1203–1209.
39. Khedr EM, Abdel-Fadeil MR, Farghali A, Qaid M. Role of 1 and 3 Hz repetitive tran-scranial magnetic stimulation on motor function recovery after acute ischaemic stroke. *Eur J Neurol.* 2009;16(12):1323–1330.
40. Takeuchi N, Tada T, Toshima M, Matsuo Y, Ikoma K. Repetitive transcranial magnetic stimulation over bilateral hemispheres enhances motor function and training effect of paretic hand in patients after stroke. *J Rehabil Med.* 2009;41(13):1049–1054.

III. INNOVATIVE THINKING

41. Halgren E, Wilson CL. Recall deficits produced by afterdischarges in the human hippocampal formation and amygdala. *Electroencephalogr Clin Neurophysiol.* 1985;61(5): 375–380.
42. Coleshill SG, Binnie CD, Morris RG, et al. Material-specific recognition memory deficits elicited by unilateral hippocampal electrical stimulation. *J Neurosci.* 2004;24(7):1612–1616.
43. Lacruz ME, Valentin A, Seoane JJ, Morris RG, Selway RP, Alarcon G. Single pulse electrical stimulation of the hippocampus is sufficient to impair human episodic memory. *Neuroscience.* 2010;170(2):623–632.
44. Suthana N, Haneef Z, Stern J, et al. Memory enhancement and deep-brain stimulation of the entorhinal area. *N Engl J Med.* 2012;366(6):502–510.
45. Buzsaki G. Theta oscillations in the hippocampus. *Neuron.* 2002;33(3):325–340.
46. McCartney H, Johnson AD, Weil ZM, Givens B. Theta reset produces optimal conditions for long-term potentiation. *Hippocampus.* 2004;14(6):684–687.
47. Hamani C, McAndrews MP, Cohn M, et al. Memory enhancement induced by hypothalamic/fornix deep brain stimulation. *Ann Neurol.* 2008;63(1):119–123.
48. Laxton AW, Tang-Wai DF, McAndrews MP, et al. A phase I trial of deep brain stimulation of memory circuits in Alzheimer's disease. *Ann Neurol.* 2010;68(4):521–534.
49. Rosen WG, Mohs RC, Davis KL. A new rating scale for Alzheimer's disease. *Am J Psychiatry.* 1984;141(11):1356–1364.
50. Hasselmo ME. Neuromodulation: acetylcholine and memory consolidation. *Trends Cogn Sci.* 1999;3(9):351–359.
51. Whitehouse PJ, Price DL, Struble RG, Clark AW, Coyle JT, Delon MR. Alzheimer's disease and senile dementia: loss of neurons in the basal forebrain. *Science.* 1982;215(4537): 1237–1239.
52. Nakano I, Hirano A. Parkinson's disease: neuron loss in the nucleus basalis without concomitant Alzheimer's disease. *Ann Neurol.* 1984;15(5):415–418.
53. Kehagia AA, Barker RA, Robbins TW. Neuropsychological and clinical heterogeneity of cognitive impairment and dementia in patients with Parkinson's disease. *Lancet Neurol.* 2010;9(12):1200–1213.
54. Turnbull IM, McGeer PL, Beattie L, Calne D, Pate B. Stimulation of the basal nucleus of Meynert in senile dementia of Alzheimer's type. A preliminary report. *Appl Neurophysiol.* 1985;48(1–6):216–221.
55. Kuhn J, Hardenacke K, Lenartz D, et al. Deep brain stimulation of the nucleus basalis of Meynert in Alzheimer's dementia. *Mol Psychiatry.* 2014. http://dx.doi.org/10.1038/mp.2014.32.
56. Freund HJ, Kuhn J, Lenartz D, et al. Cognitive functions in a patient with Parkinson-dementia syndrome undergoing deep brain stimulation. *Arch Neurol.* 2009;66(6):781–785.
57. Fenno L, Yizhar O, Deisseroth K. The development and application of optogenetics. *Annu Rev Neurosci.* 2011;34(1):389–412.
58. Boyden ES, Zhang F, Bamberg E, Nagel G, Deisseroth K. Millisecond-timescale, genetically targeted optical control of neural activity. *Nat Neurosci.* 2005;8(9):1263–1268.
59. Reijmers LG, Perkins BL, Matsuo N, Mayford M. Localization of a stable neural correlate of associative memory. *Science.* 2007;317(5842):1230–1233.
60. Liu X, Ramirez S, Pang PT, Puryear CB, Govindarajan A, Deisseroth K, Tonegawa S. Optogenetic stimulation of a hippocampal engram activates fear memory recall. *Nature.* 2012;484:381–385.
61. Ramirez S, Liu X, Lin P-A, Suh J, Pignatelli M, Redondo RL, Ryan TJ, Tonegawa S. Creating a false memory in the hippocampus. *Science.* 2013;341:387–391.
62. Conchou F, Loubinoux I, Castel-Lacanal E, Le Tinnier A, Gerdelat-Mas A, Faure-Marie N, et al. Neural substrates of low-frequency repetitive transcranial magnetic stimulation during movement in healthy subjects and acute stroke patients. A PET study. *Hum Brain Mapp.* 2009;30:2542–2557.

12

Deep Brain Stimulation for Vegetative State and Minimally Conscious State

D. Chudy[1] and V. Deletis[2,3]

[1]University Hospital Dubrava, University of Zagreb, School of Medicine, Zagreb, Croatia; [2]University of Split, Split, Croatia; [3]St Luke's-Roosevelt Hospital, New York, NY, United States

INTRODUCTION

Vegetative state (VS) is a clinical entity known as a coma vigile,[1] apallic syndrome,[2] and persistent vegetative state (PVS).[3] VS features include complete unawareness of the self and environment, usually accompanied

Innovative Neuromodulation.
DOI: http://dx.doi.org/10.1016/B978-0-12-800454-8.00012-4

by variable sleep–awake cycles, with preserved spontaneous respiration, digestion, and thermoregulation. On the other hand, patients in minimally conscious state (MCS) may from time to time follow specific commands, gestural or verbal yes/no responses, and some degree of purposeful movements. The incidence of this clinical condition for 6 months is between 5 and 25 per million population, while the prevalence is between 40 and 168 per million population.[4] According to Beaumont and Kenealy[4] the incidence and prevalence of MCS have yet to be established.

The treatment of this entity is controversial and ethically troublesome.[5] "Life-prolonging care may have negative value for some persons in a permanent MCS, who experience some minimal awareness, but have little to no hope of further recovery and little prospect of escaping a condition that is profoundly disabling and socially isolating."[6]

Historically PVS was first described by Jennett and Plum in 1972 as wakefulness without awareness.[3]

Later, the Multi-Society Task Force[7,8] defines the criteria for the diagnosis of VS as:

1. No evidence of awareness of self or environment and inability to interact with others;
2. No evidence of sustained, reproducible, purposeful, or voluntary behavioral responses to visual, auditory, tactile, or noxious stimuli;
3. No evidence of language comprehension or expression;
4. Intermittent wakefulness manifested by the presence of sleep–wake cycles;
5. Sufficiently preserved hypothalamic and brainstem autonomic functions to permit survival with medical and nursing care;
6. Bowel and bladder incontinence;
7. Cranial-nerve reflexes (pupillary, oculocephalic, corneal, vestibulo-ocular, gag) and spinal reflexes preserved to various extents.

They also reported that the recovery of consciousness from a posttraumatic PVS is unlikely after 12 months, and recovery from a nontraumatic PVS after 3 months is exceedingly rare.

In 2002, Giacino et al.[9] proposed the concept of MCS, which is characterized by inconsistent but clearly discernible behavioral evidence of consciousness and can be distinguished from coma or VS.

A Short History of DBS for VS and MCS

One of the first groups that tried to aggressively treat VS and MCS and change the level of consciousness with chronic deep brain stimulation (DBS) was Hassler et al.[10] According to their report, chronic electric stimulation started 21 weeks after the initial trauma in a patient with an apallic syndrome, using electrodes positioned in the left rostral part of thalamus and right pallidum internum. Over a period of 19 days of stimulation, a strong arousal effect was noted, along with some improvements such as spontaneous movements, however no substantial changes in level of consciousness were achieved.

McLardy et al.[11] reported in a 1964 case study done in one patient, who was comatose after neurotrauma, treated with chronic stimulation. They explored a broad range of parameters of stimulation of the upper pontine reticular formation. No improvement in the level of consciousness was observed. Sturm et al.[12] delivered chronic electric stimulation to one patient who remained in "some kind of unconsciousness" 3 weeks after clipping the tip of a basilar artery aneurysm. Bilateral stimulation was first tried with one electrode placed in left rostral part of the lamella medialis thalami and another into the right side of it. The right-sided electrode was removed because its stimulation had no effect. The effect of the left electrode, through which stimulation was delivered for a period of 7 weeks, consisted of a rise in the level of clinical responsiveness and the patient followed simple commands, even some verbal interactions were possible.

Cohadon and Richer[13] stimulated the centromedian parafascicular nuclei (CM-pf) unilaterally in 25 VS patients after neurotrauma. In 12 patients, no changes in neurological status occurred, and all of them remained in VS during the 1–10 years of follow-up. In the remaining 13 patients, recovery of some degree of consciousness was obtained. They proposed that it seems likely that DBS accelerates recovery and possibly improves the final level of consciousness. They also suggested a predictive value of the response to DBS to the recovery potential in patients with severe brain injury.

The most extensive studies concerning DBS for VS and MCS were published in several papers by the group from Nihon University.[14,15] They described selection criteria and the results of DBS in 21 VS patients and 5 MCS patients. In the VS cohort they targeted the mesencephalic reticular formation in two patients and the CM-pf complex in 19 patients. For the five patients in an MCS the CM-pf nuclei was targeted in all of them. They selected the VS and MCS patients for DBS according to their neurophysiologic evaluation. Eight of the 21 patients recovered from VS and were able to communicate through some speech or other nonverbal communication, however they continued to require some assistance with their everyday life and remained bedridden with severe disability. All five patients in MCS treated by DBS recovered from MCS but all of them required the use of a wheelchair, and only one of them could use the wheelchair without assistance.

In 2007, Schiff et al.[16] in a paper in *Nature*, assessed DBS in a single MCS patient following a 6-month double-blind alternating crossover study, reporting positive results of changing level of consciousness. We report our own work here that included evaluation and screening of 46 patients, ultimately selecting 10 for intervention (Table 12.1).

TABLE 12.1 Deep brain stimulation for vegetative state and minimally conscious state, review of the literature

Authors, year	Target	Stimulation	Duration of stimulation	Outcome	Objectives
Hassler et al. Electroenceph Clin Neurophysiol 1969;27:306–310[10]	Left thalamic lateropolar nucleus/anterior thalamic nucleus (Lpo.i) thalamic fascicle (H1), upper VA (Lpa.s) Right pallidum lamella palidi interna	Start with 50 Hz, 20 V left thalamic nuclei 8 Hz 30 V right pallidum	3–4 times daily for 15 min each time with 25 Hz to the left VA and 8 Hz to right pallidum	To MCS tracheotomy cannula could be removed after 19 days spontaneous movements of the left hand with some semibalance of purposefulness, turn head and gaze toward the voice, on 19 he pulled out the left electrode in the base of the VA	Arousal reaction opening of the eyelids with the eyes in a parallel position whereas in the absence of stimulation the patient presented a typical divergent strabismus better when stimulating the thalamus
Cohadon and Richer, Neurochirurgie 1993; 39:281–292[13]	CM-pf	Bipolar 50 Hz 5–10 mV, 5 ms duration	Daily 8–20 h	13 of 25 improved following 1–3 weeks of DBS recovery of some degree of consciousness and interpersonal relationship	Arousal reaction described as a predictive factor
Sturm et al. Acta neurochirurgica 1979; 47:235–244[12]	Rostral part of the lamella medialis thalami of the right hemisphere and toward the nucleus reticulates Polaris thalami of the left hemisphere, the right side was without effect, it was removed 4 days after implantation. (Autopsy position of the tip of the electrode in the left foramen of Monro, slightly attached to the lateral ventricular wall.)	Bipolar square wave impulses 6–10 V, 50 Hz, 500 µs of pulse duration	Percutaneous stimulation daily from 10 am to 8 pm	For weeks after the beginning of the stimulation verbal contacts were possible in the interstimulation periods, and the patient was able to sit in a chair some hours daily. Food could be administered orally. Died two months later from pneumonia	Respiratory arrest for 10–15 s thereafter. There was forced respiration for about 1 min, increased peristaltic activity occurred, reached a state of consciousness in which he was able to respond to simple commands

Reference	Target/location	Parameters	Schedule	Outcome
Yamamoto and Katayama, Neuropsychological Rehabilitation 2005; 15(3/4): 406–413[15]	CM-pf from AC PC midpoint 7–9mm posterior, 5–6mm lateral, and 0–1mm below	25Hz intensity decided according to the responses	Every 2–3h during the daytime, 30min at one session	8 of 21 in VS emerged from VS and could communicate with some speech or other responses; 7 of 8 bedridden remained unchanged
Schiff et al. Nature 2007; 448: 600–603[16]	The base of central thalamus was targeted bilaterally based on their respective anatomical distances (medial-lateral, dorsal-ventral, and rostral-caudal) with respect to the posterior commissure. The surgical approach maximized a safe trajectory through the longest length of the CL nucleus	Bipolar on right side, monopolar on left side with most dorsal two contacts as cathode; 2mA for the right and 3mA for the left DBS lead 130Hz, 90µs pulse width	Continuously for 12h a day	Single patient 38 years old in MCS improve

PATIENTS AND METHODS

A total of 46 patients were tested and 10 were selected for DBS on the basis of neurophysiologic, clinical, and imaging criteria described below (seven patients in VS and three in MCS). All 10 patients suffered from ischemic encephalopathy caused by cardiac arrest (CA). The age, gender, etiology, and time to initiation of DBS of the study population is presented in Table 12.2. The distribution of the included 10 patients in VS and MCS following anoxic injury due to CA was as follows: age from 16 to 59 years (average 35), seven were male and three female, DBS began from 2.5 to 21.5 months after injury. The distribution of the three patients in MCS was as follows: age from 16 to 28 years. We started DBS in MCS patients 65 days to 11.5 years after CA.

Patients in VS and MCS were selected on the basis of multiple tests: (1) neurophysiologic tests: somatosensory evoked potentials (SEPs), motor evoked potentials (MEPs), brain stem auditory evoked potentials (BAEPs), 12/24 hours of electroencephalography (EEG) and (2) neuroimaging: positron emission tomography (PET) and magnetic resonance imaging (MRI).

Neurophysiologic Evaluation

SEPs were elicited by stimulation of median nerves at the wrist and posterior tibialis nerves at the ankle with recording over the primary somatosensory cortex using subcutaneously placed cork screw electrodes (CS electrode INOMED GmbH, D-79331 Teningen, Germany).

MEPs were elicited by transcranial electrical stimulation (TES) with the montage C1 versus C2 according to the 10/20 EEG system. TES parameters consisted of 3–5 stimuli with a duration of 0.5 ms each (short train). These stimuli were spaced every 2 ms with a train repetition rate of 2 Hz and with an intensity of up to 120 mA. Trains were delivered through subcutaneously placed cork screw electrodes, identical to those used for

TABLE 12.2   Summary of data on vegetative state and minimally conscious state patients after anoxia treated by deep brain stimulation

	Vegetative state (VS)	Minimally conscious state (MCS)
	7 pts	3 pts
Age (years)	16–59 (mean 35)	17–23 (mean 20)
Anoxic (pts)	7	3
Sex (male M, female F)	4M, 3F	3M
Start with DBS after initial anoxic event	2.5 to 21.5 months	65 days to 11.5 years

recording SEPs. For recording of MEPs we used subdermal needle electrodes (INOMED GmbH, D-79331 Teningen, Germany) inserted into the abductor pollicis brevis and tibial anterior muscles.

Far-field short-latency BAEPs were bilaterally recorded by unilateral stimulation of each ear. Click stimuli were delivered through the ear insert while masking noise to the contralateral ear. Alternating clicks with an intensity of 100 dB and a stimulation rate of 11 Hz were used. Recordings were performed by cork screw electrodes attached to the left/right ear lobe versus fronto-parieto-central (FPZ).

Two channels of EEG were recorded with C3'/CZ and C4'/CZ montages over a 24-hour period using cork screw electrodes. The results of an automated EEG frequency spectral analysis were displayed as a compressed spectral array. The compressed spectral array of the EEG provides a clear display of the frequency spectrum of the EEG over time.

During performing neurophysiologic and neuroimaging studies the patient was slightly sedated with a combination of fentanyl, midazolam, and propofol in order to abolish myoclonic jerks and other movement- and muscle-related artifacts contaminating neurophysiologic recordings. This critical part of neurophysiologic methodology tremendously facilitated collection of data and improved their quality.

Clinical Evaluation Using Disability Rating (DR) and Coma/Near-Coma (C/NC) Scale

Patients selected for DBS were evaluated by disability rating scale (DR) and coma/near-coma (C/NC) scale[17–19] before electrode implantation, and then weekly during the first 3 months following implantation; subsequently they were evaluated once a month. The DR scale rates patients on four categories: arousability, awareness, and response to command; cognitive ability for self-care; dependence on others; and psychosocial adaptability. The DR scores range between 0 and 30 with higher scores reflecting greater disability. If DR scores were greater than 21 the C/NC categories were defined. The C/NC categories include: no coma (level 0), near coma (level 1), moderate coma (level 2), marked coma (level 3), and extreme coma (level 4).

Surgical Targeting and Procedure

An electrode was implanted stereotactically into the CM-pf nucleus of thalamic intralaminar nucleus in the left hemisphere, preferentially. However in cases with posttraumatic lesions, the electrode was placed in the better-preserved hemisphere (Fig. 12.1).

The surgery was performed under general anesthesia, and the target was determined according to the anterior and posterior commissures

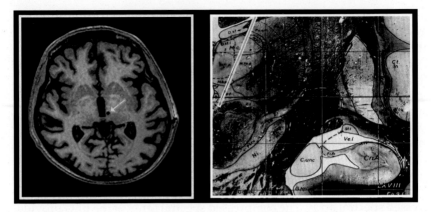

FIGURE 12.1   (Left) MRI, from the patient No. 1 (Table 12.3) with an electrode in the target-parafascicular part of left thalamic intralaminar nuclei indicated by arrow, according to the atlas coordinates from the Schaltenbrand-Wahren Atlas (Right).

shown on T2 MRI and computed tomography (CT). Contiguous T2-weighted 2-mm axial MR images were obtained the day before surgery (1.5 T Siemens AG Avanto, Erlangen, Germany).

A Leksell coordinate frame G (Elekta AB, Stockholm, Sweden) was mounted to the patient's head with the base ring, which was aligned to Reid's baseline. A CT scan was acquired with 0.7-mm slices after the placement of the Leksell frame. The calculation of target and trajectory was performed on the Frame Link Planning Stealth Station (Medtronic, Minneapolis, MN, United States). Coordinates from the Schaltenbrand-Wahren Atlas were used to approximate the target of CM-pf. The trajectory was planned to avoid passing through ventricles and sulci. An 8-mm burr hole was drilled at the entry point determined by the planned trajectory. Dynamic impedance monitoring with a radiofrequency probe 1.5 mm in diameter (Elekta AB, Stockholm, Sweden) was used to ensure that the probe did not penetrate the ventricle. The radiofrequency probe was withdrawn and the DBS 3387 electrode (Medtronic, Minneapolis, MN, United States) was immediately implanted down the same trajectory. A postoperative CT scan was obtained with the Leksell frame to confirm the position of the electrode. The Leksell frame was removed and a pulse generator Activa (Medtronic, Minneapolis, MN, United States) single channel was implanted in the chest under the skin. A postoperative MRI T1-weighted image was acquired the next day to ascertain the position of the electrode relative to the anterior-posterior commissure and ventricle wall and to confirm the absence of postoperative intracranial hemorrhage.

We began monopolar stimulation on the third postoperative day, using the contact eliciting the strongest arousal response with minimal current

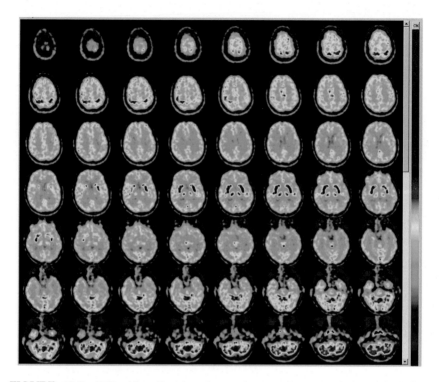

FIGURE 12.2   PET with radioactive glucose from patient No 1. (Table 12.3), before implantation of DBS. PET shows hypometabolism of glucose in most of the cortical regions with hypermetabolism within the cerebellum and basal ganglia.

using 25 Hz frequency and pulse width 90 μs. The voltage used varied among the patients from 2.5 to 3.5 V. Stimulation was applied for 30-minute periods every 2 hours during the daytime.

Entry Criteria for DBS Implantation

Neurophysiologic criteria were: presence of cortical SEP and brainstem-evoked potentials, even cortical SEPs could be abnormal (e.g., prolongation of central conduction time or small amplitude). We did not include patients with absence of BAEP. The entry criteria for EEG were desynchronized EEG during 12/24 hours of monitoring processed EEG. MRI criteria were: when MRI was pathological, to allow implantation of DBS electrode.

PET criteria were: metabolism of radioactive glucose over the cortex not worse than hypo metabolism (Fig. 12.2).

TABLE 12.3 Long-term follow up results of vegetative state and minimally conscious state patients after anoxia treated with deep brain stimulation

Pts.	Gender	Age on onset of injury	Start of DBS after injury (months)	Level of awareness before DBS (C/NC)	Level of awareness after DBS	Follow-up
1.	M	17	2.5	2.0 (1) MCS	Awareness	48
2.	F	49	6	3.6 (4) VS	2.6 (2) VS	46
3.	M	20	3	3.4 (3) VS	3.0 (3) VS	45
4.	M	23	2	1.8 (1) MCS	Awareness	45
5.	M	59	2	3.8 (4) VS	3.0 (3) VS	44
6.	M	34	7	3.0 (3) VS	Died	18
7.	F	39	7	3.8 (4) VS	Died	4
8.	M	17	137	1.0 (1) MCS	1.0 (1) MCS	38
9.	M	17	3	3.4 (3) VS	2.2 (2) VS	31
10.	F	16	4	2.6 (2) VS	Awareness	26

C/NC, Coma/near coma categories; VS, vegetative state; MCS, minimally conscious state.

RESULTS

Two patients in MCS emerged to full awareness, with the ability to interact and communicate, living independently. The first (No. 1, Table 12.3) in whom DBS began 75 days after CA, upon waking up, suffered from dysarthria, dyscalculia, and dyslexia, now partially improved after 5 months of DBS. After 5 months of stimulation the DBS system was removed, while the patient's deficits completely recovered after intense neurorehabilitation. The second patient in MCS (No. 4, Table 12.3), who began DBS 65 days after CA, experienced short-term memory impairment and emotional regression. The third patient in MCS in whom DBS was started more than 11 years after CA, showed no improvements.

One patient in VS (No. 10, Table 12.3), in whom DBS was started 4 months after CA, emerged to the level of awareness. The values of Rappaport CNC scale for each patient before DBS and at the end of follow-up are in Table 12.3. One patient (No. 6, Table 12.3) died due to pneumonia 4 months after electrode implantation and another (No. 7, Table 12.3) died from sepsis 18 months after the surgery.

Three patients had anoxic myoclonic jerks before DBS, and in all of them the myoclonus diminished several days after starting DBS of the centrum medianum pars fascicularis (CM-pf) complex.

All patients regardless of the outcome had an arousal response after turning the stimulator on. They opened their eyes (if their eyes were

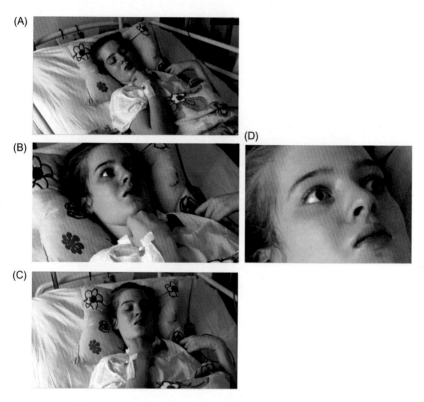

FIGURE 12.3   The arousal reaction (with pictures taken from the movie) after first trial of stimulation with implanted electrode in centrum medianum pars fascicularis complex. (A) Patient before the start of stimulation with implanted electrodes. (B) Arousal reaction (to the right, enlarged face). (C) After turning the stimulator off. Note: during stimulation mydriasis appears, with facial expression and turning the head on side. (D) Enlarged picture of the face showing facial expression. Note: this patient is not from the group of hypoxic encephalopathy, rather with a traumatic brain injury.

closed), with mydriasis and a different facial expression than before stimulation. Some of them turned their head in one direction, and had elevation of blood pressure and heart rate. One typical arousal response is presented in Fig. 12.3.

The clinical picture of patient No. 1 in the MCS with pronounced myoclonic jerks of the trunk is presented in Fig. 12.5. It is worthwhile mentioning that we discovered in screening studies that all unconscious patients, even in an early stage of VS or MCS, showed signs of cerebral atrophy (Fig. 12.2). An example is the patient in Figs. 12.4 and 12.5 (patient No. 1, Table 12.3). It is interesting to note that all seven patients who did not regain consciousness still had improved facial expression, and some of them started to swallow liquid food.

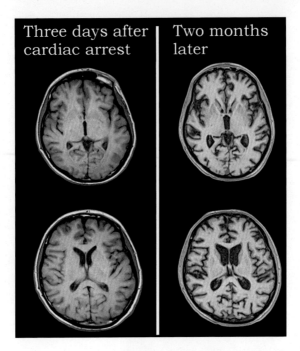

FIGURE 12.4   MRI 3 days after cardiac arrest (left) and 2 months later (right). Note brain atrophy with enlarged ventricles and pronounced sulci after 2 months in coma compared with MRI at the beginning of disease (left).

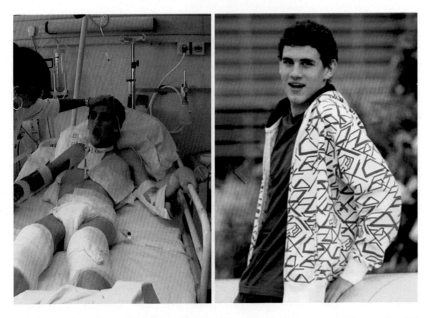

FIGURE 12.5   Patient in the MCS (left). Picture was taken during myoclonic jerks of the head and trunk. Five months after electrode implantation (right).

DISCUSSION AND CONCLUSIONS

DBS of reticular nuclei of the thalamus is targeted to treat a selected group of patients in MCS and VS. Not all patients who suffer from those conditions are candidates for this therapeutic procedure. Prior studies have tried to established selection criteria for the patients presented clinically in VS and MCS. Those criteria are: neurophysiologic, neuroradiologic, and clinical, in order to select the patients who have the best chance to regain consciousness.

The presumption is that only patients having functional integrity of the cerebral cortex could be candidates for this procedure. Therefore from the group of 46 patients in VS and MCS, we selected 10 for DBS. Three had different degrees of clinical improvement, some quite significant. For now it is unknown why only 3 of 10 patients benefited from DBS, while all 10 of selected patients fulfilled the entry criteria. Our conclusion is that we missed some critical details in those selected patients and that our entry criteria should be more elaborate, before we decide to proceed with DBS. Based on our own experience here and previous work in this area of neuromodulation, we feel it is still encouraging and more work should be performed. Ethically it is justifiable that for now we proceed with this procedure in a selected highly screened and evaluated group of VS and MCS patients, giving them a chance to improve from this grave and life-threatening condition that has minimal chance for spontaneous improvement.

References

1. Calvet J, Coll J. Meningitis of sinusoid origin with the form of coma vigil. *Rev Otoneurooptalmol.* 1959;31:443–445.
2. Kretschmer E. Das apallische Syndrom. *Z ges Neurol Psychiat.* 1940;169:292–296.
3. Jennett B, Plum F. Persistent vegetative state after brain damage. *Lancet.* 1972;1:734–737.
4. Beaumont JG, Kenealy PM. Incidence and prevalence of the vegetative and minimally conscious states. *Neuropsychol Rehabil.* 2005;15(3/4):184–189.
5. Yamamoto T, Katayama Y, Kobayashi K, Oshima H, Fukaya C, Tsubokawa T. Deep brain stimulation for the treatment of vegetative state. *Eur J Neurosci.* 2010;32:1145–1151.
6. Johnson LSM. The right to die in the minimally conscious state. *J Med Ethics.* 2011;37: 175–178.
7. The Multi-Society Task Force on PVS. Medical aspects of the persistent vegetative state (first of two parts). *N Engl J Med.* 1994;330:1499–1508.
8. The Multi-Society Task Force on PVS. Medical aspects of the persistent vegetative state (second of two parts). *N Engl J Med.* 1994;330:1572–1579.
9. Giacino JT, Ashwal S, Childs N, et al. The minimally conscious state: definition and diagnostic criteria. *Neurology.* 2002;58:349–353.
10. Hassler R, Dalle Ore G, Dieckmann G, Bricolo A, Dolce G. Behavioral and EEG arousal induced by stimulation of unspecific projection systems in a patient with post-traumatic apallic syndrome. *Electroencephalogr Clin Neurophysiol.* 1969;27:306–310.
11. McLardy T, Mark V, Scoville W, Sweet W. Pathology in diffuse projection system preventing brainstem-electrode arousal from traumatic coma. *Confin Neurol.* 1969;31(4):219–225.

12. Sturm V, Kiihner A, Schmitt HP, Assmus H, Stock G. Chronic electrical stimulation of the thalamic unspecific activating system in a patient with coma due to midbrain and upper brain stem infarction. *Acta Neurochir.* 1979;47:235–244.
13. Cohadon F, Richer E. Stimulation cérébrale profonde chez des patients en état végétatif post-traumatique, 27 observations. *Neurochirurgie.* 1993;39:281–292.
14. Tsubokawa T, Yamamoto T, Katayama Y, Hirayama T, Maejima S, Moriya T. Deep brain stimulation in a persistent vegetative state: follow up results and criteria for selection of candidates. *Brain Inj.* 1990;4:315–327.
15. Yamamoto T, Katayama Y. Deep brain stimulation therapy for the vegetative state. *Neuropsychol Rehabil.* 2005:406–413.
16. Schiff ND, Giacino JT, Kalmar K, et al. Behavioral improvements with thalamic stimulation after severe traumatic brain injury. *Nature.* 2007;448:600–603.
17. Rappaport M, Hall K, Hopkins K, Belleza T. Disability rating scale for severe head trauma. Coma to community. *Arch Phys Med Rehab.* 1982;63:118–123.
18. Rappaport M, Dougherty A, Kelting DL. Evaluation of coma and vegetative states. *Arch Phys Med Rehab.* 1992;73:628–634.
19. Rappaport M. The disability rating and coma/near-coma scales in evaluating severe head injury. *Neuropsychol Rehabil.* 2005;15:442–453.

Neuromodulation as a Bypass—Spinal Cord Injury

J. Shils[1] and J. Arle[2,3,4]

[1]Rush University Medical Center, Chicago, IL, United States;
[2]Beth Israel Deaconess Medical Center, Boston, MA, United States;
[3]Mt Auburn Hospital, Cambridge, MA, United States;
[4]Harvard Medical School, Boston, MA, United States

INTRODUCTION

Functional restoration of motor and sensory function is on the cusp of becoming a viable treatment for individuals with devastating spinal cord injury (SCI). For motor control programming, information can be obtained in three possible ways: (1) controlled movement of functional voluntary muscles via direct stimulation; (2) recording movement initiation signals and programming information from the motor cortex; and (3) recording movement activation signals directly in the spinal cord. The goal of obtaining this information is to control voluntary musculature distal to the injury or for use in other external devices. Most human trials have focused on areas 1 and 2.[1-6] Yet, direct spinal cord recording has stayed within the animal domain of research.[7] The purpose of this chapter is to discuss present work in the area of recording and stimulation in the spinal cord to *bypass* a significant SCI and enable movement via the use of implantable microelectrodes, be they microwires or microelectrode arrays placed within a more caudal region of the spinal cord. These arrays are used to both record descending motor signals and stimulate axons and/or cell bodies within the spinal cord. The recorded signals are either independent action potentials traveling in the corticospinal (CS) tract or coded signals that are normally decoded in the central pattern generator which are used to drive complex movements.

Survivable SCI occurs in around 40 cases per million.[8] About 12,500 new patients per year are diagnosed with a significant SCI with around 276,000 individuals presently in the United States with SCI.[8] Given medical breakthroughs in stabilization and palliative therapies, even patients with the most severe SCI can live many years, and this has not changed significantly since the 1980s.[8] Individuals in their 20's often live around 50 more years depending on the injury, while those in their 60's often live an additional 15 years or more depending on the level of injury.[8] Lack of SCI functional treatment is not only detrimental to a patient's health and wellbeing but also extremely costly to society,[9,10] and is emotionally and physically draining on the patients, family, and caregivers. When these injuries occur in younger patients they can lose the ability to be a productive member of society, which can affect their overall mental status, as well as the ability to independently perform simple everyday tasks such as rolling over in bed. The inability to perform these basic tasks is the cause of secondary complications, often from pulmonary and infectious causes. Even though the final goal for any SCI treatment is to regain full mobility, early interventions are motivated by the desire to restore some level of basic motor function such as rolling over in bed, bladder control, and sexual activity. It is with this motivation that researchers seek a means to regain some motor control, including work described herein where we investigated the potential of intraspinal electrophysiological recording and stimulation with microelectrode arrays for generating targeted muscle activity.

A detailed history of both the description and treatment of SCI can be found in the literature[11,12] and is briefly summarized here. The earliest description of SCI dates back to 2500 BC with a description in the Edwin Smith Papyrus of a cervical spinal injury (case 31) which the writer classifies as "an aliment not to be treated."[12] This negative outlook on treating

SCI has continued up until recently. Hippocrates around 400 BC, in discussing treatments for various congenital spinal deformities, described patients with SCI as "destined to die."[12] Galen in 150 BC performed studies on both corpses and gladiators and was the first to describe the relationship between the level of injury and the symptoms, yet he also understood, as did those before him, that there was no treatment for a traumatic SCI.[12] In the mid-600 seconds AD Paulus of Aegina was the first to hypothesis the use of traction, surgery, and decompressive surgery to treat SCI.[12] Over the next 1200 years there were sporadic descriptions of open decompressive treatments for SCI, though the majority of doctors still believed these patients had irreversible prognoses. In the 19th century more physicians attempted open reductions but were not rewarded with improved outcomes and patients still died relatively quickly. The first documented case of a positive outcome in the United States is by Alban Gilpin Smith who surgically treated a patient who had fallen off a horse with recovery of sensation,[13] in 1829.

During the latter half of the 20th century stabilization and decompression were still the mainstay of surgical interventions for SCI. Other techniques are now coming to the forefront, however, that may finally offer true restorative hope for traumatic SCI. The 1970s and 1980s saw the use of multiple chemical agents that appeared to improve outcome in SCI patients[12] and in the 1990s steroids showed a "slight but statistically significant" improvement in function.[12] Presently, treatments for SCI attempt to use genetic,[14–20] chemical,[18,19,21–23] special biomaterial constructs,[24] and electrical[18,25–28] means.

Microelectrode/Wires and Stimulation

Spinal microelectrode arrays are now well established as a neuroscience research tool for studying neural activity in the brain both in vitro and in vivo.[29] After initial work with early semiconductor-based electrodes that posed flexibility issues,[30,31] conformable and biocompatible materials have been explored for microelectrode array design.[32] Electrode arrays now are made in several variations. They can be a single stalk with multiple contacts such as the MicroProbes LMA electrodes (MicroProbes, Gaithersburg, MD, United States). They may be two-dimensional (2-D), such as the original "Utah" array (Blackrock Microsystems, Salt Lake City, UT, United States) which consists of a 10 × 10 grid with a single electrode contact on the tip.[33,34] Others are three-dimensional (3-D) arrays such as the Interuniversity Microelectronics Centre (IMEC) array (Heverlee, Belgium) consisting of multiple two-dimensional arrays of stalks that have multiple independent electrodes along their axis, providing three-dimensional coverage[35,36] or the NeuroNexus 2-D to 3-D combinations.[37] Others still, such as the Multichannel systems (Reutlingen, Germany) array, allow more conformation and are arrayed on a flat surface and overlie the structure to be recorded or stimulated.[38]

Several groups have used microwires implanted in the spinal cord of cats as a method to study the anatomy and function of the spinal cord.[1-4] For example, previous research in animals has shown that microwires can be used to perform localized stimulation in the spinal cord to demonstrate independent activation of cat hindlimb muscles and also functional combination activation, and has gone as far as to demonstrate this intraspinal microstimulation (ISMS) technique to induce walking in cats and rats with a transected spinal cord.[1-3,32,39-43] Other work has demonstrated that microelectrode recording arrays can be implanted in the spinal cord of primates and used to resolve efferent signals in the cord.[44-50] While for stimulation the focus has been on the use of microwires to either activate the motor units (alpha motor neurons (αMN)) in the lower spinal cord (ISMS) or drive the root fibers to activate the muscle directly. For ISMS the electrodes are implanted into the gray matter of the spinal cord to activate specific neural circuits within the motor pools generating coordinated muscle activity. The gray matter regions contain the motor neurons for specific muscle groups in the lower (or hind in the case of animals) limbs. The most common location is in the low thoracic and high lumbar region where the αMNs for the lower limb muscles reside. Initial studies looked at activating individual muscles via stimulation of individual αMNs. Stimulation of the motor system needs to occur below the level of the SCI. Even with present microarray technology the stimulation of individual CS tract fibers is not possible. ISMS has been employed by various groups to stimulate either lamina IX motor neuron pools[51,52] or intrinsic motor circuits in laminae III–VIII.[53,54] Lemay and Grill were able to show that circuits in these laminae (primarily laminae VII), when stimulated, generated muscle activity (recorded by EMG (electromyography)) that varied with the "limb configuration."[54] Mushahwar and Horch have shown that varying stimulation amplitude levels can cause graded individual muscle contractions when stimulating in laminae IX.[51]

More recent work has involved the stimulation around the lumbar enlargement area (where the central pattern generators are thought to be[55]) using *coded* stimulation patterns in the hopes of mimicking the signaling used by the brain. Minassian and colleagues demonstrated a frequency-related coding mechanism whereby different lower limb movement patterns were elicited with different input frequencies applied to the lumbar enlargement area in humans.[56] In their study frequencies around 2 Hz induced stimulus-related compound muscle action potential (CMAP) responses, frequencies between 5 and 15 Hz induced sustained tonic contractions, and stimulation frequencies between 25 and 50 Hz induced lower limb rhythmic activity that imitated stepping movements.[56]

RECORDING

The recording of single units (or action potentials traveling in the white matter) from the spinal cord dates to the 1950s with the work of Eccles and others using micropippettes.[57,58] Frank and Fuortes demonstrated the ability to get reliable signals in both motoneuron cell bodies as well as fibers with these techniques.[58] Fiber recording is critical in SCI patients since the level of the injury does not allow the recording from the actual αMN given they are caudal to the level of the injury site. Cell bodies for the leg tend to be between T9 and T12 with sphincter and genital cell bodies located around T12 to L1.[59] The extra-axonal spatial field generated from axonal action potentials is considerably smaller than that for cell body extracellular potentials and thus localization using microelectrodes will most likely need to triangulate on specific action potentials from multiple positioned electrodes—similar to passive phased array radar detectors. These microelectrodes may be either inserted into the white matter tracts or wrapped around the spinal cord.[60] Sahin demonstrated, using an electrode wrapped around the spinal cord of a cat, the ability to differentiate activity traveling in the CS tract using a multicontact triangulation method.[60] With four contacts he was able to get sensitivities on the order of 51%, yet this required multiple stimuli to average out noise.[60] Thus it seems that placing electrodes directly in the CS tract should increase the sensitivity and specificity.

Microarrays

Primary research using Micro-electrode arrays (MEAs) for the treatment of SCI has been focused on recording within the cranial vault in order to control tasks on either a computer monitor or external robotic systems.[5,6] Using a microelectrode array instead of a microwire for spinal cord recording and stimulation would offer considerable practical advantages. Most importantly, the electrode array would not need to be placed as precisely as a single microwire. Instead, the array could be inserted in the approximate area of interest, and then using techniques of "field recording" and triangulation could help in the localization of the critical signals. This would not just simplify the procedure but substantially reduce the risk of accidental damage to the cord caused by repositioning and/or reinsertion of a microwire. Another potential benefit of using an array is the expected robustness of the system to electrode dislocations caused by micromovements. The anatomy of the spinal cord (located behind vertebrae), presence of pia and arachnoid, and greater susceptibility of the spinal cord to serious damage make surgical implantation of neural recording and stimulation electrodes in the spinal cord a nontrivial task.

Microelectrode array-based neural recording has so far been limited mostly to cortical signals.[61,62] While impressive, this approach has been limited by the plastic nature of cortical circuits and a range of other biological and technological factors that contribute to substantial signal variability and performance instability.[63] The spinal cord, on the other hand, consists of hard-wired pathways that convey signals from cortical circuits to "circuits" (spinal cord pattern generators) in the spinal cord. Even if we consider the circuits on each end of these descending pathways to be plastic, the white matter tracts are fixed, so that placing electrodes in or around the axons in these tracts allows for recording stable signals and reducing variability. Intraspinal recording could therefore offer an alternative to cortical neuroprosthetics or brain–machine interfaces and help address the challenging problem of signal instability and lack of system robustness.

PROOF OF CONCEPT

The authors and colleagues investigated a 3-D microarray-based system on three cats. Prior to induction each animal was sedated with ketamine and midazolam and induced by a combination of ketamine and xylazine. The animal was then placed in the prone position. Continuous anesthesia including sodium pentobarbital and/or propofol was used for maintenance. End tidal CO_2 concentration was monitored and maintained at 4.0–4.5%. Blood pressure and respiration were also continually monitored. Rectal temperature was maintained at 37–39°C with the aid of a warming pad. Due to the nature of this study a total intravenous anesthetic was used to minimize the effect of anesthesia on the motor neurons. The experimental setup is shown in Fig. 13.1.

The cat's spinal cord was exposed using standard surgical techniques with incisions and laminectomies performed at the C3–C5, T3–T5, and L4–L6 levels. The dura overlying the spine was opened and secured using standard surgical techniques. The impedance of each electrode on the implanted arrays (Fig. 13.2) was measured at 1 kHz in a saline bath referenced to a stainless steel lead placed in the same normal saline bath. An array was considered acceptable as long as more than 90% of the electrodes on the array were less than 5 MΩ.

Stimulation microwires were inserted in the cervical CS tract at a medial-to-lateral angle and ventral to the root entry zone. The recording microelectrode array was then placed in the thoracic CS tract at the T5/T6 level. Array insertion speed is critical since pushing too slowly may damage the neural tissue as well as the stalk tips of the array, while pushing too fast may break the tips or cause too deep a penetration. The array was inserted using moderate but steady rate (over 1 cm/second) and relatively

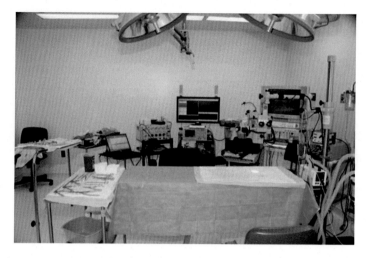

FIGURE 13.1   The OR experimental setup.

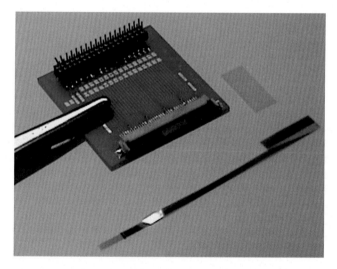

FIGURE 13.2   The microelectrode array used in this study consisted of four stalks (item farthest to right), each with eight individually addressable 35-μm IrO electrodes. The separation between each electrode was 250 μm.

constant pressure. It was placed with the array electrode columns along the length of the spinal cord (Fig. 13.3) and directed medial-to-lateral under the root entry zone. After electrode insertion the connector wire was secured using a strain relief sutured to nearby tissue and onto the skin for the duration of the experiment. There was minimal intraspinal

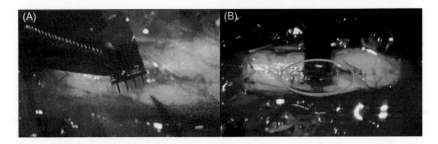

FIGURE 13.3   The recording electrode array in relation to the cat spinal cord. (A) The electrode just above the spinal cord prior to implantation into the cord. (B) The electrode implanted in the spinal cord.

bleeding during this procedure. The impedance of each electrode on the array was measured to confirm it was not damaged during the implant procedure. The array was connected to the recording system and stimulation was applied to each set of microwires.

The stimulation parameters for the cervical spinal cord stimulation and thoracic recording test consisted of a 0.5 ms single pulse with amplitude starting at 1 μA and increasing progressively as required. The spinal cord-elicited CMAPs required a train of stimuli (3–9 pulses) instead of single stimuli typically used for generating CMAP activity via direct root stimulation. The increased energy requirement, due to inhibitory effects of anesthesia on the αMN, required using temporal summation of multiple pulses, which generates a more reliable and consistent CMAP. For recoding spinal cord to spinal cord responses the single-pulse technique is acceptable for two reasons: (1) there is no need to pass through any synapses and thus the effect of anesthesia is significantly reduced and (2) a single-pulse stimulus generates much less muscle movement artifact, making the recording of the small activity in the thoracic cord much more robust. Ten trials with the anode being more cranial than the cathode, each consisting of a single stimulation pulse, with an intertrial interval of 5 seconds were performed. After this test the stimulation polarity (microwire anode and cathode) was reversed and a second set of 10 stimulation pulses were applied. All data were recorded and analyzed off-line.

A second microelectrode array was implanted inferiorly in the lumbar enlargement area. The impedance of each implant was also measured prior to implantation, similar to above. The array was implanted on one side of the conus. Testing consisted of applying a train of five stimuli through each contact using amplitudes in the 1–150 μA range and an interstimulus interval of 4 ms. The threshold for any EMG activation was noted in identified muscle groups.

The microelectrode arrays used in these studies, shown in Figs. 13.2 and 13.3, were provided by IMEC, Leuven, Belgium. The microelectrode array used in this study (Figs. 13.2 and 13.3) consisted of four stalks, each with eight individually addressable 35 µm IrO electrodes. The separation between each electrode was 250 µm. A Plexon Omniplex (Plexon, Inc., Dallas, TX, United States) neural data acquisition system was used for the recordings. A 32-channel Cadwell Cascade (Cadwell, Kennewick, WA, United States) intraoperative neuromonitoring system was used to record EMG data. A Grass Model S-88 (Natus-Grass, Warwick, RI, United States) square wave stimulator connected to the electrode via a Grass model SIU-7 constant current isolator was used to deliver all stimuli in the experiment. The stimulation microwires were 32 gage Nichrome wire (model #NW32100, Jacobs Online, Moxee, WA, United States). The EMG electrodes used were Rhythmlink model RLSND121-1-0 (Columbus, SC, United States) with 1-cm EMG leads.

RESULTS

Of the 32 electrodes placed in animal 1, 3 were found to have impedances greater than 1 MΩ and were not used in this study. The impedances were tested in a saline bath prior to insertion and again once within the spinal cord. The mean impedance was 162.4 ± 18.0 kΩ. For animal 1 small axonal responses were recorded at a latency of 816 µs (measured from the start of the first stimulus artifact to the start of the response) in the first array (Fig. 13.4). Given the 6 cm distance between the stimulation electrodes and the recording array and an estimated conduction velocity in the feline spinal cord of 69.61 m/second, these responses correspond to the appropriate area. The peak-to-peak amplitude was in the 87.5–423.8 µV range (mean 130 µV). Upon removal of the electrodes from the recording area the impedance was tested again. The mean impedance at this time was 131.1 ± 37.3 kΩ with five electrodes having impedances over 1 MΩ. For animal 2, the preimplant electrode mean impedance was 421.8 ± 68.7 kΩ and the postimplant impedance was 218.1 ± 49.4 kΩ. There were four electrodes with impedances greater than 1 MΩ, which did not change during the test. For animal 3, the preimplant electrode mean impedance was 640.7 ± 103.8 kΩ and the postimplant impedance was 502.8 ± 74.2 kΩ. In this experiment four electrodes had preimplant impedance greater than 1 MΩ but only one had high postimplant impedance.

We then conducted neural recordings with a microelectrode array implanted in the thoracic spinal cord in response to stimuli applied via microwires implanted in the cervical CS tract. The cervical stimulation was performed using two microwires (40 µm), separated by 1–2 mm, placed into the CS tract at the C6–7 cervical level. The electrodes were

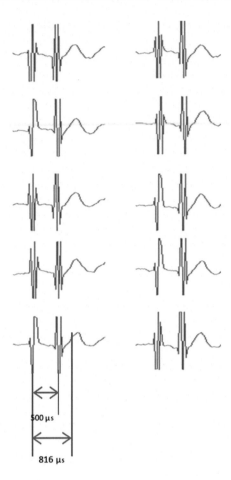

FIGURE 13.4　Recorded responses from stimulation in the spinal cord cranial to the recording electrode. The stimulation pulse was 500 μs long and the response is visible after the end of the stimulation pulse artifact. The response is 816 μs from the start of the stimulation artifact.

inserted just lateral to the midline of the spinal cord. Since the corticospinal tract is lateral and anterior to the dorsal root entry zone the stimulation electrodes were inserted to lie close to this tract. The electrodes were placed with the cranial electrode 2 mm cranial and 0.5 mm medial, approximately. Monopolar pulse train stimulation was applied at a pulse width of 0.5 ms with a minimum inter-trial interval of 5 seconds. The stimulation test current varied between 0.1 and 15 μA. We performed 10 trials for the electrodes with the cranial electrode as the anode and 10 trials for the electrodes with the caudal electrode as the anode. For animal 1 and animal 3, responses were first noted at 1–2 μA current levels.

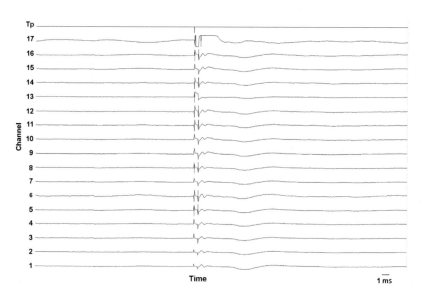

FIGURE 13.5   Recording from multiple electrode contacts in animal 1. The responses are at 862 μs from the start of the stimulation artifact.

Fig. 13.5 shows the results from animal 1. In the 10 trials, the average time of initiation of axonal anterior-posterior (AP) from the cathodic stimulus artifact was 862 μs. The distance between the stimulation and recording site was 6 cm, giving a conduction velocity of 69.61 m/second, which corresponds to previously measured values of CS conduction velocities in the cat. The distance between the two stimulus artifacts is 0.5 ms, which corresponds to the pulse width of the stimulation. For the tests in A1, with the polarities reversed (Fig. 13.6), the average time of initiation of axonal AP from the stimulation artifact was 834 μs. The distance between the stimulation and recording site was 6 cm giving a conduction velocity of 71.94 m/second, and if we correct for the 2 mm change in anodal position and use a distance of 5.8 cm, we get the conduction velocity of 69.54 m/second. No reliable recording data were obtained from animal 2 due to excessive noise in the recording system that remained untraceable even after extensive searching.

After recording from the thoracic leads, we investigated the array's ability to stimulate the ventral gray in the conus region and activate peripheral limb muscles. Thus, we sectioned the cord at the T5 level and placed stimulating electrodes in the conus region. Stimulation was applied to each electrode independently.

With the cat anesthetized, stable, and pain-free as monitored by continuous blood pressure, heart rate, respiration rate, and blood oxygenation

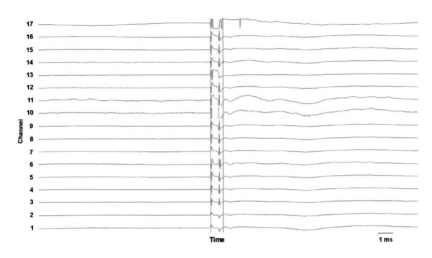

FIGURE 13.6　Recording from multiple contacts in animal with the polarities reversed from Fig. 13.5. The responses in this case are at 834 μs from the start of the stimulation artifact.

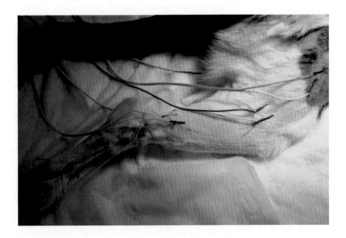

FIGURE 13.7　EMG recording electrodes placed in the sartoris, gracilis, and tibialis anterior muscles.

and to the paw squeeze test, needle EMG recording electrodes were placed, bilaterally, in six hindlimb muscles, namely biceps femoris, gastrocnemius, tibialis anterior, sartoris, gracilis, and extensor digitorum longus (Fig. 13.7). The electrodes were connected to an EMG recording system and the EMG data, sampled at 5 kHz, were recorded. Bandpass (100–1500 Hz) and line-noise (60 Hz) filters were applied to reduce unwanted artifacts, noise, and mains interference.

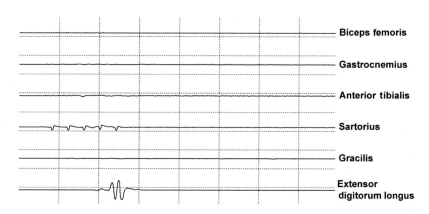

FIGURE 13.8 Example of a CMAP response in the extensor digitorum longus muscle during stimulation of electrode 1 of stalk 1 in animal 1. Scale is 5 ms per division.

Stimulation in the conus region was able to elicit CMAPs in lower limb muscles in all working electrodes. Stimulation amplitudes were in the 5–90 μA range and responses varied from the activation of a single muscle to that of multiple muscles. The differentiation of direct root or spinal cord stimulation eliciting CMAPs was difficult to determine given that some responses occurred after one or two responses in the train (see Fig. 13.12). If this occurred it was assumed that this was root stimulation based on the fact that low-threshold stimulation activated the muscle without needing the temporal summation to cause depolarization of the motor neuron under normal anesthetic conditions. Patterns indicating differential stimulation based on the location of the different microelectrodes were observed.

For animal 1, the primary activation was more related to specific stalk orientation in the spinal cord than the actual electrode. This was likely due to the columnar arrangement of myotomes in the CS tract. Thus for stalk 1 (electrodes 1 through 8) the extensor digitorum longus (Fig. 13.8 contact 1) was the primary muscle activated with sartorius and gracilis starting to activate when stimulating more dorsal electrodes (7 and 8) (Fig. 13.9, contact 8). For the electrodes on stalk 2 (electrodes 9 through 16) the sartorius muscle was the primarily activated muscle with moderate gracilis activation (Fig. 13.10, contact 9). In the most distal electrodes on this stalk the AT started to activate. For the electrodes on stalk 3 (electrodes 17 through 24) the gracilis muscle was the most prominent muscle (Fig. 13.11, contact 17). In most electrodes various other muscles were activated, but the combination was different in all electrodes. Finally, for the electrodes on stalk 4 (electrodes 25 through 32) electrode impedances were high, which in turn required much higher stimulation currents (50 μA as compared to 10

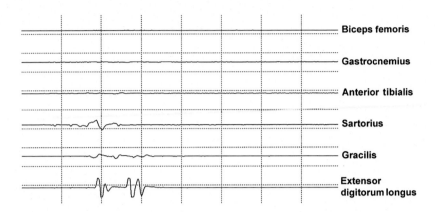

FIGURE 13.9   The CMAP response from stimulation of electrodes 7 and 8 of stalk 1 in animal 1. These more dorsal electrodes (compared to the ones shown in Fig. 13.8) activated multiple muscles compared to the single muscle of electrode 1 on the same stalk. Scale is 5 ms per division.

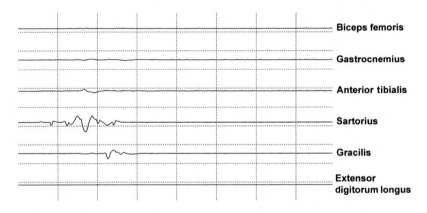

FIGURE 13.10   The CMAP response from stimulation of electrode 9 (first electrode on stalk 2), the sartorius muscle is the primary muscle compared to the electrode in Fig. 13.8. These electrodes are only 500 µm apart. Scale is 5 ms per division.

and 15 µA). This higher amplitude appeared to cause more root activation, thus the data from this stalk were not used in the analysis. In addition to electrodes 25–32 being unusable (due to high impedance), electrode 22 was also unusable after the stimulation testing phase of the experiment. For animal 1 the stimulation generating activation (discarding stalk 4 electrodes) was in the 5–15 µA range with mean 9.7 ± 3.5 µA.

For animal 2, we were only able to activate muscles with what appeared to be direct root stimulation (Fig. 13.12) as mentioned. This is based on the shorter latency of the response across all muscles (about 10 ms compared

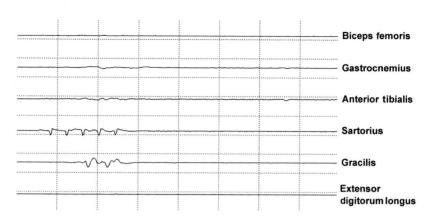

FIGURE 13.11 The CMAP response from stimulation of electrode 17 (electrode 1 on stalk 3) showing primary activation of the gracilis muscle. Scale is 5 ms per division.

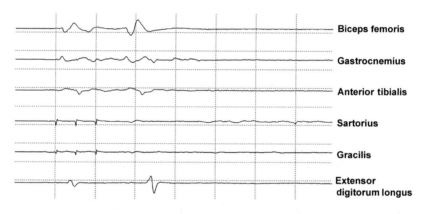

FIGURE 13.12 An example of direct root activation. Note the shorter latencies as compared to the other examples in Figs. 13.8–13.11. These were the responses obtained from animal 2. Scale is 5 ms per division.

to between 12 and 15 ms for cord responses). For animal 3, the biceps femoris and the gracilis muscle showed activation in almost all electrode stimulations. The extensor digitorum longus (EDL) was activated primarily when the electrodes on stalk 1 and the more distal electrodes of stalk 3 were stimulated, while the AT was activated on three of the electrodes on stalk 4. The electrode resolution was not as high as for A1, with two possible explanations. The first explanation involves the conversion connectors from the IMEC electrodes to the Omnetics connector for the Plexon machine. When inspecting the connectors after the procedure, some of the electrodes could have shorted out at the solder joints. Notably, 15 of the 32 electrodes had the same exact impedances after the experiment while those same electrodes had differing impedances preexperiment on a separate conversion connector. Given the resolution accuracy ($\pm 10\,k\Omega$) of the impedance meter, the second, and more likely, explanation is related to the location of the electrode. If the electrode is too medial in the spinal cord, the electrodes may be stimulating spinal cord circuits instead of fiber pathways. Given that the stimulation generating activation was in the 70–150 µA range (mean 100.4 $\pm$ 20.56 µA), which is higher than in animal 1, it is likely that stimulation affected all fibers simultaneously. One potential cause for this may be that the electrode was placed too medially in the spinal cord.

Careful observation over a 30 minutes period during each experiment demonstrated repeatable recording and stimulation properties. Since microelectrode durability is a key issue for studies of this nature, we were able to demonstrate that the electrode could be explanted and reimplanted multiple times without much degradation. We believe that the two electrodes that failed the second impedance test may have become damaged from the electrode coming in contact with the side of the saline container during testing rather than from forces imparted during implantation, implant, or explanation. The noise floor of the electrodes was on the order of 0.145 µV for the worst channel and 0.04 µV for the best channel, and all but two channels were in the 0.04 µV range. These values fall close to the recorded values, but the responses were easily distinguishable from background.

DISCUSSION

Our results have shown that a multielectrode array can be used for both stimulation and recording in the feline spinal cord. Moreover, we have shown that intraspinal stimulation with a multielectrode array can generate targeted muscle activation in the lower periphery. The choice of the feline model is based on its standard use in SCI neurophysiologic research. An alternative would be nonhuman primates, but due to the feasibility nature of this testing, cat spinal cord is considered adequate and has been demonstrated to be a good model in prior studies.[1,2,42,64] As others have shown, the general ability to perform both recording[49,50,65] and stimulation[1,2,42,64,65] from the spinal cord, the purpose of this research, demonstrates these concepts with a device containing a 3-D array of multiple electrodes spaced close together, as compared to few electrodes spaced far apart in these prior studies. A larger number of animals is therefore not deemed necessary for this proof of concept.

Electrode implantation was done by hand, but in future work more precise targeting of the CS tracts may be necessary to ensure that the electrodes are placed primarily in the region of interest. The implantation of the electrode in cat A1 required multiple attempts to obtain muscle activation from stimulation and the methodology needed for this step should be evaluated in future experiments.

The stimulation used to activate the CS tract at the cervical level was relatively large (0.9–15.0 µA). Given the size of the microwire and the stimulation amplitude, a large portion of the CS tract was likely activated, as demonstrated by the response observed in multiple recording electrodes (Figs. 13.5 and 13.6). It should also be noted that different muscle group activation when switching the polarity of this stimulation electrodes was likely due to lateral changes in the stimulation field. This result demonstrates that selective stimulation is possible, but in order to assure a greater resolution of stimulation, electrode arrays will be used to deliver the test stimuli in future experiments.

The recording data demonstrated conduction values similar to those reported in other experiments on the cat CS tract. Earlier studies[66–68] have reported conduction velocities in the cat CS tract to be between 5 and 65 m/second, which are similar to the values found in this study. It should be noted that by using the two microwires placed in the CS tract, which are relatively large compared to the size of the CS tract, we were unable to obtain much selectivity. In our future work we will use microelectrodes to obtain a higher level of spatial control.

It is interesting to note that for cat A3, three of the electrodes considered unusable at the start of the experiment (with impedance greater than 1 MΩ) had normal impedances at the end of the experiment. This was likely due to the conditioning effect whereby any oxidation or material on the electrode may dissipate with stimulation. We did not further analyze the electrode surfaces to probe whether there was any electrode damage due to stimulation, but in future experiments this analysis may be helpful or necessary.

CONCLUSION

Recording and stimulation in the spinal cord is a viable method for localizing activity and stimulating individual muscle groups. It still needs to be determined what patterning is optimal in obtaining the best functional movement of limbs below the injury. It may not be necessary to stimulate individual motor units to get sophisticated controlled movements given some recent work by Dimitrijevic et al.[55,56,69] in which they demonstrated patterned stimulation over a large spatial area causing controlled muscle coordination. Using information transmitted down the spinal cord from the brain, above the injury, may still be the best alternative given the lack of plasticity and variation of the fixed axons over time, making this "bypass" paradigm to treat SCI a potentially valuable approach in the future.

Acknowledgments

The authors would like to acknowledge Wasim Malik and Paul Pryzowski in helping with the experiments described in this chapter.

References

1. Mushahwar VK, Horch KW. Muscle recruitment through electrical stimulation of the lumbo-sacral spinal cord. *IEEE Trans Rehabil Eng*. 2000;8:22–29.
2. Mushahwar VK, Horch KW. Selective activation of muscle groups in the feline hindlimb through electrical microstimulation of the ventral lumbo-sacral spinal cord. *IEEE Trans Rehabil Eng*. 2000;8:11–21.
3. Mushahwar VK, Collins DF, Prochazka A. Spinal cord microstimulation generates functional limb movements in chronically implanted cats. *Exp Neurol*. 2000;163: 422–429.
4. Bamford JA, Mushahwar VK. Intraspinal microstimulation for the recovery of function following spinal cord injury. *Prog Brain Res*. 2011;194:227–239.
5. Hochberg LR. Turning thought into action. *N Engl J Med*. 2008;359(11):1175–1177.
6. Donoghue JP, Nurmikko A, Black M, Hochberg LR. Assistive technology and robotic control using motor cortex ensemble-based neural interface systems in humans with tetraplegia. *J Physiol*. 2007;579(Pt 3):603–611.
7. Prasad A, Sahin M. Can motor volition be extracted from the spinal cord? *J Neuroeng Rehabil*. 2012;9:41.
8. Spinal cord injury (SCI) facts and figures at a glance. The national SCI statistics Center. February 2015.
9. French DD, Campbell RR, Sabharwal S, et al. Health care costs for patients with chronic spinal cord injury in the Veterans health administration. *J Spinal Cord Med*. 2007;50(5):477–481.
10. National Spinal Cord Injury Statistical Center February *Facts and Figures at a Glance*. Birmingham, AL: University of Alabama at Birmingham; 2015.
11. Donovan WH. Donald munro lecture: spinal cord injury—past, present, and future. *J Spinal Cord Med*. 2007;30:85–100.
12. Lifshutz J, Colohan A. A brief history of therapy for traumatic spinal cord injury. *Neurosurg Focus*. 2004;16(1):1–8.
13. Knoeller SM, Seifried C. Historical perspective: history of spinal surgery. *Spine*. 2000;25(21):2838–2843.
14. Mothe AJ, Tator CH. Advances in stem cell therapy for spinal cord injury. *J Clin. Invest*. 2012;122(11):3824–3834.
15. Stenudd M, Sabelström H, Frisén Role of endogenous neural stem cells in spinal cord injury and repair. *JAMA Neuroogy*. 2015;72(2):235–237.
16. Donnelly EM, Lamanna J, Boulis NM. Stem cell therapy for the spinal cord. *Stem Cell Res Ther*. 2012;3(4) 24(1-9).
17. Kim MS, Lee HB. Perspectives on tissue-engineering nerve regeneration for the treatment of spinl cord injury. *Tissue Eng Part A*. 2014;20(13–14):1781–1783.
18. Ramer LM, Ramer MS, Bradbury EJ. Restoring function after spinal cord injury: towards clinical translation of experimental strategies. *Lancet Neurol*. 2014;13:1241–1256.
19. Festoff BW. Designing drugs that encourage spinal cord injury healing. *Expert Opin Drug Discov*. 2014;9(10):1151–1165.

20. Taha MF. Cell based-gene delivery approaches for the treatment of spinal cord injury and neurodegenerative diseases. *Curr Stem Cell Res Ther*. 2010;5:23–36.

21. Don AS, Tsang CK, Kazdoba TM, et al. Targeting mTOR as a novel therapeutic strategy for traumatic CNS injuries. *Drug Discov Today*. 2012;15-16:861–868.

22. Shen D, Wang X, Gu X. Scar-modulating treatment for central nervous system injury. *Neurosci Bull*. 2014;30(6):967–984.

23. Caron I, Papa S, Rossi F, et al. Nanovector-mediated drug delivery for spinal cord injury treatment. Wiley interdisciplinary reviews. *Nanomedicine and Nanbiotechnology*. 2014;6(5):506–515.

24. Guo JS, Qian CH, Ling EA, et al. Nanofiber scaffolds for treatment of spinal cord injury. *Curr Med Chem*. 2014;21(37):4282–4289.

25. Dimitrijevic MR, Hofstoetter US, Ladenbauer J, et al. Can the human lumbar posterior columns be stimulated by transcutaneous spinal cord stimulation? *Artif Organs*. 2011;35:257–262.

26. Dimitrijevic MR, Kakilas BA, McKay WB, Vrbova G, eds. *Restorative Neurology of Spinal Cord Injury*. New York: Oxford University Press; 2012.

27. Gerasimenko YP, Ichiyama RM, Lavrov IA, et al. Epidural spinal cord stimulation plus quipazine administration enable stepping in complete spinal adult rats. *J Neurophysiol*. 2007;98:2525–2536.

28. Zhang G, Zhang G, Rong W, et al. Oscillating field stimulation promoted spinal cord remyelination by inducing differentiation of oligodendrocyte precursor cells after spinal cord injury. *Biomed Mater Eng*. 2014;24:3629–3636.

29. Principe J, Sanchez JC, Enderle J. *Brain-Machine Interface Engineering*. Morgan & Claypool Publishers; 2007.

30. Starr A, Wise KD, Csongradi J. An evaluation of photoengraved microelectrodes for extracellular single-unit recording. *IEEE Trans Biomed Eng*. 2007;BME-20:291–293.

31. Takeuchi S, Suzuki T, Mabuchi K, et al. D flexible multichannel neural probe array. *J Micromech Microeng*. 2004;14:104–107.

32. Mushahwar VK, Horch KW. Selective activation and graded recruitment of functional muscle groups through spinal cord stimulation. *Ann NY Acad Sci*. 1998;860:531–535.

33. Vetter RJ, et al. Chronic neural recording using silicon-substrate microelectrode arrays implanted in cerebral cortex. *IEEE Trans Biomed Eng*. 2004;51:896–904.

34. Maynard EM, Nordhausen CT, Normann RA. The Utah intracortical electrode array: a recording structure for potential brain-computer interfaces. *Electroencephalogr Clin Neurophysiol*. 1997;102:228–239.

35. Neves HP, et al. Development of modular multifunctional probe arrays for cerebral applications. In: IEEE/EMBS Conference Neural Engineering, Kohala Coast, HI, USA, 2007, pp. 104–109.

36. Aarts AA, et al. A 3D slim-base probe array for in vivo recorded neuron activity. In: IEEE Engineering Medecine Biology Conference, Vancouver, BC, Canada, 2008, pp. 5798–5801.

37. Govic A, Paolini AG. In vivo electrophysiological recordings in amygdala subnuclei reveal selective and distinct responses to a behaviorally identified predator odor. *J Neurophysiol*. 2015;114:1423–1436.

38. Bisio M, Bosca A, Pasquale Emergence of bursting activity in connected neuronal subpopulations. *PLoS ONE*. 2014;9(9):e107400.

39. Yakovenko S, et al. Spatiotemporal activation of lumbosacral motoneurons in the locomotor step cycle. *J Neurophysiol*. 2002;87:1542–1553.

40. Mushahwar VK, Gillard DM, Gauthier MJ, et al. Intraspinal micro stimulation generates locomotor-like and feedback-controlled movements. *IEEE Trans Neural Syst Rehabil Eng*. 2002;10:68–81.

41. Snow S, Horch KW, Mushahwar VK. Intraspinal microstimulation using cylindrical multielectrodes. *IEEE Trans Biomed Eng*. 2006;53:311–319.

III. INNOVATIVE THINKING

42. Saigal R, Renzi C, Mushahwar VK. Intraspinal microstimulation generates functional movements after spinal-cord injury. *IEEE Trans Neural Syst Rehabil Eng.* 2004;12:430–440.
43. Guevremont L, et al. Locomotor-related networks in the lumbosacral enlargement of the adult spinal cat: activation through intraspinal microstimulation. *IEEE Trans Neural Syst Rehabil Eng.* 2006;14:266–272.
44. Goodall EV, Horch KW. Separation of action potentials in multiunit intrafascicular recordings. *IEEE Trans Biomed Eng.* 1992;39:289–295.
45. Yoshida Y, Horch K. Selective stimulation of peripheral nerve fibers using dual intrafascicular electrodes. *IEEE Trans Biomed Eng.* 1993;40:492–494.
46. Mirfakhraei K, Horch K. Classification of action potentials in multi-unit intrafascicular recordings using neural network pattern-recognition techniques. *IEEE Trans Biomed Eng.* 1994;41:89–91.
47. McNaughton TG, Horch KW. Action potential classification with dual channel intrafascicular electrodes. *IEEE Trans Biomed Eng.* 1994;41:609–616.
48. Little JW. Serial recording of reflexes after feline spinal cord transection. *Exp Neurol.* 1986;93:510–521.
49. Riddell JS, Hadian M. Field potentials generated by group II muscle afferents in the lower-lumbar segments of the feline spinal cord. *J Physiol.* 2000;522:97–108.
50. Yamamoto T, Xing T, Katayama Y, et al. Spinal cord responses to feline transcranial brain stimulation: evidence for involvement of cerebellar pathways. *J Neurotrauma.* 1990;7:247–256. Winter.
51. Mushahwar VK, Horch KW. Selective activation of muscle groups in the feline hindlimb through electrical microstimulation of the ventral lumbosacral spinal cord. *IEEE Trans Rehabil Eng.* 2000;8:11–21.
52. Lau B, Guevremont L, Mushahwar VK. Strategies for generating prolonged functional standing using intramuscular stimulation or intraspinal microstimulation. *IEEE Trans Neural Syst Rehabil Eng.* 2007;15:273–285.
53. Lemay MA, Grasse D, Grill WM. Hindlimb endpoint forces predict movement direction evoked by intraspinal microstimulation in cats. *IEEE Trans Neural Syst Rehabil Eng.* 2009;17:379–389.
54. Lemay MA, Grill WM. Modularity of motor output evoked by intraspinal microstimulation in cats. *J Neurophysiol.* 2004;91:502–514.
55. Dimitrijevic MR, Gerasimenko Y, Pinter MM. Evidence for a spinal central pattern generator in humans. *Ann N Y Acad Sci.* 1998;860:360–375.
56. Minassian K, Jilge B, Rattay F, et al. Stepping-like movements in humans with complete spinal cord injury induced by epidural stimulation of the lumbar cord: electromyographic study of compound muscle action potentials. *Spinal Cord.* 2004;42:401–416.
57. Eccles C. Synaptic potentials of motorneurons. *J Neurophysiol.* 1946;9(2):87–120.
58. Frank K, Fuortes GF. Potentials recorded from the spinal cord with microelectrodes. *J Physiol.* 1955;130:625–654.
59. Sayenko DG, Atkinson DA, Dy CJ, et al. Spinal segment-specific transcutaneous stimulation differentially shapes activation pattern among motor pools in humans. *J Appl Physiol.* 2015;118(11):1364–1374.
60. Sahin M. Selective recordings of motor signals from the corticospinal tract. Proceedings of International Functional Electrical Stimulation (Conference proceedings). 2001, Cleveland, OH, USA.
61. Hochberg LR, Bacher D, Jarosiewicz B, et al. Reach and grasp by people with tetraplegia using a neurally controlled robotic arm. *Nature.* 2012;485(7398):372–375.
62. Kim SP, Simeral JD, Hochberg LR, et al. Point-and-click cursor control with an intracortical neural interface system by humans with tetraplegia. *IEEE Trans Neural Syst Rehabil Eng.* 2011;19(2):193–203.
63. Perge JA, Homer ML, Malik WQ, et al. Intra-day signal instabilities affect decoding performance in an intracortical neural interface system. *J Neural Eng.* 2013;10(3):036004.

64. Bamford J, Putman CT, Mushahwar VK. Intraspinal microstimulation preferentially recruits fatigue-resistant muscle fibers and generates gradual force in rat. *J Physiol (Lond)*. 2005;569(3):873–884.

65. Al-Izki S, Kirkwood PA, Lemon RN, et al. Electrophysiological actions of the rubrospinal tract in the anaesthetised rat. *Exp Neurol*. 2008;212(1):2008.

66. Brookhart JM, Morris RE. Antidromic potential recordings from the bulbar pyramid of the cat. *J Neurophysiol*. 1948;11:387–396.

67. Lloyd DPC. The spinal mechanisms of the pyramidal system in cats. *J. Neurophysiol*. 1941;4:523–526.

68. Jabbur SJ Towe AL. Analysis of the antidromic cortical response following stimulation at the medullary pyramids 1961;155:148–160.

69. Minassian K, Persy I, Rattay F, Pinter MM, Kern H, Dimitrijevic MR. Human lumbar cord circuitries can be activated by extrinsic tonic input to generate locomotor-like activity. *Hum Mov Sci*. 2007;26(2):275–295.

III. INNOVATIVE THINKING

14

Neuromodulation for Psychiatric Disorders

S. Hescham, M. Tönge, A. Jahanshahi and Y. Temel

Maastricht University Medical Center, Maastricht, The Netherlands

Innovative Neuromodulation.
DOI: http://dx.doi.org/10.1016/B978-0-12-800454-8.00014-8

287

INTRODUCTION

Patients with mental disorders suffer from behavioral, affective, cognitive, and perceptual abnormalities. The World Health Organization estimated that one in four people experience mental health problems at least once in their life.[1] Consequently, mental disorders cause an enormous economic burden on societies and on quality of life of individuals and families.[2] Behavioral and/or drug therapies are effective in the majority of patients, however some patients do not respond sufficiently or experience serious side-effects of medication. In these patients surgical approaches have been proposed. In the early and mid-20th century ablative surgeries and experimental electrical stimulations were performed in patients with psychiatric indications. Deep brain stimulation (DBS) for psychiatric disorders has received increased interest after three key publications. In 1999, two of these studies were published. The first described favorable outcomes following DBS of the anterior limb of the internal capsule in four patients with obsessive-compulsive disorder (OCD).[3] The other study reported beneficial effects observed after DBS of the medial part of the thalamus in a patient with Tourette's syndrome (TS).[4] Finally, in 2005, DBS of the subgenual cingulate gyrus was described in patients with treatment-resistant depression (TRD).[5] In later years, other papers have been published on DBS for various psychiatric indications.

Here, we will update our previously published review,[6] in which we organize indications according to their clinical status, accepted or experimental, primarily focusing on DBS. Two psychiatric indications have now become accepted for DBS, OCD and TS, respectively. Other indications are still considered experimental.

ACCEPTED INDICATIONS

Obsessive-Compulsive Disorder (OCD)

OCD is a severe anxiety disorder, affecting approximately 2% of the general population[7] and is characterized by obsessive thoughts and compulsive behavior, which the patient recognizes as irrational. Symptoms include checking, washing and cleaning, counting, and a strong need for symmetry among others. These symptoms are time-consuming, might result in social isolation, and often cause severe emotional and financial distress. First-line therapy includes behavioral therapy, drug treatments, and combination of these.[8,9] However, approximately 60% of the patients do not respond adequately,[8] and 20–40% of patients remain treatment-resistant.[10,11] For these patients, DBS has been considered to help alleviate the symptoms.

DBS of the internal capsule/ventral striatum in patients suffering from refractory OCD has shown some benefits.[6] In order to investigate its potential mechanism of action when compared to a capsulotomy, Suetens and colleagues performed a positron emission tomography (PET) imaging study.[12] In total, 16 capsulotomy patients and 16 DBS patients in preoperative, postoperative, and stimulation-off states were included. The stimulation parameters were individually optimized and varied between 100 and 130 Hz, 210 and 450 ms pulse width, and 4–10.5 V. Capsulotomy and DBS led to similar metabolic changes in cortico-striato-thalamocortical (CSTC) pathways (Fig. 14.1), especially in the limbic loop consisting of the medial orbitofrontal cortex and the anterior cingulate projecting to the mediodorsal thalamus. Reduced metabolic activity was common in both interventions in the anterior cingulate, prefrontal, and orbitofrontal cortices, although metabolic changes were more pronounced in capsulotomy than in DBS and also extended to areas outside the CSTC. Metabolic activity was largely reversed in DBS patients when stimulation was turned off. Both treatment strategies resulted in significant improvements in the yale-brown obsessive-compulsive scale (Y-BOCS) and the Hamilton rating scale for depression (HRSD) scores when compared to preoperative states.[12]

Another study found a significant and continuous improvement in quality of life scores both in early (8 months postoperative) and late

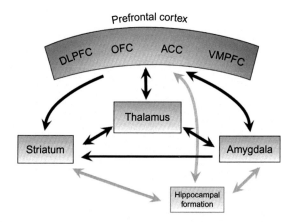

FIGURE 14.1   Cortico-striato-thalamocortical circuit (CSTC). Schematic diagram of the CSTC, which is implicated in the pathophysiology of OCD. In DBS for OCD, activity within this circuit is thought to be modulated by high-frequency stimulation. DLPFC, dorsolateral prefrontal cortex; ACC, anterior cingulate cortex; OFC, orbitofrontal cortex; VMPFC, ventromedial prefrontal cortex. Arrowheads indicate direction of neural input. Black lines represent connections among the major structures implicated in DBS for OCD; gray lines indicate additional connections. *Source: Adapted from Bourne SK, Eckhardt CA, Sheth SA, Eskandar EN. Mechanisms of deep brain stimulation for obsessive compulsive disorder: effects upon cells and circuits. Front Integr Neurosci. 2012;6:29.*[13]

(3–5 years postoperative) periods in 16 OCD patients with nucleus accumbens (NAc) DBS at 130 Hz, maximum of 5 V, and 90 μs pulse width. The patients' perception of the quality of life improvement at 3–5 years after surgery was 90%, additionally 39.5% were attributed to physical and psychological factors and 16% for the environmental domain. The social domain did not change between baseline and follow-ups. These data suggest that the improvement in OCD is not restricted to the disease symptoms, but also influences a patient's overall quality of life.[14] The authors also corroborate the relapse and rebound effects of OCD symptoms following acute cessation of DBS. Not only did Y-BOCS scores decrease by 50%, but Hamilton anxiety and depression levels even worsened by 40% when compared to presurgical states. In this study, improvements in quality of life disappeared with an acute cessation of DBS.[15]

The subthalamic nucleus (STN) has also been suggested as a potential target for OCD. Following beneficial effects reported in a well-designed clinical trial,[16] Chabardes et al. reported a 50–75% improvement in Y-BOCS scores at 6 months follow-up in four OCD patients who underwent limbic STN DBS at 130 Hz, 90 μs pulse width, and 1.2–4 V.[17] Interestingly, also the anteromedial internal globus pallidus has shown to produce favorable effects. In four TS patients with prominent OCD symptoms anteromedial internal globus pallidus DBS (high-frequency, 60–90 μs pulse width, and about 4 mA) resulted in significant alleviation of symptoms. These data suggest the anteromedial internal globus pallidus as a possible new target for intractable OCD, at least in patients with comorbid TS. The authors encourage further investigations of this nucleus as a DBS target to confirm long-term benefits in patients suffering solely from OCD.[18]

The American Society for Stereotactic and Functional Neurosurgery, the Congress of Neurological Surgeons, and the American Association of Neurological Surgeons established a guideline based on the available literature for DBS surgery in OCD. According to this guideline, there is Level I evidence for the use of bilateral STN DBS and Level II evidence for the use of bilateral NAc DBS surgery in medically refractory OCD. Unilateral DBS in either target, however, has been found to be insufficient in medically refractory OCD.[19]

Tourette's Syndrome (TS)

TS is a neuropsychiatric disorder with a typical onset in childhood, characterized by motor and vocal tics.[20] Among US children aged 6–17 years, approximately 0.2% suffer from TS.[21] In the majority of cases, frequency and severity of tics diminish considerably during adulthood, however, some patients continue to exhibit identifiable tics. Patients with mild symptomatology might benefit from psychotherapy, but when symptoms interfere with daily life activities, typical and atypical neuroleptics

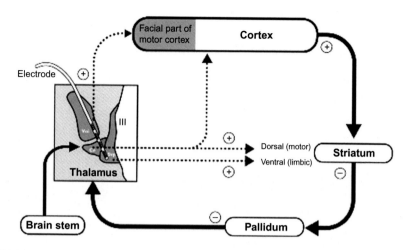

FIGURE 14.2 Schematic representation illustrating the target of stimulation. Dotted lines represent the output, hypothetically reduced by the stimulation, toward the main output structures of the targeted nuclei. Ce, centromedian nucleus; Svp, substantia periventricularis; Voi, nucleus ventrooralis internus; III, third ventricle. *Source: Adapted from Visser-Vandewalle V, Temel Y, Boon P, et al. Chronic bilateral thalamic stimulation: a new therapeutic approach in intractable Tourette syndrome. J Neurosurg. 2003; 99(6):1094–1100.*[22]

have been prescribed. For patients refractory to medication, neuromodulation techniques have produced beneficial effects.

For DBS, the two most commonly accepted targets are the centromedian-parafascicular thalamic nucleus (Fig. 14.2) and the internal globus pallidus. In line with this, a recent study has shown that bilateral centromedian-parafascicular thalamic nucleus DBS at about 150 Hz, 3.6 V, and 90–210 μs pulse width reduced motor and sonic tics in three out of five patients after 3 months. Also, symptoms of depression and anxiety improved.[23] Similar results were reported by Ackermans and colleagues, although the authors highlighted adverse effects related to oculomotor function and energy levels.[24]

Lately, the application of scheduled rather than continuous DBS has gained increased attention. The safety and preliminary efficacy of scheduled centromedian DBS for TS has been the subject of one recent study.[25] In five patients, a scheduled DBS paradigm was applied in which stimulation pulse trains were adjusted individually for a certain period of time (e.g., 2 seconds on and 10 seconds off; from 10:00 to 22:00 h). The most robust changes observed across these five patients were visible improvements in motor and vocal tics. Although in the present paradigm no subject achieved greater than 50% tic reduction, this study provides important planning information of how DBS therapy can be improved in TS patients. The advantages of scheduled over continuous stimulation are battery life improvements, possibly less stimulation-induced tolerance, and a more scientific and physiological approach to address the paroxysmal symptoms of TS.[25]

EXPERIMENTAL

Addiction/Substance Dependence

Substance dependence is a chronic relapsing disorder involving compulsive seeking and intake of drugs, resulting in withdrawal syndromes when access to the drug is prevented. Most drugs of abuse target the brain's reward system, and several structures involved in the circuitry of addiction are confirmed to be part of the reward pathway. Several possible targets for neuromodulation have been under investigation in attempts to treat addiction: NAc, lateral hypothalamus, amygdala, lateral habenula, dorsal striatum, prefrontal cortex, and STN.[26]

The NAc, however, remains the most widely used of these DBS targets. Recently, the effect of 130 Hz, 4.5 V, and 90 μs pulse width NAc DBS was described in five patients with alcohol addiction.[27] In these patients, NAc DBS was tolerated without substantial side-effects. All patients experienced significant and continuous improvement of cravings. Two patients even remained completely abstinent during the 4-year follow-up. The authors have also recorded local field potentials of the NAc and applied surface electroencephalography while patients performed neuropsychological tasks and found that the NAc plays a pivotal role in processing alcohol-related cues.[27]

With regard to heroin addiction, NAc DBS has also been found to alleviate cravings as well as ameliorate depressive and anxious symptoms in a pilot study of two patients.[28] The patients remained abstinent during 2 years and the overall quality of life was improved. Because both patients reported the occasional consumption of other psychotropic substances, the authors highlighted the importance of psychotherapy accompanying DBS in mental disorders. This study was used to justify the launch of a larger clinical trial (NCT01245075).

Alzheimer Disease

The most common form of dementia is Alzheimer disease (AD), which is defined as a condition of severely impaired cognitive functioning in various domains with a substantial negative effect on patients, families, and caregivers. The age-standardized prevalence of people aged 65 years or older of population-based studies in Europe suggests that 4.4% suffer from AD.[29] In the United States, a study of a national representative sample of people aged more than 70 years provided a prevalence for AD of 9.7%.[30] Current pharmacological treatment is only mildly and temporarily beneficial. Consequently the development of effective treatment for AD remains a major unmet need. Neuromodulation techniques have, however, shown innovative and promising outcomes.

Stimulation of the fornix, innovative as a tract target rather than a nucleus or mixed target, has shown benefits in AD and additionally indicated that the nucleus basalis of Meynert can be used as a potential target.[6] Since then, more evidence has evolved confirming beneficial effects for both target regions. It was reported recently, that in two AD patients with best clinical response bilateral fornix DBS of 130 Hz, 3–3.5 V, and 90 μs pulse width increased hippocampal volume.[31] This hippocampal volume change strongly correlated with hippocampal metabolism and a volume change in the fornix and mammillary bodies, suggesting a circuit-wide effect of stimulation. In addition, a recent animal study suggests that fornix DBS enhances acetylcholine and not glutamate levels in the hippocampus (Fig. 14.3).[32]

In a case study, fornix DBS of 130 Hz, 2.5 V, and 240 ms pulse width induced an increased metabolic effect on mesial temporal structures and reduced the progression of memory loss in one AD patient, in a 1-year postsurgical follow-up.[33] The authors, however, raised the awareness that out of 110 recruited patients, only nine fulfilled the strict inclusion criteria. In the end, *only one patient* agreed to undergo DBS surgery. This number appears to be very low considering the devastating effects of the disease and the lack of benefit of current therapies, highlighting how much work needs to be done additionally in educating patients and caregivers about their options.

A first phase I trial of nucleus basalis of Meynert DBS in AD has recently been published.[34] In this study, six mild–moderate AD patients were implanted with DBS electrodes and stimulated with 20 Hz, 2.5 V, and 90 μs pulse width. After assessing the Alzheimer's Disease Assessment scale-cognitive subscale it was found that four out of six patients responded to the therapy at 11 months follow-up. Because no severe side-effects were observed, the authors concluded that nucleus basalis of Meynert DBS is at least safe and feasible.[34]

Depression

The most common psychiatric disorder is major depression. It is ranked the fourth leading cause of societal burden of all diseases.[35] Standard therapies include pharmaco- and psychotherapy, but a large proportion of patients do not achieve enduring symptom remission. Approximately 20% of these patients enter a condition of TRD. DBS within the subgenual cingulate gyrus[5] and the nucleus accumbens[36] are both currently being investigated as potential treatment targets for TRD.

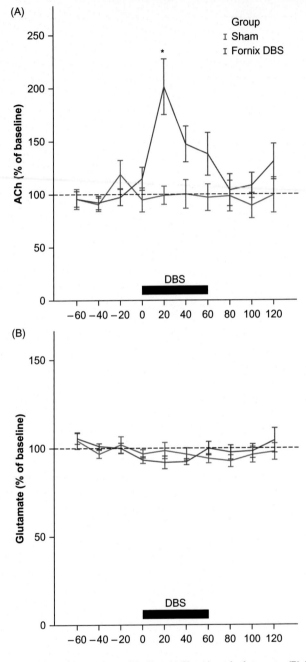

FIGURE 14.3 Microdialysate acetylcholine (ACh; A) and glutamate (B) levels of the dorsal hippocampus in anesthetized fornix DBS and sham rats. Horizontal bar indicates stimulation period. ACh levels were significantly elevated in the fornix DBS group after 20 min of stimulation. No difference in glutamate levels was detected between fornix DBS and sham. Data points are mean ± SEM values expressed as a percentage of baseline. Mean raw values for baseline ACh were 0.324 nM ± 0.023 and for glutamate 3.05 μM ± 0.24. * $p < 0.05$, repeated measures ANOVA for fornix DBS versus sham rats. *Source: Adapted from Hescham S, Jahanshahi A, Schweimer J, et al. Fornix deep brain stimulation enhances acetylcholine levels in the hippocampus. Brain Struct Funct. 2015.*

A preliminary trial compared NAc and caudate nucleus as DBS targets for TRD in four patients.[37] Stimulation parameters for both targets were 130 Hz, 60 µs pulse width, and 4–8 V. In order to retain the ability to stimulate the two different targets along the same trajectory, directional leads were used, in which electrodes spaced 4 mm apart can be activated independently. After 5 months of NAc DBS, none of the patients were responders or remitters, although the authors observed a fluctuant decrease in the HRSD scores for three patients. After switching to caudate stimulation for 4 months, no improvement was observed. However, during the 6-month extension phase, NAc DBS produced a significant response in three out of four patients. This response was accompanied by a decrease in glucose metabolism in the posterior cingulate gyrus, left frontal lobe, superior and medial gyrus, and bilateral cerebellum. An increase in metabolism was observed in the bilateral superior and left medial gyrus of the frontal lobe and the right anterior cingulate gyrus. The authors concluded that the NAc is likely a more promising target than the caudate,[37] but they also highlighted the overall postimplant timeframe that needs to be considered in evaluating results.

Recently, Lozano et al. published a multicenter, open-label, prospective study including 21 subcallosal cingulate gyrus (SCC) DBS patients with 12 months of follow-up. Average stimulation settings were 130 Hz, 95 µs pulse width, and 4.8 mA. HRSD scores were investigated in these follow-ups and a 50% reduction of HRSD scores was revealed in 57%, 48%, and 29% of patients at 1, 6, and 12 months, respectively.[38] This was intriguing, yet disappointing that initial promising effects seemed to fade so significantly within only 12 months. Another study indicated that longer pulse width (270–450 µs) may play a role in stimulus optimization in SCC DBS. Longer pulse durations produce larger current spread, suggesting that we do not yet know the most optimal stimulation parameter to embark on large-scale randomized sham-controlled trials.[39]

In the Berlin Deep Brain Stimulation Depression Study, six treatment-resistant depressive patients were implanted with bilateral SCC DBS electrodes. While two of six patients remained remitted in 24–36 weeks follow-up, four patients failed to respond.[40] Belrim et al. concluded from these recent outcomes that SCC DBS for depression seems more beneficial only in the early postoperative (6 months) period.[41]

A recent multicenter, prospective, randomized trial of ventral capsule/ventral striatum DBS for depression, sponsored by Medtronic, failed to show significant improvement in the stimulation group when compared to the sham stimulation group 16 weeks after implantation of the device. Similarly, another study sponsored by St. Jude Medical (BROADEN study) also showed less than 17.2% improvement in 6 months follow-up (lower than proposed success rates). Both studies were discontinued.[42]

While some of these results have been tantalizing, as of this writing, effectively treating major depression with DBS remains elusive. Other targets being explored include: medial forebrain bundle, inferior thalamic peduncle, lateral habenular complex, STN, and the rostral cingulate gyrus.[43]

NEUROMODULATION IN OTHER PSYCHIATRIC INDICATIONS

The major psychiatric disorders in which neuromodulation has been applied are described above. Previously, we have reviewed the effects of DBS in schizophrenia, attention deficit hyperactivity disorder (ADHD), autism spectrum disorder, and aggressiveness.[6] We now report the latest findings for schizophrenia and also include emerging indications such as anorexia nervosa (AN) and posttraumatic stress disorder (PTSD).

Schizophrenia

Schizophrenia is a mental disorder often classified into positive and negative symptoms with a lifetime prevalence of 0.4% worldwide.[44] Positive symptoms are characterized by delusions, hallucinations, and disordered thoughts, while negative symptoms include flat expressions, lack of motivation, and anhedonia.[45] Antipsychotic medication can mainly reduce the positive symptoms of schizophrenia. However, about 20% of patients are treatment-resistant and up to 75% of the patients experience recurrent relapse.[46]

Only a single case study reported the application of unilateral NAc DBS in a 51-year-old woman with intractable OCD and residual symptoms of schizophrenia.[47] Stimulation parameters were 130 Hz, 4.5 V, and 60 µs pulse width. In this particular case, DBS resulted in a substantial reduction of obsessions and compulsions as well as an improvement of psychosocial functioning after 6 months, 1- and 2-year follow-up. Based on these promising results, a clinical trial was recently launched in Canada and is currently recruiting patients (NCT01725334). The study will include three patients for NAc/ventral striatum DBS and another three for VTA DBS. Both targets have been found to be hypoactive in patients primarily suffering from the negative symptoms in schizophrenia.

Anorexia Nervosa

AN is a debilitating and potentially lethal (when resistant to treatment) psychiatric disorder, with a nonresponse rate to medical treatment of approximately 20–33%.[48,49] In a case study it was found that DBS of the right subgenual cingulate area with intermittent stimulation, 2 minutes on and 1 minute off, at 130 Hz, 91 μs pulse width, and 5 mA improved symptoms in comorbid AN. The patient was a 56-year-old female with severely disabling chronic recurrent depression suffering from AN since she was 17. DBS was able to recover her eating disorder and the patient was able to maintain a body mass index (BMI) of 19.1 kg/m^2 for over 2 years.[49] Another case study reported findings of unilateral DBS of the left ventral capsule/ventral striatum with 120 Hz, 120 μ s pulse width, and 7.5 V in a 52-year-old female patient suffering from intractable OCD and concomitant AN. DBS led to an improvement of OCD symptoms and induced a BMI of about 19 kg/m^2. The authors attempted to further improve her symptoms and added another DBS electrode into the ventral caudate. Unexpectedly, generalized anxiety, mood, and OCD symptoms worsened, and she had a concurrent 6 kg weight loss. With the acute cessation of ventral caudate DBS, her symptoms improved again.[50]

DBS to treat AN as a primary disorder has been addressed in two studies. In the first study, four young female patients with a BMI between 10 and 13.33 kg/m^2 underwent bilateral DBS of the NAc and were stimulated with 180 Hz, 90 μs pulse width, and 6–8 V. After approximately 3 years of continuous stimulation, all patients showed an average weight gain of 65% and an average BMI of 18.4–22.1 kg/m^2.[51] The second study is a phase I trial in which six female patients with refractory AN received SCC DBS at 130 Hz, 90 μs pulse width, and 5–7 V for 9 months. The BMI of the patients ranged between 11.1 and 15.1 kg/m^2 preoperatively. After 9 months DBS showed therapeutic effects in 50% of the patients. Three patients increased their BMI to 16–21 kg/m^2, while the remaining patients did not change from their baseline BMI.[52]

Posttraumatic Stress Disorder

PTSD is a psychiatric disorder in which 30% of patients are refractory to medical treatment, widely consisting of selective serotonin reuptake inhibitors. In a rat model of PTSD, amygdala DBS of 160 Hz, 2.5 V, and 120 μs pulse width has been suggested to treat the cause of PTSD, based on the idea that the disorder involves a hyperactive amygdala function.[53] These data led to the initiation of a prospective, randomized controlled pilot trial on six severe PTSD combat veterans refractory to conventional medication.[54] The basolateral amygdala will also be targeted in these patients. The preliminary results of this study, however, have not been reported, yet.

CONCLUSION

Patients with severe psychiatric disorders not responsive to pharmacotherapy, behavioral therapy, or combinations of both, are being considered as candidates for neuromodulation therapies. Currently, the most widely used chronic neuromodulation therapy is DBS. DBS has been explored in a number of different psychiatric disorders, as well as in well-designed clinical trials and in a few case reports/series. There is good evidence for a beneficial outcome of DBS in patients with severe OCD and TS. For other indications, based on the current level of evidence, DBS should be considered experimental. Ongoing clinical trials are likely to provide more conclusive insights.

An interesting and rather unexpected development comprises the unfavorable outcomes of two large trials of DBS for major depressive disorder, despite promising results in case series published earlier in major scientific journals. Our concern is that the clinical application of neuromodulation outpaces the scientific evidence supporting or discouraging the application of this approach. The field needs further understanding of the cell- and circuit-based pathophysiology as well as the mechanisms of action of DBS.[55,56]

In line with this, a few studies have already attempted to scrutinize mechanisms of action by means of PET imaging. In OCD, for instance, the benefits of internal capsule DBS over capsulotomy have been suggested to be related to the specificity of metabolic changes within the limbic pathways.[12] In a different study, functional magnetic resonance imaging results have shown that NAc DBS in OCD patients was able to normalize the dysfunctional NAc–frontal cortex connection to regain activity levels of healthy controls.[57]

Two features make DBS favorable over ablative surgery. First, the reversible nature of DBS allows for investigation of new targets without the morbidity of permanent side-effects. Second, the programmable nature of DBS allows neurosurgeons to improve efficacy through reprogramming. Advances in the field of neuromodulation include directionally segmented DBS leads, allowing control over the direction of current flow, as well as adaptive DBS consisting of a closed-loop feedback system, both of which are explored elsewhere in this text. With a robust scientific knowledge on the mechanisms of action of DBS, adaptive and directional DBS might constitute a future therapeutic approach in psychiatric disorders.

References

1. Bebbington P. The World Health Report 2001. *Soc Psychiatry Psychiatr Epidemiol.* 2001;36(10):473–474.
2. World Health Organization. *The Global Burden of Disease: 2004 Update.* World Health Organisation; 2008.
3. Nuttin B, Cosyns P, Demeulemeester H, Gybels J, Meyerson B. Electrical stimulation in anterior limbs of internal capsules in patients with obsessive-compulsive disorder. *Lancet.* 1999;354(9189):1526.

4. Vandewalle V, van der Linden C, Groenewegen HJ, Caemaert J. Stereotactic treatment of Gilles de la Tourette syndrome by high frequency stimulation of thalamus. *Lancet.* 1999;353(9154):724.

5. Mayberg HS, Lozano AM, Voon V, et al. Deep brain stimulation for treatment-resistant depression. *Neuron.* 2005;45(5):651–660.

6. Temel Y, Hescham SA, Jahanshahi A, et al. Neuromodulation in psychiatric disorders. *Int Rev Neurobiol.* 2012;107:283–314.

7. Rasmussen SA, Eisen JL. The epidemiology and clinical features of obsessive compulsive disorder. *Psychiatr Clin North Am.* 1992;15(4):743–758.

8. Kellner M. Drug treatment of obsessive-compulsive disorder. *Dialogues Clin Neurosci.* 2010;12(2):187–197. Epub 2010/07/14. eng.

9. Hollander E. Obsessive-compulsive disorder: the hidden epidemic. *J Clin Psychiatry.* 1997;58(suppl 12):3–6. Epub 1997/01/01. eng.

10. Simpson HB, Foa EB, Liebowitz MR, et al. A randomized, controlled trial of cognitive-behavioral therapy for augmenting pharmacotherapy in obsessive-compulsive disorder. *Am J Psychiatry.* 2008;165(5):621–630. Epub 2008/03/05. eng.

11. Skoog G, Skoog I. A 40-year follow-up of patients with obsessive-compulsive disorder [see comments]. *Arch Gen Psychiatry.* 1999;56(2):121–127. Epub 1999/02/20. eng.

12. Suetens K, Nuttin B, Gabriels L, Van Laere K. Differences in metabolic network modulation between capsulotomy and deep-brain stimulation for refractory obsessive-compulsive disorder. *J Nucl Med.* 2014;55(6):951–959. Epub 2014/04/12. Eng.

13. Bourne SK, Eckhardt CA, Sheth SA, Eskandar EN. Mechanisms of deep brain stimulation for obsessive compulsive disorder: effects upon cells and circuits. *Front Integr Neurosci.* 2012;6:29.

14. Ooms P, Mantione M, Figee M, Schuurman PR, van den Munckhof P, Denys D. Deep brain stimulation for obsessive-compulsive disorders: long-term analysis of quality of life. *J Neurol Neurosurg Psychiatry.* 2014;85(2):153–158. Epub 2013/05/30. eng.

15. Ooms P, Blankers M, Figee M, et al. Rebound of affective symptoms following acute cessation of deep brain stimulation in obsessive-compulsive disorder. *Brain Stimul.* 2014;7(5):727–731. Epub 2014/08/05. eng.

16. Mallet L, Polosan M, Jaafari N, et al. Subthalamic nucleus stimulation in severe obsessive–compulsive disorder. *N Engl J Med.* 2008;359(20):2121–2134.

17. Chabardes S, Polosan M, Krack P, et al. Deep brain stimulation for obsessive-compulsive disorder: subthalamic nucleus target. *World Neurosurg.* 2013;80(3–4) S31. e1-8. Epub 2012/04/04. eng.

18. Nair G, Evans A, Bear RE, Velakoulis D, Bittar RG. The anteromedial GPi as a new target for deep brain stimulation in obsessive compulsive disorder. *J Clin Neurosci.* 2014;21(5):815–821. Epub 2014/02/15. eng.

19. Hamani C, Pilitsis J, Rughani AI, et al. Deep brain stimulation for obsessive-compulsive disorder: systematic review and evidence-based guideline sponsored by the American Society for Stereotactic and Functional Neurosurgery and the Congress of Neurological Surgeons (CNS) and endorsed by the CNS and American Association of Neurological Surgeons. *Neurosurgery.* 2014;75(4):327–333. quiz 33. Epub 2014/07/23. eng.

20. Mink JW. Basal ganglia dysfunction in Tourette's syndrome: a new hypothesis. *Pediatr Neurol.* 2001;25(3):190–198. Epub 2001/10/06. eng.

21. Bitsko RH, Holbrook JR, Visser SN, et al. A national profile of Tourette syndrome, 2011-2012. *J Dev Behav Pediatr.* 2014;35(5):317–322.

22. Visser-Vandewalle V, Temel Y, Boon P, et al. Chronic bilateral thalamic stimulation: a new therapeutic approach in intractable Tourette syndrome. *J Neurosurg.* 2003;99(6): 1094–1100.

23. Schoenberg MR, Maddux BN, Riley DE, et al. Five-months-postoperative neuropsychological outcome from a pilot prospective randomized clinical trial of thalamic deep brain stimulation for tourette syndrome. *Neuromodulation.* 2014 Epub 2014/09/25. Eng.

III. INNOVATIVE THINKING

24. Ackermans L, Duits A, van der Linden C, et al. Double-blind clinical trial of thalamic stimulation in patients with Tourette syndrome. *Brain*. 2011;134(Pt 3):832–844.

25. Okun MS, Foote KD, Wu SS, et al. A trial of scheduled deep brain stimulation for Tourette syndrome: moving away from continuous deep brain stimulation paradigms. *JAMA Neurol*. 2013;70(1):85–94.

26. Pelloux Y, Baunez C. Deep brain stimulation for addiction: why the subthalamic nucleus should be favored. *Curr Opin Neurobiol*. 2013;23(4):713–720. Epub 2013/03/30. eng.

27. Voges J, Muller U, Bogerts B, Munte T, Heinze HJ. Deep brain stimulation surgery for alcohol addiction. *World Neurosurg*. 2013;80(3–4) S28.e1-31. Epub 2012/07/25. eng.

28. Kuhn J, Moller M, Treppmann JF, et al. Deep brain stimulation of the nucleus accumbens and its usefulness in severe opioid addiction. *Mol Psychiatry*. 2014;19(2):145–146.

29. Lobo A, Launer LJ, Fratiglioni L, et al. Prevalence of dementia and major subtypes in Europe: a collaborative study of population-based cohorts. Neurologic Diseases in the Elderly Research Group. *Neurology*. 2000;54(11 suppl 5):S4–S9. Epub 2000/06/15. eng.

30. Plassman BL, Langa KM, Fisher GG, et al. Prevalence of dementia in the United States: the aging, demographics, and memory study. *Neuroepidemiology*. 2007;29(1–2):125–132. Epub 2007/11/03. eng.

31. Sankar T, Chakravarty MM, Bescos A, et al. Deep brain stimulation influences brain structure in Alzheimer's disease. *Brain Stimul*. 2014;8(3):645–654.

32. Hescham S, Jahanshahi A, Schweimer J, et al. Fornix deep brain stimulation enhances acetylcholine levels in the hippocampus. *Brain Struct Funct*. 2015

33. Fontaine D, Deudon A, Lemaire JJ, et al. Symptomatic treatment of memory decline in Alzheimer's disease by deep brain stimulation: a feasibility study. *J Alzheimers Dis*. 2013;34(1):315–323. Epub 2012/11/22. eng.

34. Kuhn J, Hardenacke K, Lenartz D, et al. Deep brain stimulation of the nucleus basalis of Meynert in Alzheimer's dementia. *Mol Psychiatry*. 2014;20(3):353–360.

35. Richards D. Prevalence and clinical course of depression: a review. *Clin Psychol Rev*. 2011;31(7):1117–1125. Epub 2011/08/09. eng.

36. Schlaepfer TE, Cohen MX, Frick C, et al. Deep brain stimulation to reward circuitry alleviates anhedonia in refractory major depression. *Neuropsychopharmacology*. 2007;33(2):368–377.

37. Millet B, Jaafari N, Polosan M, et al. Limbic versus cognitive target for deep brain stimulation in treatment-resistant depression: accumbens more promising than caudate. *Eur Neuropsychopharmacol*. 2014;24(8):1229–1239. Epub 2014/06/22. eng.

38. Lozano AM, Giacobbe P, Hamani C, et al. A multicenter pilot study of subcallosal cingulate area deep brain stimulation for treatment-resistant depression. *J Neurosurg*. 2012;116(2):315–322. Epub 2011/11/22. eng.

39. Ramasubbu R, Anderson S, Haffenden A, Chavda S, Kiss ZH. Double-blind optimization of subcallosal cingulate deep brain stimulation for treatment-resistant depression: a pilot study. *J Psychiatry Neurosci*. 2013;38(5):325–332. Epub 2013/03/27. eng.

40. Merkl A, Schneider GH, Schonecker T, et al. Antidepressant effects after short-term and chronic stimulation of the subgenual cingulate gyrus in treatment-resistant depression. *Exp Neurol*. 2013;249:160–168. Epub 2013/09/10. eng.

41. Berlim MT, McGirr A, Van den Eynde F, Fleck MP, Giacobbe P. Effectiveness and acceptability of deep brain stimulation (DBS) of the subgenual cingulate cortex for treatment-resistant depression: a systematic review and exploratory meta-analysis. *J Affect Disord*. 2014;159:31–38. Epub 2014/04/01. eng.

42. Morishita T, Fayad SM, Higuchi MA, Nestor KA, Foote KD. Deep brain stimulation for treatment-resistant depression: systematic review of clinical outcomes. *Neurotherapeutics*. 2014;11(3):475–484. Epub 2014/05/29. eng.

43. Delaloye S, Holtzheimer PE. Deep brain stimulation in the treatment of depression. *Dialogues Clin Neurosci*. 2014;16(1):83–91. Epub 2014/04/16. eng.

44. McGrath J, Saha S, Chant D, Welham J. Schizophrenia: a concise overview of incidence, prevalence, and mortality. *Epidemiol Rev.* 2008;30:67–76.

45. Torres-Gonzalez F, Ibanez-Casas I, Saldivia S, et al. Unmet needs in the management of schizophrenia. *Neuropsychiatr Dis Treat.* 2014;10:97–110.

46. Smith T, Weston C, Lieberman J. Schizophrenia (maintenance treatment). *Am Fam Physician.* 2010;82(4):338–339.

47. Plewnia C, Schober F, Rilk A, et al. Sustained improvement of obsessive-compulsive disorder by deep brain stimulation in a woman with residual schizophrenia. *Int J Neuropsychopharmacol.* 2008;11(8):1181–1183. Epub 2008/08/14. eng.

48. Oudijn MS, Storosum JG, Nelis E, Denys D. Is deep brain stimulation a treatment option for anorexia nervosa? *BMC Psychiatry.* 2013;13:277. Epub 2013/11/02. eng.

49. Israel M, Steiger H, Kolivakis T, McGregor L, Sadikot AF. Deep brain stimulation in the subgenual cingulate cortex for an intractable eating disorder. *Biol Psychiatry.* 2010;67(9):e53–e54.

50. McLaughlin NC, Didie ER, Machado AG, Haber SN, Eskandar EN, Greenberg BD. Improvements in anorexia symptoms after deep brain stimulation for intractable obsessive-compulsive disorder. *Biol Psychiatry.* 2013;73(9):e29–e31.

51. Wu H, Van Dyck-Lippens PJ, Santegoeds R, et al. Deep-brain stimulation for anorexia nervosa. *World Neurosurg.* 2013;80(3–4) S29, e1-10.

52. Lipsman N, Woodside DB, Giacobbe P, et al. Subcallosal cingulate deep brain stimulation for treatment-refractory anorexia nervosa: a phase 1 pilot trial. *Lancet.* 2013;381(9875):1361–1370.

53. Stidd DA, Vogelsang K, Krahl SE, Langevin JP, Fellous JM. Amygdala deep brain stimulation is superior to paroxetine treatment in a rat model of posttraumatic stress disorder. *Brain Stimul.* 2013;6(6):837–844. Epub 2013/07/10. eng.

54. Koek RJ, Langevin JP, Krahl SE, et al. Deep brain stimulation of the basolateral amygdala for treatment-refractory combat post-traumatic stress disorder (PTSD): study protocol for a pilot randomized controlled trial with blinded, staggered onset of stimulation. *Trials.* 2014;15:356.

55. Hamani C, Temel Y. Deep brain stimulation for psychiatric disease: contributions and validity of animal models. *Sci Transl Med.* 2012;4(142):142rv8.

56. Temel Y, Jahanshahi A. Treating brain disorders with neuromodulation. *Science.* 2015;347(6229):1418–1419.

57. Figee M, Luigjes J, Smolders R, et al. Deep brain stimulation restores frontostriatal network activity in obsessive-compulsive disorder. *Nat Neurosci.* 2013;16(4):386–387.

Index

Note: Page numbers followed by "*f*" and "*t*" refer to figures and tables, respectively.